SUCCESS ON THE WARDS

SUCCESS
ON THE
WARDS

250
RULES FOR
CLERKSHIP SUCCESS

SAMIR P. DESAI MD
RAJANI KATTA MD

FROM THE AUTHORS OF THE SUCCESSFUL MATCH

PUBLISHED BY

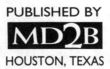

HOUSTON, TEXAS

www.MD2B.net

Success on the Wards: 250 Rules for Clerkship Success is published by MD2B, PO Box 300988, Houston, TX 77230-0988.

www.MD2B.net

NOTICE: The authors and publisher disclaim any personal liability, either directly or indirectly, for advice or information presented within. The authors and publishers have used care and diligence in the preparation of this book. Every effort has been made to ensure the accuracy and completeness of information contained within this book. The reader should understand, however, that most of the book's subject matter is not rooted in scientific observation. The recommendations made within this book have come from the authors' personal experiences and interactions with other attending physicians, residents, and students over many years. Since expectations vary from medical school to medical school, clerkship to clerkship, attending physician to attending physician, and resident to resident, the recommendations are not universally applicable. No responsibility is assumed for errors, inaccuracies, omissions, or any false or misleading implication that may arise due to the text.

Printed in the United States of America

978-0-9725561-9-4

Dedication

To Teja and Shaan
And to our
families.

It takes more than just two individuals to write a book. We would like to thank our families for making all of this possible.

A portion of the proceeds from this book is donated to organizations supporting health and literacy.

About the Authors

Samir P. Desai, M.D.

Dr. Samir Desai serves on the faculty of the Baylor College of Medicine in the Department of Medicine. He is actively involved in medical student and resident education, a member of the Clerkship Directors in Internal Medicine, and the recipient of teaching awards. He is an author and editor, having written twelve books that together have sold over 100,000 copies worldwide.

In 2009, he co-authored *The Successful Match: 200 Rules to Succeed in the Residency Match,* a well regarded and highly acclaimed book that has helped thousands of residency applicants match successfully. His commitment to helping medical students reach their professional goals led him to develop the website, www.TheSuccessfulMatch.com. The website's mission is to provide residency applicants with a better understanding of the residency selection process.

With Dr. Rajani Katta, he writes a regular column for the Student Doctor Network called "The Successful Match." Dr. Desai keeps residency applicants abreast of key information at The Successful Match blog (www.TheSuccessfulMatch.blogspot.com). He is also the founder of www.ImgAssist.com, a website providing guidance to international medical graduates (IMGs) seeking residency positions in the United States.

His other books include the best-selling *Clinician's Guide to Laboratory Medicine: Pocket.* This resource, widely used by students, residents, and other healthcare professionals, offers a unique step-by-step approach to lab test interpretation.

After completing his residency training in Internal Medicine at Northwestern University in Chicago, Illinois, Dr. Desai had the opportunity of serving as chief medical resident. He received his M.D. degree from Wayne State University School of Medicine in Detroit, Michigan, graduating first in his class.

Rajani Katta, M.D.

Dr. Rajani Katta is an Associate Professor in the Department of Dermatology at Baylor College of Medicine. She has authored over 40 scientific articles and chapters, and lectured extensively both nationally and locally on dermatology and contact dermatitis to students, residents, and physicians. She serves as the course director for dermatology in the basic science years, and has served as the clerkship director for the dermatology rotation. In these capacities, she has seen firsthand the importance of outstanding clinical evaluations in securing a position in a competitive specialty, and her insight in this area has helped students seeking these types of competitive positions.

Having advised many students over the years regarding the dermatology match process, she was determined to become expert in this area and share her knowledge, insight, and perspective. In 2009, she co-authored *The Successful Match: 200 Rules to Succeed in the Residency Match*. This book has quickly become the best-selling title in this field. She also contributes regularly to www.studentdoctor.net with a recurring column on topics specific to the residency match, including a series of interviews with decision-makers.

After graduating with honors from Baylor College of Medicine and completing her internship in Internal Medicine, she completed her dermatology residency at the Northwestern University School of Medicine.

Contents

Chapter 1

Introduction

Rule # 1   You came to medical school to be a great doctor. That process begins now.

Why did you become a doctor? There may be a number of reasons, but the most important one is the same across the board: to take care of patients. You will read startling amounts of information during medical school, and your training will include many procedures and new techniques, but all of it is in the service of patient care. You are here to make each and every individual patient better.

That process starts now.

It is an amazing privilege to take care of patients. You can read about a disease all that you want, but to be able to speak to and examine a patient with that disease is an unsurpassed learning experience. It is an incredible responsibility as well. You will be asking patients the most intimate and intrusive types of questions. You will be asking patients to offer their arm for a needle, to disrobe for an exam, to let you literally poke and prod at their body. In return, you are responsible for protecting them from harm, and for healing them.

Starting as a medical student, and progressing to a respected physician, is a long, difficult, and intense process. It takes years of education, and years of training. The privileges granted to physicians are remarkable. In return, you have a great responsibility. Your education is in the service of patient care. You have a responsibility to make the most of that education.

What does it take to be a great doctor? There is an impressive body of research devoted to medical student education, and to the factors and interventions that ensure good doctors. Medical educators work hard to ensure that students master these different facets of the practice of medicine.

Why are clerkships so important to the process of producing great doctors?

1

The areas emphasized in clerkships are those that are integral to becoming a great physician.

Patient care requires the daily use of many skills. On a daily basis, a physician may need to:

Obtain an accurate medication history.

Detect a heart murmur.

Create a differential diagnosis for the patient with abdominal pain.

Interpret an elevated alkaline phosphatase.

Formulate a management plan for the patient with a myocardial infarction.

Communicate that plan through oral discussions and written documentation.

Utilize the talents of an entire health care team to maximize patient care.

Manifest their concern for the patient in every interaction.

Clerkships teach students how to accomplish these difficult, vital skills.

If you don't learn certain skills in medical school, you may never learn them.

Clinical clerkships provide the foundation of successful patient care. They represent a critical time in your education. If you want to become proficient in exam skills, you have to learn now. These aren't skills you can learn from reading a textbook. You need to evaluate patients with these findings, and you need to have a teacher that can demonstrate these findings. You need to be able to ask questions freely in order to learn all the finer points of physical exam skills. This isn't something you can easily do as a resident, and certainly not as a board-certified physician. If you don't know how to assess jugular venous distention by the end of medical school, you may never learn.

While you would assume that medical school teaches you everything you need to know to function well as a resident, that isn't true for all students, particularly those who take a passive approach to learning or those who focus their education on textbook learning. You need to maximize your learning experiences and teaching opportunities on the wards. Passive learning has real consequences.

In one eye-opening study, internal medicine residents were tested on cardiac auscultatory skills. They listened to 12 prerecorded cardiac events. American residents demonstrated poor proficiency, with mean identification rates of only 22%.[1] In another study of resident skills, ECG proficiency was measured. Surprisingly, 58% of residents wrongly diagnosed complete heart block, and only 22% were certain of their diagnosis of ventricular tachycardia.[2] In a study of radiologic proficiency, participants included mainly residents, with some students. In x-rays representing emergency situations, pneumothorax was misdiagnosed by 91% of participants overall, while a misplaced central venous catheter was missed by 74%.[3]

Skills in patient examination, interpretation of tests, synthesis of information, and medical decision-making are honed through years of practice. Clerkships are only the first step, but provide an invaluable education, with supervisors there to demonstrate, to model, and to teach skills. The best medical students regard clerkships as a unique and invaluable learning experience, difficult to replicate in residency or later through seminars and conferences.

If you don't learn it now, you may have problems as a resident.

Medical school is the time to learn and develop your clinical skills. It's also the time to develop and hone the learned attributes and attitudes that predict success as a physician. In a study of residents with problematic behavior, investigators sought to determine if there were prognostic indicators in their medical school evaluations.[4] The short answer is yes.

Students whose evaluations indicated that they were timid, had problems in organization, displayed little curiosity, and had difficulty applying knowledge clinically, among other types, were more likely to become problem residents. The authors "found a rather robust multilevel correlation between residents who have problems, major or minor, during or after residency, and negative statements, even subtle ones, in the dean's letter." The predictive statements noted in the dean's letter included:

Very nervous, timid initially / Displayed little curiosity / Had difficulty applying knowledge clinically / He came across as confrontational / Maybe somewhat overconfident for his level of training / Lack of enthusiasm and problems in organization / Needs to read more on her own / Lots of effort, uneven outcome

Difficulties during clerkships may predict difficulties as a physician, including disciplinary actions by the State Medical Board.

Clerkships are the foundation of successful patient care. During clerkships, medical students also develop and hone the attributes and attitudes that are required of successful physicians. These are referred to collectively as medical professionalism. "The specific attributes that have long been understood to animate professionalism include altruism, respect, honesty, integrity, dutifulness, honour, excellence and accountability."[5] – Dr. Jordan Cohen, president emeritus, Association of American Medical Colleges

If you don't hone these traits during medical school, you may have problems as a physician. Unprofessional behavior in medical school is a possible predictor of future disciplinary action. A particularly notable study was performed by Dr. Maxine Papadakis, associate dean for student affairs at the UCSF School of Medicine. She and her team examined the medical school records of 235 graduates of three medical schools. Each of these physicians had been disciplined by one of 40 state medical boards over a 13-year period. The disciplined physicians were three times more likely than a control group to have negative comments about their professionalism documented in their medical school record.[6]

Another study sought to identify the domains of unprofessional behavior in medical school that were associated with disciplinary action by a state medical board.[7] Three domains of unprofessional behavior were significantly associated with future disciplinary action: poor reliability and responsibility, poor initiative and motivation, and lack of self-improvement and adaptability.

Your core clerkship grades may either limit or expand your future career options.

The skills and traits reflected in core clerkship grades are considered so important to future success as a resident that residency programs use these grades as a major criteria in the selection process. Program directors are decision-makers in the residency selection process. In a survey of over 1,200 residency program directors across 21 medical specialties, grades in required clerkships were ranked as the # 1 factor used in the selection process.[8]

Studies across multiple specialties have supported the predictive nature of clerkship grades. In one study, researchers sought to determine which residency selection criteria had the strongest correlation with performance as an orthopedic surgery resident. The authors concluded that the "number of honors grades on clinical rotations was the strongest predictor of performance."[9] In a study of physical medicine and rehabilitation residents, "clinical residency performance was predicted by clerkship grade honors."[10] In one study of internal medicine residents, performance as a resident was significantly associated with the internal medicine clerkship grade.[11]

In the next 400 plus pages, we review each of the areas that students need to master in clerkships. The book contains a great deal of in-depth content across a range of areas vital to medical student success. It's also arranged to ensure ease of use. The first sections serve as straightforward how-to guides for each of the core clerkships. If you're starting your Pediatrics clerkship, and aren't sure how to write the daily patient progress note, Chapter 4 walks you through that process. If you're starting the Ob/Gyn clerkship, and don't know how to write a delivery note, Chapter 6 provides a template and sample note that details exactly what you'll need to include. The latter chapters provide more wide-ranging content. If you'll be presenting in rounds for the first time, you can turn to the chapter on oral case presentations and review the features you'll need to include. If you are committed to fully protecting your patients from the hazards of hospitalization, Chapter 8 Patients includes several tables that outline the steps that medical students can take, even at their level, to protect their patients. Chapter 22 reviews the impact of collaborative care on patient outcomes, and provides recommendations that students can implement.

The recommendations presented here are based on discussions with numerous faculty members, residents, and students, as well as our own experiences. We've also focused our efforts on evidence-based advice. This evidence-based advice is based on our review of the substantial medical literature in the area of medical student education. The book includes over 400 references from the relevant literature.

Over the next 400 plus pages, you'll learn how to maximize your education during core clerkships, as well as your performance. Your success on the wards will become the foundation of outstanding patient care.

Patients

We begin this chapter with one of the most famous quotes in the history of medicine. "First, do no harm." From ancient times onwards, medical practice has posed dangers to patients. In modern times, those dangers are shockingly common. Medical error is thought to be the third leading cause of death in the US.[12] Those errors include the unbelievable: one report described an average of 27 cases in one year, per New York hospital, of invasive procedures performed on the wrong patient.[13] Some of those dangers have become so commonplace that we consider them routine. When a patient develops a hospital-related infection, we document it as a nosocomial infection and treat the infection without questioning why it occurred. However, many of those infections are preventable, and should never have occurred at all. In this chapter, you'll learn a number of specific measures that medical students can implement to protect their patients, from the use of standardized abbreviations to ensuring that patients receive venous thromboembolism prophylaxis when indicated. We outline how medical students can identify the hazards of hospitalization, thus ensuring that you can act to mitigate those hazards. We review nosocomial infections, and how you may be a culprit through your hands, your clothing, and even your stethoscope.

We also review the type of skills that ensure that patients feel comfortable with your care. The best medical care necessitates that patients trust their physicians and have confidence in both their abilities and the fact that the physician cares about the patient, not just the illness. In this chapter, our focus is on the patient, and how medical students can improve the care provided to patients. We outline steps that students can take, even at their level, to protect their patients from physical harm. We emphasize the different ways in which medical students can enhance patient care, patient education, and patient counseling. On a daily basis, you have the opportunity and the power to enhance the care provided to your patients.

Internal Medicine Clerkship

The field of internal medicine (IM) has a broad impact on all fields of medicine. "Learning about internal medicine – the specialty providing comprehensive care to adults – in the third year of medical school is an important experience, regardless of what specialty the medical student ultimately pursues," says Dr. Patrick Alguire, the Director of Education and Career Development at the American College of Physicians.[14] Through this clerkship, you will hone your skills in history and physical examination, diagnostic test interpretation, medical decision-making, and management of core medical conditions. These skills are important ones for all physicians, even if you ultimately decide to enter radiology, pathology, emergency medicine, or another field. Overall, internal medicine does stand as the most frequently chosen specialty in the residency match. In 2010, over 3,000 allopathic and osteopathic medical students matched into an internal medicine residency program.

Your IM clerkship grade can impact your career. It's a factor in the residency selection process for all specialties, not just internal medicine. In a survey of over 1,200 residency program directors across 21 medical specialties, grades in required clerkships were ranked as the # 1 factor used in the selection process.[8] "Do well in your clerkship," writes the Department of Medicine at the University of Washington. "Yes, this is obvious – and easier said than done – but it's also important. Most residency programs look closely at the third-year clerkship grade when selecting applicants."[15]

Many medical students find this clerkship formidable. A lack of knowledge isn't the main factor. The main factor is a lack of preparation for your many responsibilities. How do I evaluate a newly admitted patient? What do I need to include in a daily progress note? What information do I need to include in a comprehensive write-up? How do I present newly admitted patients to the attending physician?

In this chapter, templates and outlines are included for each of these important responsibilities. You'll also find a number of tips and suggestions on how to maximize your learning and performance during this rotation. You'll find detailed information that will help you effectively pre-round, succeed during work rounds, deliver polished oral case presentations, create well-written daily progress notes, and generate comprehensive write-ups.

For students interested in a career in internal medicine, this chapter also details how to strengthen your application. You'll learn how to identify potential mentors and obtain strong letters of recommendation. You'll learn about recommended electives and sub-internships, as well as specifics that detail how to maximize the impact of your application.

Surgery Clerkship

The surgery clerkship provides significant exposure to common surgical problems, and allows you to evaluate the specialty as a potential career choice. Although the bulk of your education will take place on the general surgery service, most rotations provide the opportunity to explore several surgical subspecialties. A surgical clerkship education is very valuable, whether or not you choose to practice in a surgical field. Primary care physicians must be familiar with the evaluation and management of patients in the pre-operative and post-operative settings. An understanding of core surgical principles is important across many fields, including ones such as anesthesiology, dermatology, and emergency medicine.

From a personal standpoint, you or a family member is likely to undergo surgery in your lifetime, and you'll find that an understanding of the pre-operative, operative, and post-operative stages will be valuable.

Regardless of your chosen career, your surgery clerkship grade will be a factor used in the residency selection process, due to an emphasis on core clerkship grades in the residency selection process. In a survey of residency program directors across 21 medical specialties, grades in required clerkships were ranked as the # 1 factor used in the selection process.[8] The University of Colorado Department of Surgery writes that "most surgery programs look very favorably on an 'Honors' grade in your MS3 surgery clerkship rotation and may factor in the grades you received in your Medicine and Ob/Gyn rotations."[16] It's not easy to honor the clerkship. In a survey of medical schools across the country, Takayama found that only 27% of students achieve the highest grade in the surgery clerkship.[17]

Many students approach the surgery clerkship with considerable anxiety. In one study, students were most concerned about fatigue, long hours, workload, insufficient sleep, lack of time to study, mental abuse (getting yelled at or relentless pimping), and poor performance.[18] Unfamiliarity with the operating room environment was also concerning.

In the Surgery Clerkship chapter, we provide tips for operating room success, a checklist for thorough pre-rounding, a step-by-step guide to presenting patients, and time-saving templates for the pre-op, post-op, and op notes. This information will maximize your education as well as your performance.

In 2010, approximately 2,500 allopathic and osteopathic medical students matched into general surgery or a related surgical specialty, such as orthopedic surgery, otolaryngology, plastic surgery, or urology. This chapter includes recommendations for those students interested in pursuing general surgery as a career. When should you do a sub-internship? Should you do an away elective? What are considered negatives in a residency application? These questions, and others, are answered.

Pediatrics Clerkship

During the pediatrics clerkship, students will gain experience and skills in the evaluation and management of common medical problems in infants, children, and adolescents. The Department of Pediatrics at the University of South Alabama writes that "there are few areas in medicine where knowledge of pediatrics will not be necessary."[19] In pediatrics, there is an emphasis on family-centered care. Learning how pediatricians deliver family-centered care will be of benefit, regardless of your medical specialty choice. The Institute for Patient- and Family-Centered Care writes that families "are essential to patients' health and well-being and are allies for quality and safety."[20]

As a core clerkship grade, your performance in Pediatrics is important to residency programs in other specialties. In a survey of over 1,200 residency program directors, grades in required clerkships were ranked as the # 1 factor used in the selection process.[8] In a survey of medical schools across the country, Takayama found that only 29% of students achieve the highest grade in the pediatrics clerkship.[17]

Dr. Andrew Bremer, a pediatric endocrinologist and assistant professor in the Department of Pediatrics at Vanderbilt University, is the author of the *Pediatrics Clerkship: 101 Biggest Mistakes And How To Avoid Them*. He writes that "the pediatrics clerkship is different in many respects from other core clerkships and students are often uncertain of how best to navigate the transition from adult to pediatric care. The challenges of learning how to interact with pediatric patients, take and perform the pediatric history and physical exam, and present patients during rounds presents a steep learning curve for students in the first few weeks of the clerkship."[21]

In the Pediatrics Clerkship chapter, you'll find templates and outlines to help you fulfill your daily responsibilities and tasks. You'll learn how to effectively pre-round, succinctly and accurately present new and established patients, and develop comprehensive write-ups using our checklist. Do you know what elements to include in the neonatal, growth, and developmental histories? This chapter details those elements.

In the 2010 NRMP Match, over 1,900 allopathic and osteopathic students matched into pediatrics. For those of you interested in pediatrics as a career, this chapter provides insight into the pediatric residency selection process. You'll learn how to ask for letters of recommendation, establish a relationship with a mentor, and choose fourth year electives. Should you do an away elective? Will your USMLE Step 1 score be a cause for concern? This section reviews those questions and others.

Family Medicine

According to the Society of Teachers of Family Medicine, the family medicine clerkship provides "essential patient care knowledge and skills necessary for generic medical school development, regardless of ultimate career choice."[22] The family medicine clerkship teaches students the role of the family physician in the delivery of primary care in the United States. You will learn how to evaluate and manage patients with a wide variety of acute and chronic medical problems.

The experiences in the family medicine clerkship are important to your growth as a physician, regardless of specialty. Physicians in most specialties care for patients in the outpatient setting. Since family medicine clerkships are largely outpatient rotations, you will see medicine as it's practiced in the ambulatory setting. The clerkship will show you how family physicians "identify, prioritize, and manage the multiple medical problems of many patients in time limited visits," writes Dr. Robert Taylor, professor of family medicine at the Oregon Health & Science University.[23]

Through this clerkship, you will hone your skills in interviewing, examination, and clinical problem-solving. These skills are important ones for all physicians, even if you ultimately decide to enter anesthesiology, urology, or another field.

The family medicine clerkship is a core rotation, and your clerkship grade will be a factor in the residency selection process, regardless of your specialty choice. In a survey of medical schools across the country,

Takayama found that only 34% of students achieve the highest grade in the family medicine clerkship.[17] In the 2010 NRMP match, over 1,400 allopathic and osteopathic applicants secured positions in family medicine residency programs.

Obstetrics and Gynecology Clerkship

All medical students benefit from an increased knowledge of women's health. The Department of Obstetrics and Gynecology at Yale University writes that "physicians of all specialties will care for female patients who present with reproductive health issues, whether it is a teen seeking contraception, a young athlete with amenorrhea, a pregnant woman with an autoimmune disease, a patient with type II diabetes and abnormal uterine bleeding, or a post-menopausal woman with breast cancer and symptoms of hypoestrogenemia."[24]

Although only 5% of U.S. medical school graduates enter the specialty, the obstetrics and gynecology clerkship is a core clerkship, and therefore this grade will be utilized in the residency selection process of any field. According to the Department of Obstetrics and Gynecology at University of California Davis, "USMLE scores and clerkship grades (especially in ob/gyn, surgery, and internal medicine) are considered factual data and ranked high."[25] However, honoring the rotation is challenging. "Obstetrics and gynecology is a difficult field, and it takes a truly outstanding student to earn an Honors grade in the clerkship," writes Dr. Yasuko Yamamura, clerkship director of the University of Minnesota obstetrics and gynecology rotation.[26] In a survey of medical schools across the country, Takayama found that only 29% of students achieve the highest grade in the obstetrics and gynecology clerkship.[17]

In the Obstetrics and Gynecology chapter, you'll find outlines and templates that will enable you to complete the daily responsibilities unique to the field, including templates for the delivery note, obstetric admission history and physical exam, and postpartum notes following vaginal delivery and Cesarean section. Do you know what LOP, TOA, or IUGR stand for? This chapter reviews the commonly used abbreviations in obstetrics and gynecology.

The chapter ends with recommendations for students who wish to pursue obstetrics and gynecology as a career. Dr. Vicki Mendiratta, clerkship director of the UCSF obstetrics and gynecology clerkship, writes that the "3rd year is an excellent time to review your credentials to date" and to "make reasonable recommendations regarding your residency options."[27] You'll learn the data on student qualifications from the 2010 NRMP match. You'll also learn specific ways to strengthen your residency application, as well as suggestions on how to identify a mentor and schedule electives.

Psychiatry Clerkship

Psychiatric disease is highly prevalent, and physicians in all specialties need to be familiar with a variety of psychiatric diseases. The skills learned in this core clerkship are essential for all students, irrespective of specialty choice. All physicians must ensure that patients with psychiatric disease are recognized, diagnosed, and treated correctly. In fact, most patients with psychiatric illness initially present to primary care physicians and specialists, not psychiatrists. "It is known that among outpatients attending specialist clinics, about 15% of those given a diagnosis have an associated psychiatric disorder, and an average of 20 – 30% of those given no medical diagnosis have a psychiatric disorder."[28]

While less than 5% of U.S. medical school graduates match into the field, your psychiatry clerkship grade will be used as a factor in the residency selection process for all fields, as all place considerable value on core clerkship grades. In a survey of medical schools across the country, Takayama found that only 35% of students achieve the highest grade in the psychiatry clerkship.[17]

Even for students who've completed a number of clerkships, the psychiatry clerkship poses unique challenges, and can be anxiety-provoking. Dr. Kimberly McLaren is an assistant professor of psychiatry at the University of Washington and the author of the book, *Psychiatry Clerkship: 150 Biggest Mistakes And How To Avoid Them*. She states that a variety of factors contribute to this apprehension, including the need to learn a new psychiatric "language," as well as the need to learn how to interact with psychiatric patients.[29] In this field, students must leave the comfort zone of the medical-style interview and examination. "Medical students rotating through psychiatry often feel like tourists in a strange country. A new language and new customs confront them at every turn," writes Dr. Glen Gabbard, professor of psychiatry at the Baylor College of Medicine.[29]

In the Psychiatry Clerkship chapter, you'll learn how to present patients and complete write-ups. You may already be knowledgeable about these tasks, but presentations and write-ups in psychiatry are completely different from those in other specialties. In one study, major problem areas identified in medical student psychiatry write-ups included inadequate gathering of developmental histories, omission of sexual histories, brief mental status descriptions, and no attempts at developing a biopsychosocial formulation.[30] In this chapter, you'll find outlines and templates to guide you through the unique facets of psychiatric examinations and documentation. Checklists for the mental status exam highlight for students unique specifics, such as psychomotor activation, affect, perception, and sensorium. Other outlines help in the creation of a biopsychosocial formulation, as well as the multi-axial DSM diagnosis.

If you're interested in psychiatry as a career, this chapter also provides a number of recommendations for strengthening your application, including suggestions for identifying a mentor, scheduling electives, and obtaining strong letters of recommendation.

The New Rotation

"The clinical years, especially the third year, are in some ways a very harsh experience. It is frightening to feel you are ignorant in a setting where sick people are depending on you for care... You worry about making a mistake. You worry about hurting someone. On a different level, you worry about making a fool of yourself, about looking stupid on rounds."[31]

— From *A not entirely benign procedure: four years as a medical student* by Perri Klass MD.

Transitioning from one rotation to another is stressful. Just when students determine which behaviors, actions, and attitudes are valued and rewarded, it's time to rotate to the next clerkship. Every new rotation represents new responsibilities, a new team, a new physical environment, and an entirely new facet of medicine. These factors all impact student performance at the start of every single new rotation. In this chapter, you'll learn the basics: the resources you'll need to accomplish your work, as well as suggestions on how to learn the chart, the electronic medical record, and your physical environment.

We provide concrete recommendations on how to remain in control of all the data and tasks related to patient care. This is a challenge for even experienced physicians. In an observational time and motion study, doctors were interrupted nearly seven times per hour, and alarmingly, "doctors failed to return to 18.5% of interrupted tasks."[32]

In this chapter, you'll learn how to adapt to your new role and responsibilities quickly and how to integrate professionally into your new team and environment. You will learn the questions that should be asked of every new resident, intern, and attending, as well as ways to make the best possible first impression. When your team recognizes your potential, and rewards you with increased responsibility, you can begin to make meaningful contributions to patient care.

Admitting Patients

Admitting a patient to a hospital would appear to be a straightforward process, and yet it can be remarkably complex. Evaluating the patient, formulating a diagnosis, creating a therapeutic plan, accurately conveying that plan to the entire patient care team, and ensuring that it's carried out properly by all the multiple individuals involved in patient care is a complex process. It's a process with many steps, each of which can go wrong.

As a medical student, your goal is to function as the patient's intern, as well as become the team's expert on this patient. As the expert on the patient, you play a vital role in ensuring the best patient care, and it starts with the first minutes of admission. Evaluations must be thorough, and they must be accurate, and yet this often proves challenging. Start with something as seemingly straightforward as the medication history. When researchers evaluated agreement between the patient and physician regarding their medications (defined as congruence) they found a rate of only 58% for residents.[33]

You can ask about a patient's medications, but you won't always get the correct answer. Some patients rely on memory, while others bring in a typed list of their medications. Others may bring in their brown bag or plastic grocery bag full of medication bottles and hand them over to you. In any of these cases, you won't just be able to copy information about drug names and dosages from the list or bottles. In this section, you'll learn the process and the questions you need to ask to ensure complete accuracy.

Every component of the patient history is essential to reaching an accurate diagnosis. In one study, 76% of diagnoses made by clinicians were suggested or established by the history.[34] While integral to patient care, obtaining an accurate history can be difficult. One study looked at medical students who self-assessed their communication skills with simulated patients.[35] Eliciting information was found to be the most frequently noted weakness, cited by 35% of participants. Faculty members who work with poorly performing students note several specific problems with history taking. "Many low-scoring students focused prematurely, failing to ask open-ended questions or adequately characterize the chief complaint. Respondents also observed students being too focused on the history of present illness, omitting or incompletely exploring the pertinent past medical, social, or family history, particularly as they related to the chief complaint."[35]

In this chapter, you'll learn the potential pitfalls in evaluating patients. You'll learn how to avoid these pitfalls, and ensure both thorough and accurate patient evaluations.

We provide a step by step approach to the evaluation of a newly admitted patient, starting from the patient information template, to obtaining prior medical records, to reviewing pre-admission clinical data, to the formulation of your assessment and plan.

Finally, we review the admission orders. You'll learn the checklist that is required whenever you write any new or updated medication order. In one study, researchers found that prescribing errors were common and contributed to over half of all significant adverse but preventable drug events.[36] These are preventable drug events, and if we as a profession are committed to seeing that number reduced, we need to focus on prescribing errors. You'll learn the concrete steps that you can take to reduce these errors, from double-checking dosage calculations, to checking for renal impairment, to always checking for drug-drug interactions, and to special considerations with verbal orders. We also outline dangerous abbreviations. Examples include Q.D., which may be misread as QID. In such a case, a patient might receive a medication four times daily instead of the intended once daily. Another example is the use of μg [micrograms] which may be mistaken for mg [milligrams]. Older faculty have been using these abbreviations for decades. While still in use in some institutions, these abbreviations are dangerous enough that many institutions are committed to seeing that they are eradicated.

Laboratory Tests

The state of lab testing in America can be summarized succinctly:

Physicians waste a lot of money on lab tests.

Many of us don't know enough about lab testing.

This ignorance can lead to medical errors.

The Centers for Disease Control wrote that "medical education on laboratory testing is inadequate. Despite the integral role of laboratory testing in the practice of medicine, formal teaching of laboratory medicine is a relatively neglected component of the medical school curriculum."[37]

The end result is that medical school graduates often enter practice with significant deficiencies in this area. This has significant consequences. The misinterpretation of test results may significantly impact patient care, increasing morbidity and mortality due to missed diagnoses or wrong diagnoses.

From a monetary standpoint, according to the U.S. Congressional Budget Office, approximately $700 billion per year is spent on diagnostic tests that <u>do not improve</u> health outcomes.[38]

Although lab testing in modern medicine is integral to patient care, many physicians have received relatively little formal instruction in either the ordering of lab tests or their interpretation. Major medical textbooks, often utilized resources in patient care, may not help. Dr. George Lundberg, Editor in Chief Emeritus of Medscape and Former Editor of *JAMA*, wrote that "guidance on diagnostic testing in medical textbooks often consist of little more than listings of tests that may be abnormal in a given disease. Both the number and complexity of diagnostic tests have increased rapidly, requiring physicians to have not only considerable knowledge of the properties of individual tests but also a strategy for their sequential interpretation."[39]

Yet this area is of vital importance. Lab test abnormalities are extremely common. In a study of patients admitted to the general medicine service at a city hospital, 29% of the tests obtained were abnormal.[40]

In another study of patients admitted to an inpatient psychiatry unit, 25% had an abnormal LDH, while 14% had an abnormal alkaline phosphatase.[41] These numbers highlight the fact that no matter what field of medicine you practice, you must learn how to interpret and manage abnormal lab tests.

The fact that your deficiencies in this area can harm your patient brings more urgency to the issue. Dr. Laposata, director of laboratory medicine at Vanderbilt University Hospital, wrote that "medical error from incorrect laboratory test selection and result interpretation is rapidly becoming a more serious problem as the test menu becomes larger and more complex."[42] Reviews of malpractice claims have shown that incorrect interpretation of laboratory test results is a major cause of missed or delayed diagnoses.[43] Even errors in specimen collection can impact the patient, as when the sample is hemolyzed or when the tubes are filled in the incorrect order.

This is clearly an area of vital importance for medical students. Multiple organizations, including the Clerkship Directors of Internal Medicine,

Society of General Internal Medicine, and the Academy of Clinical Laboratory Physicians and Scientists have identified the selection and interpretation of appropriate diagnostic or lab studies as key competencies for medical students.[44, 45]

In this chapter, we introduce the principles of laboratory medicine. You will learn about lab test errors, and how to recognize and prevent them. You'll learn the step-by-step approach to the interpretation of lab tests. Lastly, we include a sample algorithm that demonstrates this approach to lab test interpretation, reproduced from the *Clinician's Guide to Laboratory Medicine: Pocket*, a guide authored by Dr. Desai.

Attending Rounds

Attending rounds are a formal meeting of the team that are led by the attending physician. During rounds, team members discuss the patients on the team in order to establish the diagnostic and therapeutic plan. Your main interaction with the attending will take place during this time.

Rounds present a great educational opportunity, and just by listening to the specifics of patient care recommendations you'll learn a great deal. However, rounds also serve an evaluative function. Since you'll interact most often with your attending during rounds, your participation in rounds is one of the main ways your attending will assess your progress. Therefore, this participation has a significant impact on your clinical evaluation.

For an accurate evaluation of your performance, attendings need their students to participate in rounds. However, the literature shows that medical students often function as a passive audience. In fact, one study revealed that students talked only 4% of the time.[46] This poses real difficulties for students; this reticence may be interpreted as a lack of knowledge or a lack of interest. In one study evaluating problem students, among 21 types the "excessively shy, nonassertive" student was the second most frequently encountered problem type in obstetrics and gynecology, the fourth in surgery, and the fifth in internal medicine, pediatrics, and psychiatry.[47]

You need to be prepared during rounds. This involves evaluating your patient fully, knowing all of the clinical data, and becoming an expert on the patient's diagnoses. This allows you to prepare for both the clarifying and probing questions that will be asked during rounds. While data shows that a significant percentage of these questions involve simple recall, one study showed that nearly 20% of questions "required analysis of data or the demonstration of deeper thinking processes."[48] Often these are open-ended questions such as "What do you think about...?", "What would you do at this point?", and "What if this patient were 70 instead of 35?" For example, Dr. Samuels, a faculty member at the Penn State University College of Medicine, engages students by "asking them questions...what are you thinking...how do these two go together...if this were different what would you do?"[49]

In this chapter, you'll learn effective techniques that will enable you to answer these questions. You will be introduced to the RIME method of evaluation, developed originally by Dr. Louis Pangaro, and learn how this method can help you answer higher order questions.[50]

You'll learn the basics as well: how to ensure that bedside rounds are conducted properly. Throughout this chapter, you will learn how to interact with attendings, and how to make the most of their teaching. These rules will enhance your clinical education as well as your overall rotation performance.

Oral Case Presentation

During an oral case presentation [OCP], students will formally "present" a patient to the team. Oral communication skills are vital in patient care, and the development of these skills is emphasized during core clerkships. Poor skills have the potential to directly impact patient care. In a study of malpractice claims, researchers found that incomplete or inaccurate transfer of clinical information frequently occurred between residents and attending physicians. Transfer of information resulted in a patient care error in 32% of cases.[51]

Poor communication skills also impact a student's evaluation. Faculty and resident ratings account for the majority of a student's grade in core rotations. These ratings include comments on specific skills, such as a student's ability to take a history and perform a physical examination. However, attendings rarely or infrequently observe students in these areas. In fact, in a survey of medical students at the end of their third year, 51% reported never having a faculty member observe them while taking a history.[52] Therefore, many faculty draw conclusions about a student's ability in these areas from the quality of the oral case presentation (OCP).

Pulito wrote that "in the clinic setting, for example, if a student presents a patient to an attending and is verbally facile, succinctly describing a focused history and physical examination, the inference may be drawn that the student expeditiously obtained the relevant history and performed an appropriate examination."[53]

In recent years, organizations such as the Association of American Medical Colleges (AAMC), Clerkship Directors of Internal Medicine (CDIM), and the Accreditation Council for Graduate Medical Education (ACGME) have emphasized the importance of communication skills. In fact, the AAMC considers the development and acquisition of communication skills a core learning objective for medical students.

In this chapter, you will learn how to effectively transfer important clinical information between team members. You'll learn the mechanics of the OCP, including proper format, components, transitions, and level of detail. You'll learn about the different facets of oral presentations that affect their quality, including volume, pace, tone, and nonverbal communication. You'll learn specific techniques to decrease anxiety. In short, you'll learn how to deliver high quality oral case presentations, the type that facilitate patient care, improve team efficiency, become a valuable learning experience, and best reflect your excellence in patient care.

Write-up

Communication skills are of vital importance in patient care, and the development of written communication skills is emphasized heavily in core clerkships. The American Association of Medical Colleges issued a report stating that schools must ensure that, prior to graduation, students "have the ability to communicate effectively, both orally and in writing, with patients, patients' families, colleagues, and others with whom physicians must exchange information in carrying out their responsibilities."[54]

Studies of medical errors have found that documentation errors are common and dangerous. In a chart review of resident physician progress notes in a neonatal intensive care unit, researchers found discrepancies in 61.7% of notes with respect to weight, vascular lines, or medications.[55] Discrepancies in the documentation of medications were found in 27.7% of notes, including omission of information as well as documentation of inaccurate information.

The accuracy of student documentation has also been studied. Senior medical students were videotaped examining standardized patients.[56] The patient encounter was then compared to the information documented by students in the patient note. Researchers found that only 4% of the notes accurately reflected what occurred during the encounter. The problems identified included under-documentation, over-documentation, and inaccurate documentation.

In another study, Jefferson Medical College researchers had students examine standardized patients.[57] While the students documented their findings, patients completed checklists identifying the history and physical exam elements performed by students. When students' notes and patients' checklists were compared, an under-documentation rate of 29% was found, a rate similar to experienced physicians.

Recognizing the importance of written communication, the USMLE Step 2 Clinical Skills Examination evaluates the ability of students to *document* the findings of encounters with standardized patients.

The written case presentation, or write-up, is a detailed account of the patient's clinical presentation. Its major purpose is to help you develop the written communication skills needed to take care of patients, specifically the ability to communicate patient information in an organized and succinct way.

During rotations, you'll be asked to prepare write-ups on the patients you admit. Your write-ups may be placed in the medical record, along with those of the resident and attending. Student write-ups, because they are usually more detailed than any other evaluation, are often referenced by other physicians. Their importance in patient care should not be underestimated.

In your future career, you'll find that any written documentation obtained from a physician encounter can also be used for billing, in epidemiological research, and as evidence during malpractice litigation.

You may be required to submit one or more write-ups to your attending or clerkship director as part of your clerkship grade. This highlights another purpose of the student write-up: it serves an important evaluative function. The website www.usmle.org describes an interesting aspect of medical education on the wards: "During recent field trials, 20 percent of the fourth-year students who completed a survey said they had been observed interacting with a patient by a faculty member two or fewer times. One in 25 said they had never been observed by a faculty member."[58]

If you aren't observed while taking care of patients, how can attendings evaluate your ability to perform a thorough history and physical? The oral case presentation and written case presentation become proxies for direct observation.

When you submit your write-up, reviewers will evaluate your ability to perform a comprehensive patient evaluation and appropriately record the results of this evaluation. In addition to your ability to collect information, reviewers will assess additional skills. Kogan and Shea wrote that "Assessment of the write-up is believed to be important because it evaluates a student's ability to collect information; identify, prioritize, and evaluate problems; demonstrate clinical reasoning; develop management plans; and communicate through a written record. These are important clinical skills that students are expected to be proficient in prior to graduation."[59]

In this chapter, we review each section of the write-up, and review the specifics of each section. You will learn the proper order and format of the write-up, starting with subjective data, moving to objective data, then the assessment, and finally the plan, with evidence of your reasoning and references included. You'll learn all the information that must be included in the history of present illness, as well as information on how to create a thorough problem list. You'll also learn a step-by-step approach to creating a high quality assessment and plan, including a discussion of the differential diagnosis and the inclusion of appropriate references from the current medical literature.

Outpatient Setting

You'll spend a substantial period of your third year in the outpatient setting. According to the report "Medical Schools in the United States, 2008-2009", published by *JAMA*, students spent varying amounts of time in the ambulatory setting during required third year clerkships, ranging from 23% in surgery to 91% in family medicine.[60] Fifty-four schools had a separate ambulatory care clerkship, during which nearly the entire time was spent in the ambulatory setting.

The ability to rotate in an outpatient setting provides distinct opportunities. In a study comparing the experiences of third year students in the ambulatory versus inpatient setting, students in the outpatient rotation "felt more like doctors, more responsible for patients, and more able to know and help their patients." They also reported better relationships with their teachers.[61]

Experience in outpatient medicine is also required training for the USMLE CS exam. The USMLE Clinical Skills (USMLE Step 2 CS) exam is required for graduates of US medical schools. The exam simulates a typical day in the outpatient setting, lasting eight hours and requiring focused examinations of patients with a variety of presenting complaints.

The absolute best way to prepare for this type of exam is to hone your skills as a physician in the outpatient setting.

At the same time, outpatient medicine poses a number of unique challenges. For medical students used to the luxury of time in the inpatient setting, the clinic with its need for thoroughness and efficiency, along with speed, is a major challenge. Operating under time constraints requires a change in your approach, starting with the need for focused histories and exams, as well as concise presentations. Just as challenging, you'll have to learn how to formulate assessments and plans based solely on these focused exams, as you typically won't have the results of laboratory tests.

In this chapter, you'll learn the questions to ask your preceptor at the start of the rotation, and how best to quickly orient yourself to the new setting. You'll learn how to begin an outpatient visit, and how to focus on the correct patient issues, which is more challenging than one would suspect. In a videotaped analysis of histories performed by senior medical students, 24% of all students did not ascertain the patient's main problems.[62]

Education in the outpatient setting can hone a student's assessment skills. In a study of the surgery clerkship, researchers found that students have greater opportunities to develop their critical thinking skills in the outpatient setting.[63] When compared to the inpatient setting, students in the clinic were more often the first to elicit the history (59.6 vs 4.3% of cases), perform the physical exam (70.2 vs 8.7% of cases), and generate the hypotheses (29.8 vs 2.2% of cases). This chapter will help you with these skills. You'll learn how to focus your exam, how to present succinctly, and how to analyze the focused and often incomplete data obtained from a single outpatient encounter.

Evaluations

"Different doctors…achieve competency in remarkably similar ways, despite working in disparate fields. Primarily, they recognize and remember their mistakes and misjudgments, and incorporate those memories into their thinking. Studies show that expertise is largely acquired not only by sustained practice but by receiving feedback that helps you understand your technical errors and misguided decisions."

— By Jerome Groopman MD
author of *How Doctors Think*[64]

Feedback is a critical tool in medicine. Physicians utilize feedback from patients, from colleagues, and from their own observations of patient outcomes in order to improve patient care. In clerkships, the main purpose of formal evaluations is to provide valuable feedback that students can act upon to improve patient care.

Clerkship evaluations are also used to grade students. These grades, and comments on evaluation forms, are taken seriously by residency programs. In our companion book, *The Successful Match*, we review all the factors that form the basis of residency selection. The most important factor is grades in required clerkships.

There is a growing body of literature devoted to the study of accurate evaluation. Evaluating a student's performance on a clinical rotation is challenging. In the basic sciences, the process is straightforward, as the evaluation is completely objective: what score did the student receive on the exam? In clinical rotations, subjective factors become much more important.

How do medical schools evaluate students' clinical performance? A number of methodologies are utilized, including written examinations and review of required assignments (write-ups). However, faculty and resident ratings are used in almost all U.S. core clerkships, and typically account for the majority of a student's grade.

This chapter will help you understand all the factors that impact these ratings. You'll learn about the evaluation form, and the use of formal feedback. You'll learn the ways in which you can use this knowledge to improve your provision of patient care and increase your chances of clerkship success. You'll also learn about the inherent difficulties in subjective evaluations, and how you can ensure that these issues don't affect your evaluation.

You'll learn about the variability that may occur even when evaluating the same performance. In one study of over 200 faculty internists, participants watched a videotape of a resident performing a work-up of a new patient.[65] When faculty rated the clinical skills of the resident, significant disagreement was found. With one resident, 5% rated the overall clinical performance as unsatisfactory, 5% rated it as superior, 26% rated it as marginal, and 64% rated it as satisfactory. Investigators concluded that evaluators base their ratings on different criteria and standards, and may assign different weights to these criteria.

In this chapter, you'll learn about each of these different criteria that are used in the subjective evaluations of clerkship performance. You'll learn about the major impact of oral case presentations and formal patient write-ups on your clerkship performance. You'll learn about factors that can cloud your evaluation, such as central tendency, recency bias, and primacy bias, and the measures that you can take to avoid a rating error.

You'll also learn how to seek formal feedback, how to ask for specific feedback, and how to utilize these to improve your clinical performance. You'll learn to prepare for negative feedback which, while essential for growth, can be distinctly uncomfortable. Your response to feedback gives others a sense of your professionalism, and therefore is important.

No matter what field of medicine you plan to go into, your grades in each and every clerkship have the potential to impact your future career options. While the final clerkship grade is important, individual comments made on the evaluation form may also impact your future career choices. While MSPE comments are generally positive, negative comments are included. In an analysis of nearly 300 MSPEs, negative comments included:[66]

"His most annoying attribute, he failed to show appropriate respect for his colleagues."

"She did not turn in write-ups on time and was felt by many to be defensive in the face of constructive criticism."

Throughout this chapter, you'll learn about the factors that impact your evaluation, and how you can ensure evaluations that accurately reflect your provision of outstanding patient care.

Written Exam

In terms of ensuring that you have the most potential career options, standardized examinations do matter. Core clerkship grades are a major factor in the residency selection process, and the end of rotation exam factors into this grade. While it varies from rotation to rotation, the written exam typically accounts for 20 to 40% of a student's clerkship grade.

In general, a superb performance on the written exam won't make up for a poor performance on the wards. Clinical evaluations are still most important. However, even if you earn outstanding clinical evaluations, simply obtaining a passing exam score may not be sufficient to achieve a clerkship grade of honors. In some rotations, you have to exceed a certain exam score or percentile to be considered for an overall clerkship grade of honors.

Studying for the written exam should begin on Day # 1 of the rotation, especially with short rotations that may last only a few weeks. Clerkship days often start early and end late, leaving little time to study. In the basic sciences, students get used to coasting in the first few weeks, and then doing their heavy studying closer to exam time. Clinical rotations don't allow for that type of preparation, as the workload is heavy throughout the rotation.

Exam preparation involves three main facets: the hands-on process of patient care, didactic lectures, and extensive reading. Providing care for your patients, learning from their real-life examples of typical medical histories and physical exam findings, and having those experiences reinforced and strengthened by teaching from your residents and attending is an invaluable learning experience. A number of studies have shown that student performance on NBME subject examinations improves with increasing clerkship experience.[67, 68, 69, 70] In a study of over 1,800 students from 17 U.S. medical schools, caring for more patients per day was associated with higher NBME internal medicine exam scores. Most clerkship directors felt that students should follow 3-4 patients at a time.[71]

Exam preparation will include extensive reading, and should include textbooks as well as the medical literature. In-depth reading about each of your patients is very effective, especially when this type of active learning is done correctly. In this chapter, you'll learn the questions that should guide your reading on each patient. With every single problem on the patient's problem list, you'll need to review a number of aspects, including symptoms, differential diagnoses, how to differentiate these diagnoses, the tests used to confirm the diagnosis, the prognosis, and pathogenesis, among others.

We also provide concrete recommendations for taking the exam. You should first determine if the exam will be an essay, multiple choice, or a standardized exam. If your clerkship uses the NBME (National Board of Medical Examiners) subject examination, you can review the content of the exam at www.nbme.org. At their website, the NBME has made available the content of each subject examination, including the percentage of questions that will come from different areas.

Rotation Success

You never just want to be the medical student on the team. You want to be recognized as a vital member of the health care team, making significant contributions to the care of your patient.

Providing excellent patient care is your number one goal in medical school. Receiving recognition for that excellence is a related topic, and one that encompasses additional factors. In order to succeed on a rotation, you need to learn how to quickly adapt to a new culture and new responsibilities.

Some new clerks make the mistake, early on, of focusing exclusively on learning how to perform patient care tasks. However, your team members are also concerned with many other aspects of patient care. These include your ability to work effectively with other team members, your ability to learn new subject material, your communication skills with patients and the medical team, and your overall work ethic. Many of these traits are the same that patients will use to evaluate your skills and effectiveness.

In this chapter, you'll learn how to effectively convey these additional traits. You'll learn that it's acceptable to make the "right" kind of mistakes, which are those associated with the learning process. You'll learn how to avoid the wrong type of mistakes, which are those associated with professionalism.

The ability to anticipate potential outcomes is important in medical care. Many medical students can adequately respond to a change in a patient's condition by modifying the plan. However, excellent medical students anticipate. In any admission, there are only three potential outcomes: the patient may improve, stay the same, or worsen. Outstanding students anticipate a plan for each of these outcomes.

We discuss the traits required of all practicing physicians, including integrity, credibility, and initiative. In the real-life situations of patient care, you will be challenged, and you need to be prepared. In a survey of students at Johns Hopkins University School of Medicine, 13 to 24% admitted to cheating during the clinical years of medical school.[72] Examples included "recording tasks not performed" and "lying about having ordered tests."

For many of these traits, evaluations are, of necessity, highly subjective. We provide examples of how you can demonstrate, in a concrete fashion, each of these traits. In one example, the Association of Professors of Gynecology and Obstetrics encourage students to "take initiative. 'How can I help out? I'll write the note on that patient' goes a long way to make the team function better and gives the residents more time to teach you."[73] Another suggestion is to "teach the team. Volunteer to help the team by reading about topics in depth and by sharing what you have learned with the group."

Attendings

Have the physical exam skills of physicians deteriorated over the years? It's widely believed that they have. This may be related to an increased dependence on lab testing and radiologic imaging, as well as clinical skills training in medical school and residency. According to Dr. Sal Mangione, director of the physical diagnosis curriculum at Jefferson Medical College, too little time is spent during medical school learning these skills. "Surveys have indicated that less than 16% of attending time may be spent at the patient's side."[74]

These issues have real consequences. In one eye-opening study, over 300 internal medicine residents were tested on cardiac auscultatory skills. They listened to 12 prerecorded cardiac events. It was found that their proficiency was poor, with mean identification rates of only 22% in American residents.[1]

We devote a full chapter to attending physicians. Your teachers on the wards, attendings have a great deal of knowledge and experience that they can impart. This type of education, based on the care of actual patients, is completely different from anything you'll learn in textbooks. Clinical clerkships are a critical time in your education. If you want to become proficient in exam skills, you have to learn now. These aren't skills you can learn from reading a textbook. You need to evaluate patients with these findings, and you need to have a teacher that can demonstrate these findings. You need to be able to ask questions freely in order to learn all the finer points of physical exam skills. This isn't something you can easily do as a resident, and certainly not as a board-certified physician. If you don't know how to assess jugular venous distention by the end of medical school, you may never learn.

The best attendings have an ability to model and teach patient care that is unforgettable, and in this chapter we provide suggestions on how to work with attendings known to be great teachers. In one study, researchers determined that "attending faculty's clinical teaching ability has a positive and significant effect on medical students' learning."[75] They found that ratings of teaching ability were strong predictors of students' performance on the end-of-clerkship NBME subject examination.

The attending physician is the leader of the team. His or her primary goal is to ensure that the patients assigned to the team receive the best possible care. The attending is also responsible for providing a solid educational experience for the resident, intern, and medical students. They may also have significant influence over your future career. They are responsible for clerkship evaluations, and these are considered by many program directors to be the best indicators of potential for residency success.

In order to be an outstanding physician, you must provide outstanding patient care. However, you typically won't be observed by the attending during direct patient care. Since your interactions will often be limited to attending rounds, your excellence in patient care must be conveyed by other methods. These involve being well-read on your patients' problems, delivering solid oral patient presentations, turning in thoughtful and thorough patient write-ups, and giving outstanding talks.

In this chapter, you'll learn specific recommendations that help maximize your medical education and ensure the best working relationship with your attending. This includes specifics on increasing participation in attending rounds and techniques of active listening. We also highlight areas that can prove problematic for students. Recognition of these problems can hopefully help prevent these issues. In one study, residents and attendings were asked to comment on "problem" students. Frequent problems included bright with poor interpersonal skills, excessively shy or non-assertive, over-eager, cannot focus on what is important, disorganized, and a poor fund of knowledge.[76]

Working as a Team

Physicians never care for patients alone. It takes a team of health care professionals working together effectively to provide the best patient care, and research has increasingly found that collaborative care improves outcomes. In response to this growing literature, organizations, including the Institute of Medicine and Accreditation Council for Graduate Medical Education, have urged medical schools to educate students about the roles of non-physician providers. As a third year student, you'll spend most of your time with the intern, resident, and attending. However, your team also includes nurses, social workers, pharmacists, physical therapists, lab technicians, and other professionals. Your success as a physician depends on maximizing the combined efforts of each of these health care professionals. The most successful physicians live this daily.

Research has shown that collaborative relationships between team members leads to improved patient outcomes. In a study done in the intensive care unit, Knaus found that greater interaction of staff in different disciplines was associated with lower patient mortality.[77] In a study of surgical patients, relational coordination across disciplines was associated with reduced pain and shorter length of stays among total hip and knee arthroplasty patients.[78]

Despite this knowledge, in practice, collaboration and communication between professionals often doesn't occur. In one study of randomly selected hospitalized patients, nurses and physicians were interviewed.[79] Nurses reported communicating with physicians only 50% of the time. The authors wrote that "there was no agreement between nurses and physicians on planned tests or procedures for the day in 25% and 11% of instances, respectively. There was no agreement between the nurses and physicians on planned medication changes for the day in 42% of instances." In chapter 22, we review the benefits of collaboration with all members of the healthcare team, including nursing professionals.

You'll work most closely with your nuclear team, which consists of an attending, resident, interns, and students. Maximizing the effectiveness of your nuclear team involves significant teamwork. The teaching you receive from these professionals may be formal or informal, and is invaluable, and we review ways to maximize this teaching.

In one study, interviews with attendings and residents were conducted to determine what behaviors make students "good" or "bad" clerks. Supervisors viewed behavior as positive when students acted "for the sake of patient care, for the sake of their own learning, or for the sake of their own team."[80] Behavior was considered negative if students were thought to be shirking responsibility or "acting for the sake of appearance." In this chapter, we provide advice on how to work effectively with all team members. You'll learn practical measures that you can take to maximize the effectiveness of the team, and you'll learn how to prepare for and manage the inevitable conflict that occurs when a team is working together so closely in an intense environment.

Giving Talks

The typical medical student talk, which we've sat through many times, usually follows this script:

> Introduction: "The subject of my talk is pulmonary embolism."
>
> Content: unrealistically extensive overview of a massive topic relying heavily on major medical textbooks
>
> Conclusion: "Well, I guess that's all I have."

It's easy to make that talk significantly more impressive and memorable.

> Introduction: *"Substantial and unacceptable."* Those were the words of Dr. Kenneth Moser, referring to the morbidity and mortality rate of venous thromboembolism ...[81] A major issue in reducing these high rates is enhancing early diagnosis. In my talk today, I'll review recent advances in diagnostic techniques of pulmonary embolism."
>
> Content: in-depth review of a focused topic utilizing references from the recent medical literature
>
> Conclusion: "As the recent literature has shown, the diagnosis of pulmonary embolism may clearly be challenging. As in the case of our patient Mr. Smith, however, a combination of diagnostic methods leads to improved sensitivity."

Being asked to give a talk is a common and anxiety-provoking student experience. Medical students are often asked to give a talk to the team, usually pertaining to an issue that arises during rounds. While this is usually an anxiety-provoking, or even dread-inducing experience, preparing and presenting a talk is a great opportunity to demonstrate your knowledge and grasp of clinical issues. Your stellar performance can definitely impress the team. While you can't control what an attending might ask during rounds, you do have complete control over your talk. With sufficient preparation and practice, you should be able to deliver an outstanding talk.

In this chapter, you'll learn specific recommendations to improve the quality and impact of your talks. You'll learn the importance of choosing the correct topic. In a study of medical student talks, students were informed to avoid overviews or large topics.[82] As an example, rather than talking about pneumonia, students were asked to focus on a particular aspect of pneumonia. Despite this recommendation, faculty evaluations noted that 35% of presentations were too broadly focused.

You'll learn how to perform an audience analysis, including the questions that ensure a talk tailored to the audience's level of expertise and learning needs, as well as the types of resources to utilize. You'll read a number of styles of introductions, as well as concluding statements, that capture an audience's interest. These introductory and concluding statements are all ones that you can easily incorporate into any topic. You'll learn techniques that enhance the quality of your speaking and the quality of your audiovisual aids. You'll learn how to reduce the anxiety common to public speaking, and you'll learn specific techniques on how to respond to questions, an anxiety-provoking situation for even experienced speakers.

References

[1]Mangione S. Cardiac auscultatory skills of physicians-in-training: a comparison of three English-speaking countries. *Am J Med* 2001; 110(3): 210-6.

[2]Berger J, Eisen L, Nozad V, D'Angelo J, Calderon Y, Brown D, Schweitzer P. Competency in electrocardiogram interpretation among internal medicine and emergency medicine residents. *Am J Med* 2005; 118(8): 873-80.

[3]Eisen L, Berger J, Hegde A, Schneider R. Competency in chest radiography. A comparison of medical students, residents, and fellows. *J Gen Intern Med* 2006; 21(5): 460-5.

[4]Brenner A, Mathai S, Jain S, Mohl P. Can we predict "problem residents"? *Acad Med* 2010; 85(7): 1147-51.

[5]Cohen J. Professionalism in medical education, an American perspective: from evidence to accountability. *Med Educ* 2006; 40(7): 607-17.

[6]Papadakis M, Teherani A, Banach M, Knettler T, Rattner S, Stern D, Veloski J, Hodgson C. Disciplinary action by medical boards and prior behavior in medical school. *N Engl J Med* 2005; 353(25): 2673-82.

[7]Teherani A, Hodgson C, Banach M, Papadakis M. Domains of unprofessional behavior during medical school associated with future disciplinary action by a state medical board. *Acad Med* 2005; 80(10 Suppl): S17-20.

[8]Green M, Jones P, Thomas J. Selection criteria for residency: results of a national program directors survey. *Acad Med* 2009; 84(3): 362-7.

[9]Dirschl D, Dahners L, Adams G, Crouch J, Wilson F. Correlating selection criteria with subsequent performance as residents. *Clin Orthop Relat Res* 2002; 399: 265-71.

[10]Amos D, Massagli T. Medical school achievements as predictors of performance in a physical medicine and rehabilitation residency. *Acad Med* 1996; 71(6): 678-80.

[11]Fine P, Hayward R. Do the criteria of resident selection committees predict residents' performances? *Acad Med* 1995; 70(9): 834-8.

[12]Starfield B. Is US health really the best in the world? *JAMA* 2000; 284: 483-5.

[13]Institute of Medicine. *To Err is Human: Building a Safer Health System.* Washington, DC: National Academy Press; 2000.

[14]What medical students need to know about the internal medicine rotation. http://www.acponline.org/pressroom/ess_clerk.htm. Accessed January 30, 2011.

[15]University of Washington Medicine Clerkship Website. http://depts.washington.edu/medclerk/drupal/pages/Careers-Internal-Medicine. Accessed January 28, 2011.

[16]Univeristy of Colorado Department of Surgery. http://www.ucdenver.edu/academics/colleges/medicalschool/education/studentaffairs/studentgroups/SurgicalSociety/Pages/FAQ.aspx. Accessed January 30, 2010.

[17]Takayama H, Grinsell R, Brock D, Foy H, Pellegrini C, Horvath K. Is it appropriate to use core clerkship grades in the selection of residents? *Curr Surg* 2006; 63(6): 391-6.

[18]Pettitt B. Medical student concerns and fears before their third-year surgical clerkship. *Am J Surg* 2005; 189(4): 492-6.

[19]Univeristy of South Alabama Pediatrics Clerkship Handbook. http://www.usouthal.edu/peds/reshome/documents/PEDIATRICCLERKSHIPHANDBOOK4.10.pdf. Accessed January 30, 2011.

[20]Institute for Patient- and Family-Centered Care. http://www.ipfcc.org/advance/topics/primary-care.html. Accessed January 30, 2011.

[21]Bremer A, Goldstein B, Nirken M, Desai S. *Pediatrics Clerkship: 101 Biggest Mistakes And How To Avoid Them*. Houston; MD2B: 2005.

[22]The Family Medicine Clerkship Curriculum. http://www.stfm.org/documents/fmcurriculum(v3).pdf. Accessed January 30, 2011.

[23]Taylor R. *Fundamentals of Family Medicine: The Family Medicine Clerkship Textbook*. New York; Springer-Verlag: 2003.

[24]Yale University Department of Obstetrics and Gynecology. http://medicine.yale.edu/obgyn/education/medstudents/index.aspx. Accessed January 30, 2011.

[25]University of California Davis Department of Obstetrics and Gynecology. www.ucdmc.ucdavis.edu/gme/ppts/residency_advice_1.pps. Accessed January 30, 2011.

[26]University of Minnesota Department of Obstetrics and Gynecology. http://www.obgyn.umn.edu/education/medstudent/clerkship/home.html. Accessed January 30, 2011.

[27]University of Washington Department of Obstetrics and Gynecology. http://depts.washington.edu/obgyn/clerkship/electives.html. Accessed January 30, 2011.

[28]World Psychiatric Association. http://www.wpanet.org/detail.php?section_id=8&content_id=109. Accessed January 30, 2011.

[29]McLaren K, Martin C, Hebig P. *Psychiatry Clerkship: 150 Biggest Mistakes And How To Avoid Them*. Houston: MD2B; 2005.

[30]Roman B, Trevino J. An approach to address grade inflation in a psychiatry clerkship. *Acad Psychiatry* 2006; 30(2): 110-5.

[31]Klass P. *A not entirely benign procedure: four years as a medical student*. New York; Kaplan Publishers: 2010.

[32]Westbrook J, Coiera E, Dunsmuir W, Brown B, Kelk N, Paoloni R, Tran C. The impact of interruptions on clinical task completion. *Qual Saf Health Care* 2010; 19(4): 284-9.

[33]Bikowski R, Ripsin C, Lorraine V. Physician-patient congruence regarding medication regimens. *J Am Geriatr Soc* 2001; 49(10): 1353-7.

[34]Peterson M, Holbrook J, Hales D, Smith N, Staker L. Contributions of the history, physical examination, and laboratory investigation in making medical diagnoses. *West J Med* 1992; 156: 163-5.

[35]Hauer K, Teherani A, Kerr K, O'Sullivan P, Irby D. Student performance problems in medical school clinical skills assessments. *Acad Med* 2007; 82(10 Suppl): S69-S72.

[36]Bates D, Cullen D, Laird N, et al. Incidence of adverse drug events and potential adverse drug events. Implications for prevention. *JAMA* 1995; 274(1): 29-34.

[37]Division of Laboratory Systems, Centers for Disease Control and Prevention. Patient-centered care and laboratory medicine: national status report: 2008-2009 update. https://www.futurelabmedicine.org/ reports%5CLaboratory_Medicine_National_Status_%20Report_08-09_Update--Patient-Centered_Care.pdf. Published May 2009. Accessed May 18, 2010.

[38]Controlling Health Care Costs while Promoting the Best Possible Health Outcomes. http://www.acponline.org/advocacy/where_we_stand/policy/ controlling_healthcare_costs.pdf. Accessed on January 30, 2011.

[39]Wong E, Lincoln T, Lundberg G. Ready! Fire!...Aim! An inquiry into laboratory test ordering. *JAMA* 1983; 250 (18): 2510-13.

[40]Ferguson R, Kohler F, Chavez J, Puthumana J, Zaidi S, Shakil H. Discovering asymptomatic biochemical abnormalities on a Baltimore internal medicine service. *Md Med J* 1996; 45(7): 543-6.

[41]Arce-Cordon R, Perez-Rodriguez M, Baca-Baldomero E, Oquendo M, Baca-Garcia E. Routine laboratory screening among newly admitted psychiatric patients: is it worthwhile? *Psychiatr Serv* 2007; 58(12): 1602-5.

[42]Laposata M. CDC Website. http://wwwn.cdc.gov/cliac/pdf/Addenda/cliac0906/ AddendumL.pdf. Accessed January 30, 2011.

[43]Gandhi T, Kachalia A, Thomas E, Puopolo A, Yoon C, Brennan T, et al. Missed and delayed diagnoses in the ambulatory setting: a study of closed malpractice claims. *Ann Intern Med* 2006; 145: 488-96.

[44]Clerkship Directors in Internal Medicine (CDIM) and Society of General Internal Medicine (SGIM). Core Medicine Clerkship Guide: A Resource for Teachers and Learners, Version 3.0. http://www.im.org/Resources/Education/Students/ Learning/Documents/OnlineCDIMCurriculum.pdf. Published 2006. Accessed May 18, 2010.

[45]Smith B, et al. Educating medical students in laboratory medicine: a proposed curriculum. *Am J Clin Pathol* 2010; 133(4): 533-42.

[46]Foley R, Smilansky J, Yonke A. Teacher-student interaction in a medical clerkship. *J Med Educ* 1979; 54(8): 622-6.

[47]Hunt D, Caroline J, Tonesk X, Yergan J, Siever M, Loebel J. Types of problem students encountered by clinical teachers on clerkships. *Med Educ* 1989; 23: 14-8.

[48]Williamson K, Ya-Ping K, Steele J. Gunderman R. The art of asking: teaching through questioning. *Acad Radiology* 2002; 9(12): 1419-22.

[49]Taylor E, Tisdell E, Gusic M. Teaching beliefs of medical educators: perspectives on clinical teaching in pediatrics. *Med Teach* 2007; 29: 371-6.

[50]Pangaro L. A new vocabulary and other innovations for improving descriptive in-training evaluations. *Acad Med* 1999; 74: 1203-7.

[51]Singh H, Thomas E, Petersen L, Studdert D. Medical errors involving trainees. A study of close malpractice claims from 5 insurers. *Arch Intern Med* 2007; 167(19): 2030-6.

[52]Howley L, Wilson L. Direct observation of students during clerkship rotations: a multiyear descriptive study. *Acad Med* 2004; 79 (3): 276-80.

[53]Pulito A, Donnelly M, Plymale M, Mentzer R Jr. What do faculty observe of medical students' clinical performance. *Teach Learn Med* 2006; 18(2): 99-104.

[54]Association of American Medical Colleges. Learning Objectives for Medical Student Education: Guidelines for Medical Schools (MSOP Report). Washington, DC: Association of American Medical Colleges; 1998.

[55]Carroll A, Tarczy-Hornoch P, O'Reilly E, Christakis D. Resident documentation discrepancies in a neonatal intensive care unit. *Pediatrics* 2003; 111: 976-80.

[56]Szauter K, Ainsworth M, Holden M, Mercado A. Do students do what they write and write what they do? The match between the patient encounter and patient note. *Acad Med* 2006; 81 (10 Suppl): S44-7.

[57]Worzala K, Rattner S, Boulet J, Majdan J, Berg D, Robeson M, Veloski J. Evaluation of the congruence between students' postencounter notes and standardized patients' checklists in a clinical skills examination. *Teach Learn Med* 2008; 20(1): 31-6.

[58]USMLE website. http://www.usmle.org/news/cse/step2csfaqs1103.htm. Accessed December 23, 2009.

[59]Kogan J, Shea J. Psychometric characteristics of a write-up assessment form in a medicine core clerkship. *Teach Learn Med* 2005; 17(2): 101-6.

[60]Barzansky B, Etzel S. Medical schools in the United States, 2008-2009. *JAMA* 2009; 302(12): 1349-55.

[61]Kalet A, Earp J, Kowlowitz V. How well do faculty evaluate the interviewing skills of medical students? *J Gen Intern Med* 1992; 7(5): 499-505.

[62]Rutter D, Maguire G. History-taking for medical students. *Lancet* 1976; 2(7985): 558-60.

[63]Boehler M, Schwind C, Dunnington G, Rogers D, Folse R. Medical student contact with patients on a surgery clerkship: is there a chance to learn? *J Am Coll Surg* 2002; 195(4): 539-42.

[64]Groopman J. *How doctors think?* New York; Houghton Mifflin Company: 2007.

[65]Noel G, Herbers J, Caplow M, Cooper G, Pangaro L, Harvey J. How well do internal medicine faculty members evaluate the clinical skills of residents? *Ann Intern Med* 1992; 117(9): 757-65.

[66]Shea J, O'Grady E, Wagner B, Morris J, Morrison G. Professionalism in clerkships: an analysis of MSPE commentary. *Acad Med* 2008; 83 (10 Suppl): S1-4.

[67]Manley M, Heiss G. Timing bias in the psychiatry examination of the National Board of Medical Examiners. *Acad Psych* 2006; 30: 116-9.

[68]Reteguiz J, Crosson J. Clerkship order and performance on Family Medicine and Internal Medicine National Board of Medical Examiners exams. *Fam Med* 2002; 34: 604-8.

[69]Hampton H, Collins B, Perry K, Meydrech E, Wiser W, Morrison J. Order of rotation in third year clerkships: influence on academic performance. *J Reprod Med* 1996; 41: 337-40.

[70]Cho J, Belmont J, Cho C. Correcting the bias of clerkship timing on academic performance. *Arch Pediatr Adolesc Med* 1998; 152: 1015-8.

[71]Griffith C, Wilson J, Haist S, Albritton T, Bognar B, Cohen S, Hoesley C, Fagan M, Ferenchick G, Pryor O, Friedman E, Harrell H, Hemmer P, Houghton B, Kovach R, Lambert D, Loftus T, Painter T, Udden M, Watkins R, Wong R. Internal medicine clerkship characteristics associated with enhanced student examination performance. *Acad Med* 2009; 84(7): 895-901.

[72]Dans P. Self-reported cheated by students at one medical school. *Acad Med* 1996; 71(1 Suppl): S70-72.

[73]The Obstetrics and Gynecology Clerkship: Your Guide to Success," the Association of Professors of Gynecology and Obstetrics. http://www.apgo.org/binary/Clerkship%20Primer%20Online%20Version.pdf. Accessed January 20, 2011.

[74]Kelly C. Good diagnostic skills should begin at the bedside. *ACP Internist.* February 2001. http://www.acpinternist.org/archives/2001/02/diagnostics.htm. Accessed January 30, 2011.

[75]Stern D, Williams B, Gill A, Gruppen L, Woolliscroft J, Grum C. Is there relationship between attending physicans' and residents' teaching skills and students' examination scores? *Acad Med* 2000; 75(11): 1144-6.

[76]Hunt D, Caroline J, Tonesk X, Yergan J, Siever M, Loebel J. Types of problem students encountered by clinical teachers on clerkships. *Med Educ* 1989; 23: 14-8.

[77]Knaus W, Draper E, Wagner D, Zimmerman J. An evaluation of outcome from intensive care in major medical centers. *Ann Intern Med* 1986; 104: 410-8.

[78]Gittell J, Fairfield K, Bierbaum B, et al. Impact of relational coordination on quality of care, postoperative pain and functioning, and length of stay: a nine-hospital study of surgical patients. *Med Care* 2000; 38: 807-19.

[79]O'Leary K, Thompson J, Landler M, Kulkarni N, Haviley C, Hahn K, Jeon J, Wayne D, Baker D, Williams M. Patterns of nurse-physician communication and agreement on the plan of care. *Qual Saf Health Care* 2010; 19(3): 195-9.

[80]Lavine E, Regehr G, Garwood K, Ginsbury S. The role of attribution to clerk factors and contextual factors in supervisors' perceptions of clerks' behaviors. *Teach Learn Med* 2004; 16(4): 317-22.

[81]Moser KM: Venous thromboembolism. *Am Rev Respir Dis* 1990 Jan; 141(1): 235-49.

[82]Kernan W, Quagliarello V, Green M. Student faculty rounds: a peer-mediated learning activity for internal medicine clerkships. *Med Teach* 27(2): 140-4.

Chapter 2

Internal Medicine Clerkship

Rule # 2   **The field of internal medicine has a broad impact on all fields of medicine.**

"Learning about internal medicine – the specialty providing comprehensive care to adults – in the third year of medical school is an important experience, regardless of what specialty the medical student ultimately pursues," says Dr. Patrick Alguire, the Director of Education and Career Development at the American College of Physicians.[1] Through this clerkship, you will hone your skills in history and physical examination, diagnostic test interpretation, medical decision-making, and management of core medical conditions. These skills are important ones for all physicians, even if you ultimately decide to enter radiology, pathology, emergency medicine, or another field.

Your internal medicine (IM) clerkship grade can impact your career. It's a factor in the residency selection process for all specialties, not just internal medicine. In a survey of over 1,200 residency program directors across 21 medical specialties, grades in required clerkships were ranked as the # 1 factor used in the selection process.[2] "Do well in your clerkship," writes the Department of Medicine at the University of Washington.[3] "Yes, this is obvious – and easier said than done – but it's also important. Most residency programs look closely at the third-year clerkship grade when selecting applicants."

Many medical students find this clerkship formidable. A lack of knowledge isn't the main factor. The main factor is a lack of preparation for your many responsibilities. How do I evaluate a newly admitted patient? What do I need to include in a daily progress note? What information do I need to include in a comprehensive write-up? How do I present newly admitted patients to the attending physician?

In this chapter, templates and outlines are included for each of these important responsibilities. You'll also find a number of tips and suggestions on how to maximize your learning and performance during this rotation. You'll find detailed information that will help you effectively preround, succeed during work rounds, deliver polished oral case presentations, create well-written daily progress notes, and generate comprehensive write-ups.

For students interested in a career in internal medicine, this chapter also details how to strengthen your application.

About the rotation

The internal medicine clerkship is usually two to three months in duration. Depending on your school, you may spend the entire rotation at one hospital, or you may rotate through several affiliated institutions. While largely an inpatient experience, you'll also have opportunities to practice outpatient medicine, either through regularly scheduled outpatient clinics or a dedicated month-long outpatient block. The clerkship will expose you to not only general internal medicine, but also to subspecialties, including cardiology, pulmonology, gastroenterology, nephrology, endocrinology, hematology, oncology, infectious disease, rheumatology, and allergy.

Typical day

Here's what a typical day on the internal medicine clerkship looks like (inpatient setting):

6:30 – 7:30 AM	Pre-rounds
7:30 – 9:00 AM	Work rounds
9:00 – 10:00 AM	Patient care tasks
10:00 – 12:00 NOON	Attending rounds
NOON – 1:00 PM	Noon conference
1:00 - ?	Patient care tasks (+ student conferences)

What should you carry with you?

- Stethoscope
- Penlight
- Reflex hammer
- Tuning fork
- Eye chart
- Tongue blades
- Calculator
- Ophthalmoscope
- Watch with second hand for pulse measurement

Your Team

During your clerkship, you'll work as a team to take care of your assigned patients. The team usually consists of the following individuals:

Attending physician

The attending physician is typically a faculty member at the medical school (clinical or academic) who has been assigned to be the leader of the team. The attending's primary goal is to ensure that the patients assigned to the team receive the best possible care. Providing a solid educational experience for residents, interns, and medical students is also an important goal. The attending is responsible for evaluating all team members. The team's contact with the attending is usually limited to attending rounds, a period of time during the day in which the entire team meets.

Resident

The resident physician is a house officer who, at the minimum, has completed an internship. Second in charge, the resident (along with intern), under the guidance of the attending, formulates a treatment plan for the patients assigned to the team. The resident then makes sure that the interns and medical students implement this plan. The resident is also responsible for teaching the junior members of the team. The extent of teaching varies, and may consist of didactic lectures or pimping.

Intern

By definition, internship refers to the first year of residency training that follows medical school graduation. Next to medical students, interns are the most junior members of the team. They are responsible for executing the treatment plan. Interns have a lot on their plate, which is why they need to function quickly and efficiently to accomplish the day's patient care activities.

You will interact the most with the intern, since he or she will also follow the patients assigned to you. When issues arise in the management of your patient's condition(s), you should first discuss them with your intern. Although many interns love to teach, this isn't always possible, given the many demands on their time. On a daily basis, some of their responsibilities include scheduling tests and procedures, checking lab test results, entering orders, drawing blood, and writing daily progress notes.

Pre-rounds

Your day will typically begin with pre-rounds, in which you'll see your patients alone. The goal is to identify any new events in the patient's course. This information will be presented to the resident and intern during work rounds (morning walk rounds).

What to do during pre-rounds

- Review the chart for any new progress notes that may have been placed after you left the hospital.
- Review the patient's orders, looking for any new orders that may have been written after you left the hospital.
- Speak with the intern (i.e. cross-covering intern) who was taking care of your patient while your team was out of the hospital. See if any new events occurred in your patient's hospital course. If this isn't possible, touch base with your intern, who will get sign-out from the cross-covering intern.
- Speak with the nurse involved in your patient's care to see if he or she has any concerns or issues.
- Speak with the patient. Ascertain the following:
  - Has the patient's overall condition improved, stayed the same, or worsened?
  - Does the patient still have the same symptoms? If so, have these improved, stayed the same, or worsened?
  - Does the patient have any new symptoms?
  - Does the patient have any new concerns? Questions?
- Examine the patient.
  - Write down the most recent vital signs (BP, HR, RR, temperature), maximum temperature (Tmax), and if pertinent, O_2 sat, weight, blood glucose checks, and Ins/Outs. Also note any trends in the temperature, BP, or HR. If vital signs haven't been taken recently, do so yourself.
  - Check the IV. Note the type of intravenous fluids hanging and the rate of administration.
  - Perform a brief physical exam: focus on the area of interest (if the patient has a foot ulcer, examine the foot). At a minimum, you should also perform a heart, lung, abdomen, and lower extremity exam, irrespective of the reason for hospitalization.
- Check on the results of lab and diagnostic tests: labs, ECG, radiographs, other.
- Gather your thoughts and formulate your assessment and plan for each problem.
- Get ready to present this information to the resident and intern during work rounds.

ls: 10 Tips for Success

rrive early. Give yourself enough time to see your patients) that you can gather the necessary information without being rushed. An extra cushion of time is especially helpful when the patient had an eventful night, which creates considerable information to gather and sort through.

Tip # 2 Write down all information so that you can accurately convey it to your team in work rounds. Writing it down in an organized manner also helps with the patient's progress note.

Tip # 3 A review of the chart for any new progress notes is a must. This is one of the keys to getting up to speed on your patient's hospital course. Read all new progress notes, including those left by nurses.

Tip # 4 Always look at the orders. New orders may be written after you leave the hospital. Often these orders aren't documented in the progress notes.

Tip # 5 Your intern may know things about your patient that you don't. They receive report (sign-out) from the cross-covering intern, who cares for your patient when your team is out of the hospital. Always ask your intern if they know anything about your patient that you don't.

Tip # 6 Perform a heart, lung, abdomen, and lower extremity exam on every patient, irrespective of the reason for the patient's hospitalization.

Tip # 7 Always check the computer for the most up-to-date lab test results. Don't rely on the chart because it often takes time for the most recent results to be placed in the patient's chart.

Tip # 8 Some lab test results take days to return. Check on pending test results every morning.

Tip # 9 Think about the data you've gathered. Actively processing the data will help you formulate an assessment and plan.

Tip #10 Before leaving the hospital for the day, read any new progress notes that may have been added to the chart. This shortens the time needed for the next day's pre-rounds.

Work Rounds

During work rounds, also known as morning or resident walk rounds, the team (usually without the attending) travels from room to room, seeing each of the patients on the service. At times, depending on the institution, other healthcare professionals may join rounds. These may include pharmacists, dieticians, social workers, and nurses. The most junior member of the team (junior medical student, subintern, intern) following the patient is required to update the team on the patient's progress. This update includes any significant events that have occurred overnight and the results of any lab or diagnostic testing. The information you present will help the team formulate a diagnostic and therapeutic plan.

8 Questions to Ask Your Resident before Your First Work Rounds

Question # 1   Where will work rounds begin?

Question # 2   What information should I gather for work rounds?

Question # 3   What time does work rounds start?

Question # 4   How much time do I have for my work rounds presentation?

Question # 5   How would you like me to present newly admitted patients?

Question # 6   How would you like me to present established patients?

Question # 7   In what order should I present the information?

Question # 8   How detailed should my work rounds presentation be?

Step-by-Step Approach for the Work Rounds Presentation

Step 1: Start with a short summary of the patient to remind the team of his or her problems. Give the patient's name, age, gender, and chief complaint or working diagnosis/reason for being in the hospital.

Mr. Smith is a 64-year old white male who was admitted two days ago with shortness of breath and diagnosed with COPD exacerbation

Step 2: Present the subjective data, which should include the patient's current status and any events or complaints that have occurred or developed since yesterday's rounds.

He states that his night was uneventful. He continues, however, to have shortness of breath without significant improvement from the day of admission. He denies fever, cough, or chest pain.

Step 3: Present the objective data, beginning with the most recent vital signs, including temperature, blood pressure, heart rate, respiratory rate, and pulse oximetry (mention the amount of oxygen patient is receiving). Also mention the maximum temperature in the last 24 hours. Express the vitals with ranges. Also mention the total fluid input and output, blood glucose checks over the last 24 hours, and daily weights if pertinent to the patient.

Current respiratory rate, pulse, temperature, and blood pressure are 18, 84, 99, and 130/80, respectively. Maximum temperature of 99. The blood pressure has ranged from 118/75 to 135/85.

Step 4: Present the physical exam findings from your most recent exam. Always present the heart, lung, abdominal, and lower extremity exam (be brief). Also include findings pertinent to the patient's problem. If the patient was admitted with delirium, you need to perform a mental status exam.

Physical exam is remarkable for prolonged expiratory phase and scattered expiratory wheezes throughout both lung fields. Heart exam reveals a regular rate and rhythm. Abdominal and lower extremity exams are unremarkable.

Step 5: Present the laboratory test results. Include only new lab test results, if they are back. Present the pertinent or changed lab values, not unchanged or normal values. Old results may be presented if needed.

All laboratory test results are normal except for the serum BUN and creatinine, which are 30 and 1.5, respectively. Admission values were 15 and 1.0, respectively.

Step 6: Present the results of any other diagnostic studies or i. ı. tests. Include only the results of new studies or tests.

Chest x-ray performed yesterday revealed no evidence of pneumonia or pneumothorax.

Step 7: Discuss each of the patient's problems in descending order of importance. Provide an assessment for each problem followed by the management plan.

Problem # 1 is COPD exacerbation. He has been receiving albuterol and atrovent nebs every 8 hours. Despite this therapy, his condition has not improved. The plan is to increase frequency of the neb treatments to q4 hours and add intravenous solumedrol at a dose of 60 mg q6 hours. I will continue to check in on him every few hours.

Problem # 2 is HTN. He has been normotensive over the past 24 hours. The plan is to continue his antihypertensive regimen of hydrochlorothiazide and felodipine.

ʒs: 10 Tips for Success

ʒuᴉnб   37

/s be on time. There is a lot to accomplish, and if
ϱ late you put the team behind schedule.

ᴗᵣᵢᴇᵣ oral patient presentations are preferred during work
rounds. Ask your resident how much time you have to
present the information. Don't exceed your allotted time.

Tip # 3   Know the order of the work rounds presentation. Don't
deviate from the expected order.

Tip # 4   Bring any new studies, such as ECGs, with you to rounds.
This saves the team time, and increases efficiency.

Tip # 5   As the day's plan for each patient is defined during work
rounds, add each task to your to-do list. Don't rely on
memory.

Tip # 6   Your team would like to hear your own assessment and
plan for the patient because it reflects your thinking
process. Don't defer to the intern for this discussion.

Tip # 7   After discussing the day's plan for your patient, make sure
you understand the reasoning behind the plan. Ask
questions if you need to.

Tip # 8   Residents often teach during work rounds. They often pass
along important pearls of information, which may very well
be the answers to your attending's questions later in the
day.

Tip # 9   Listen carefully to all patient presentations, even if you
aren't directly following the patient. You'll maximize your
medical education.

Tip # 10   Students are graded on enthusiasm. One way to
demonstrate interest is to ask informed questions.

Evaluating the New Patient when On Call

"On call" denotes the time period when you admit new patients onto the service. Call structure varies according to the medical institution, but in general ward teams admit anywhere from 5-10 patients when on call. Call can either be during the day or night. Call is an outstanding educational experience, and it allows you to evaluate new and interesting patients.

Step 1: Have a patient information template available to collect all data. This helps you organize the information for write-ups and oral case presentations.

Step 2: See if there are previous medical records on your patient. In some hospitals, you have to call and request medical records. In others, electronic records are readily available.

Step 3: Before seeing the patient, review the emergency room or clinic notes which prompted the admission.

Step 4: See the patient and perform a *complete* history and physical exam. It's preferable to perform this evaluation separate from the housestaff.

Step 5: Gather lab test results, ECGs, and imaging test results. Interpret the studies yourself before reading the reports. Add these results to your patient template.

Step 6: Use the information from the history, physical examination, and other data, including labs and imaging, to create a complete problem list.

Step 7: Prioritize the problem list in descending order of importance and generate a differential diagnosis for each active problem. Ask yourself:

-What is the most likely diagnosis and why?
-What is the differential diagnosis?
-What further evaluation is needed to support my working (likely) diagnosis?
-What treatment should I recommend?

The answers to these questions will help you create your own assessment and plan.

Step 8: Present the information and offer your assessment and plan to the resident. Use the information from your patient template to help you present an organized H & P. Ask the resident for feedback, especially about your assessment and plan.

Step 9: Write the admission orders if permitted.

Step 10: Read in depth about your patient's specific issues.

On Call: 10 Tips for Success

Tip # 1   Learn your on call responsibilities. At the beginning of your rotation, meet with your resident and intern to learn what's expected of you.

Tip # 2   Prepare for call by bringing all necessary items. This includes a change of clothes, personal hygiene items, snacks, and books.

Tip # 3   When the resident informs you of a new patient admission, write down the patient's essential information. Note the full name, medical record number, and location on a patient card or note card.

Tip # 4   Patients often can't remember everything about their medical history, so having information from the medical record, when available, can be extremely useful for filling in the gaps.

Tip # 5   If you can't obtain a reliable history from the patient, don't stop there. Attempt to contact family members. If the patient lives in a nursing home, call the nursing home. If the patient was recently discharged from another hospital, call the medical records department at that hospital to have the discharge summary or records sent to you.

Tip # 6   Find out what was done for the patient in the ER or clinic prior to your involvement. Be familiar with the evaluation performed there, including the lab and diagnostic studies obtained and the medications and therapies administered. In order to provide the best possible care, it is essential that you know this information. Your attending will ask for it during your oral case presentation.

Tip # 7   Interpret all lab and diagnostic studies on your own. Then ask your intern or resident to review the studies with you. Also review imaging tests with the radiologist so you have a better understanding of the findings.

Tip # 8   If time permits, present the case to your intern. They may provide you with tips and hints on what the resident or attending may ask about your patient.

Tip # 9   If patients or family members ask you specific questions about the treatment plan or prognosis, defer the answers to your intern or resident.

Tip # 10   When you complete your work, don't just leave without offering to help other team members. The on call day is busy and stressful for the entire team. Any assistance that you provide will be appreciated.

Writing Admit Orders

ABC - VANDALISM is a popular mnemonic to help remember the contents of the admission orders.

Admit to: location, service, attending physician

Because: admitting diagnosis/problem

Condition: good, fair, poor, serious/guarded, critical

Vitals: parameters, frequency

Allergies: medication allergies

Nursing: blood glucose checks, foley to gravity, intake/output, daily weights, patient positioning/turning, wound care, nasogastric tube, precautions

Diet:

Activity: bed rest, bed rest with bathroom privileges/bedside commode, up in chair, walk with help, up ad lib

Labs: e.g. CBC in the AM

Intravenous
fluids: composition, rate of administration, quantity

Studies: e.g. ECG in the AM, CT Scan of the Chest

Medications: dosage, route of administration, frequency

Checklist for Internal Medicine Write-Up

The write-up, or written case presentation, is a detailed account of the patient's clinical presentation. You were probably introduced to the process of writing a case presentation during your physical diagnosis course. During the Internal Medicine clerkship, you will be asked to submit write-ups on patients you admit. One of the major purposes of the write-up is to help you develop the written communication skills needed to take care of patients. These are skills that will serve you and your patients well throughout your medical career. For many attendings, the oral case presentation and patient write-up are two major determinants of a student's clerkship grade. Below is a checklist you can use to ensure your write-up is complete.

Chief Complaint (CC)

____ Chief complaint is included.
____ Source of the history is included.

History of Present Illness (HPI)

____ First sentence includes the necessary and relevant information: age, gender, chief complaint, duration of chief complaint, relevant PMH.
____ HPI is presented in a chronological fashion beginning with when patient was at baseline or usual state of health.
____ Chief complaint is defined properly: location, quality or character, frequency, onset, course, duration, severity, radiation (of pain), precipitating factors, alleviating factors, associated symptoms.
____ Description of how the symptom has affected the patient and his or her life: physically, emotionally, social relationships, others
____ Includes what the patient thinks has caused the problem as well as the patient's concerns
____ Addresses why the patient sought medical attention now rather than earlier
____ Elements of the PMH, social history, and family history that are relevant to the HPI are incorporated.
____ Information from the review of systems pertinent to the chief complaint is included.

Past medical history (PMH)

____ Complete with sufficient detail for each diagnosis, including date of diagnosis, how the diagnosis was made, past studies done for evaluation, dates of any surgeries or hospitalizations, therapy previously received, current therapy, and current status of the problem.

Medications

___ Includes dose, route, and frequency of each medication
___ Includes over the counter and herbal preparations and PRN
medications
___ Medications being given for the same condition are grouped together

Allergies

___ Includes nature of adverse reaction

Social History

___ Occupation
___ Marital status
___ Tobacco, alcohol, and substance abuse
___ Living situation
___ Functional status

Family History

___ Includes state of health of parents, siblings, children
___ Lists age of family members at the time of diagnosis with important
conditions
___ Explores family history of CAD, DM, HTN, and cancer beyond first
degree relatives

Review of systems (ROS)

___ All systems are included.
___ Each system is explored in sufficient depth.
___ ROS does not include information already given in HPI.

Physical examination

___ Description of patient's general appearance
___ Includes vital signs (O_2 saturation, orthostatics if pertinent)
___ Physical examination does not include any judgments or
interpretations (e.g. wheezing consistent with asthma)
___ Complete, including the following that are commonly omitted from the
exam:
- Skin examination
- Thyroid examination
- Lymph node survey beyond just "neck
nodes"
- Neck veins
- Distal pulses
- Liver span

- Rectal exam (if not done, offer reason)
- Mental status
- Cranial nerves
- Strength/sensation
- Cerebellar function
- Reflexes

Laboratory and other studies

___ All lab and diagnostic test results are reported.
___ Basic lab test results are reported first.

Problem list

___ All active medical problems are included.
___ All abnormalities in the physical exam are included.
___ All abnormal lab test results are included.

Assessment & Plan

___ Begins with summary statement with key history, physical exam, and lab data.
___ Assessment & Plan is problem-based rather than systems or organ-based.
___ Problems are listed in descending order of importance.
___ Assessment is provided for every problem.
___ Differential diagnosis is offered for major problems.
___ Differential diagnosis includes potentially life-threatening causes of the patient's symptoms.
___ Diagnostic and therapeutic plan is included for every problem, along with rationale

General

___ Write-up is legible, and free of spelling or grammatical errors
___ Medical abbreviations are recognized as appropriate
___ References are included

For more detailed information on completing the patient write-up, see Chapter 16.

Presenting newly admitted patients

The day after you evaluate a new patient is the post-call day. On post-call days, the attending expects formal presentations on newly admitted patients. You are responsible for presenting your patients. Before presenting, you should learn your attending's preferences. A step-by-step method of presenting newly admitted patients is described below.

Step 1: State the patient's full name, room number, and medical record number (if needed to identify the patient at the hospital).

Step 2: State the chief complaint in the patient's own words.

Step 3: State the history of present illness (HPI) in chronological order:

First sentence should include patient's age, gender, and relevant past medical history. What is relevant past medical history? An example: if the patient's chief complaint is chest pain, you should include major cardiac risk factors in the first line, since one of your considerations is angina or myocardial infarction. "Patient is a 54-year old white male with PMH significant for hypertension and diabetes who presents with one day history of chest pain." If the same patient had a history of acne, it wouldn't be included in the first line, because it isn't relevant to the chief complaint of chest pain.

Never use days of the week when conveying the HPI. Instead, use the words "prior to admission." If the patient tells you his chest pain started on Thursday and it's now Saturday, don't say that the pain started on Thursday. Instead, state that the pain started two days prior to admission.

Last sentence of the HPI should end with "and that prompted the patient to present to the hospital."

Step 4: Provide complete past medical history (PMH)

Step 5: Provide complete past surgical history (PSH)

Step 6: List medications. Include dosage, frequency, and route if attending prefers this information. Include herbal and over-the-counter medications; if the patient isn't taking any, state so.

Step 7: List allergies, along with the reaction.

Step 8: Provide relevant social history

Step 9: Provide relevant family history

Step 10: Provide review of systems. You should do a complete review of systems. Even though it should be complete, your attending may not wish to hear the entire ROS because it takes too much time. Ask their preference.

Step 11: Provide the physical exam

- Start with the general appearance and vital signs, which should be your own.
- You should do a complete exam. Even though it should be complete, your attending may not wish to hear the entire exam. Ask their preference.

Step 12: Provide laboratory test results

- Make sure you have all the results
- Before presenting, check to see if any new results have returned
- If your patient has abnormal test results, make sure you have the old results for comparison.

Step 13: State ECG findings, if applicable to patient. Bring the ECG to rounds

Step 14: State chest x-ray and/or other imaging test results. Bring the chest x-ray or other imaging tests to rounds

Step 15: Provide an assessment and plan. For every problem on the problem list, there should be an assessment and plan.

For further information, see Chapter 15 on Oral Case Presentations.

Step-by-Step Approach to Presenting Established Patients

Presenting patients who have been in the hospital for some time (established patients) differs from presenting newly admitted patients. Whereas the new patient presentation requires more details on all aspects of the history, physical, assessment, and plan, the oral presentation on an established patient focuses on providing an update on the patient's hospital course.

Step 1:   Always start with a one-line statement that includes the patient's name and why the patient is here. This reminds the audience of the patient.

Mr. Jones is a 55-year old man with diabetes and a history of peptic ulcer disease who was admitted yesterday with melena.

Then proceed with the rest of your presentation using the SOAP format. This stands for Subjective, Objective, Assessment and Plan.

Step 2:   Present all the "Subjective" data. A common preference is to start with how the patient is currently doing and then present a summary of events since you last discussed the patient. Some students include any new information or recommendations from consultants in this summary.

The patient is currently doing well with no complaints. He denies any further episodes of melena. GI evaluated the patient yesterday and is planning to do an EGD this morning.

Step 3:   Report all the "Objective" Data. This includes the vital signs, the physical exam, and results of labs and studies.

First, present the vital signs, using numbers. Don't say, "Vital signs are stable." Don't forget to mention the blood glucose, daily weight, and oxygen saturation, if applicable. Also pay attention to trends, particularly in the vital signs and in the lab values.

He has been afebrile with Tmax 99 and Tcurrent 98.6. His blood pressure is currently 140/80 with a pulse of 70. Respirations are 12. His blood glucose has been 108 and 115, and is 120 this morning.

Next, present the physical exam. You don't have to present a detailed and thorough physical exam again, such as the one you presented when the patient was first admitted to the hospital. Instead, present a focused physical exam, always including the general appearance, heart, lung, abdomen, and extremity exam. If they are unremarkable and unchanged since admission, a common preference is to say that they are unchanged since admission. If there are remarkable findings, then describe them.

On exam, the patient appears well. His heart, lung, and abdominal exams are unchanged since admission. He still has trace pre-tibial edema on his bilateral lower extremities and the left foot ulcer appears worse today. There is worsening erythema…

When presenting labs, don't present old test results unless they're pertinent. Present the latest lab results. This is another area where noting trends is very important. The team needs to know how the pertinent lab values have changed, which helps indicate if the condition is improving or worsening.

Step 4:   Present the assessment and plan of established patients by starting with a one line summary of the patient and reason for admission. Present the assessment and plan as you would with a new patient; however, the emphasis should be on presenting follow up information and on the plan of action.

Step-by-Step Approach to Writing the Daily Progress Note

You will be expected to write a daily progress note for every patient you follow. You are "following" a patient if you are participating in his or her care. The purpose of the daily progress note is to update readers of the patient's hospital course since the last progress note was written.

Meet with the resident or intern at the beginning of the rotation to discuss how the daily progress note should be written. Even if you know how to write a progress note, realize that residents often have their own preferences.

Step 1: Follow the proper order. Daily progress notes should be written using the SOAP format. SOAP is an acronym for "**s**ubjective, **o**bjective, **a**ssessment, and **p**lan."

Order of the daily progress note

Date and time of the progress note
Title (level of training, type of note)
Subjective statement
Medication list
Physical examination
Laboratory/diagnostic test results
Assessment and plan
Signature

Step 2: In the subjective portion of the note, describe the patient's complaints. For example, if the patient was hospitalized for abdominal pain, comment on whether it is still present and, if so, how it has changed. Also include any pertinent positives and negatives. New patient complaints should be listed here as well.

Step 3: Depending on the attending, medications may be listed.

Step 4: In the objective section of the note, begin with the physical exam. Always include the patient's general appearance and vital signs. After reporting the vital signs, list the 24-hour intake and output (I & O), daily weight, IV fluid rates, and other objective values (i.e. accuchecks) that pertain.

Step 5: After reporting the physical exam, move on to the laboratory and other diagnostic data. Always begin with lab test results. Generally, only lab test results that have returned since the previous day's progress note require inclusion. If results are pending at the time the note is written, indicate that the status is pending. When the results return later, the information can be charted in the form of an addendum.

Step 6: Results of other diagnostic studies should follow the lab test results: ECG, chest x-ray.

Step 7: Finish your note with the assessment and plan. Most attendings prefer that the assessment and plan be written in a problem list format. In this format, the patient's medical problems are listed in descending order of importance. Keep the following points in mind:

- Be as specific as possible in your labeling of problems. For example, if your patient was admitted with shortness of breath and the etiology was unclear, shortness of breath would be acceptable to list as the problem. However, if you have determined that the shortness of breath is due to COPD exacerbation, then COPD exacerbation should be the listed problem.
- For each problem, offer an assessment
- Following the assessment, document the plan. The plan may consist of further diagnostic testing and/or changes in management.

Sample Daily Progress Note

S: SOB with walking to the bathroom but no longer SOB at rest. No orthopnea or PND overnight. Swelling in legs continues to improve.

O: BP 128/79 (range 115/72 – 138/82)   P 68 (range 62 – 78)   R 14
T 97 (Tmax 98.9)
Weight 102.3 kg (103.6 kg yesterday)   I/O 2200cc/3600cc
Fingerstick blood sugars 101 - 121

Gen: Alert and oriented X 3, NAD
CV: RRR, + S3, no murmurs or rubs
Resp: Clear to auscultation bilaterally
Abd: + BS, NT, ND
Ext: + 1 pitting edema to knees bilaterally

Lab test results (5/17 6:30 AM results):

Serum chemistry: Na^+ 141, K^+ 4.4, Cl^- 105, HCO_3^- 27, BUN 25, creatinine 0.9, glucose 129 (high)

Complete blood count: WBC 6.2, Hgb 14.8, Hct 42.3, platelet count 176, MCV 93.6, RDW 13.4

A/P: Patient is a 47-year old male with CHF, DM, HTN, and GERD who was hospitalized with CHF exacerbation.

1. CHF exacerbation

   Overall, condition is improving – patient has less SOB and edema, weight is decreasing. Will continue intravenous furosemide, low Na diet, strict I/O, and daily weight. Echo done four years ago demonstrated findings consistent with diastolic heart failure. Will repeat echo today to assess for any change in heart function.

2. Diabetes mellitus

   Review of blood glucose values over the past 24 hours shows good glycemic control with FSBS ranging between 101 and 121. Will continue current insulin regimen and make adjustment to dosage as necessary based on FSBS.

3. Hypertension

   Blood pressure has been well controlled over the past 24 hours with no readings above 138/82. Will continue metoprolol therapy

4. GERD

   No symptoms since admission. Continue omeprazole.

Rule # 3   Strategize now if you're interested in internal medicine as a career.

During or following their internal medicine clerkship, many students decide to pursue a career in internal medicine or one of its subspecialties. In the 2010 NRMP Match, 2,722 U.S. seniors secured positions in categorical internal medicine residency programs.[4]

Of U.S. senior applicants who matched in 2007, the mean USMLE Step 1 score was 222.[5]

Of U.S. senior applicants who matched in 2007, 12.6% were members of the honor organization AOA.[5]

How hard is it to secure a position in an internal medicine residency program?

In the 2010 NRMP Match, 4,999 positions were offered. Close to 55% of these positions were filled by U.S. senior medical students.[4] Therefore, for U.S. applicants, it is indeed a buyer's market, and most students are able to secure a position at their top choice.

However, getting into a top tier internal medicine residency program remains very difficult, and a well-thought-out strategy for success is required if you covet one of these positions. According to the Clerkship Directors of Internal Medicine, "students who match at top internal medicine programs often have sustained superior clinical performance on their clerkships and fourth-year rotations, obtained Alpha Omega Alpha (AOA) Honor Medical Society status, scored well on the United States Medical Licensing Examination Step I and Step II, and secured strong letters of recommendation."[6]

When should I ask for a letter of recommendation?

If your internal medicine attending physician has been impressed with the quality of your work, ask for a strong letter of recommendation at the end of your clerkship. There's no need to wait until the fourth year of medical school, when it's time to submit applications. According to the Department of Medicine at the University of Washington School of Medicine, "faculty get many requests for letters, and we are happy to do them – but they are much better if written soon after working with a student. If you work closely with one of the faculty during your clerkship, and they give you good verbal feedback at the end of the block, it's fine to ask if they would be willing to write a letter for you (if they say yes, thank them, and tell them you will send them an email soon)."[3]

DId you know...

Internal Medicine residency programs require students applying for preliminary (one-year) or categorical (three-year) positions to submit a Department of Medicine letter. Also known as the "Chairman's letter," this letter is written by the chairman or his or her designee.

How can I strengthen my application for residency?

The process begins with an accurate and objective analysis of your background, accomplishments, and credentials. Since we are often not the best judges of the strength of our candidacy, it's preferable to seek the opinion of faculty involved in the residency selection process. The chairman, program director, or clerkship director at your school would be ideal faculty members to approach.

Tip # 1

If you're considering a career in internal medicine, identify an advisor who can help you explore the specialty further, plan your fourth-year electives, and develop your application strategy.

These individuals will have advised students with profiles similar to yours over a period of many years, and will therefore be readily able to estimate your chances at different programs. Of obvious importance is your performance on the USMLE, junior core clerkship grade in internal medicine, and subinternship grade. However, residency programs are also interested in your letters of recommendation, Dean's letter, leadership potential, research experience, volunteerism, and interpersonal skills. According to Dr. Karen Hauer, internal medicine clerkship director at UCSF, distinguishing accomplishments in the areas of research, leadership, curriculum work, advocacy, and policy can enhance the application.[7]

Did you know...

While USMLE scores are used in the residency selection process, the way in which these scores are used will vary from program to program. At some internal medicine residency programs, a cut off or threshold score will be used to screen applicants. Only applicants exceeding the score will be considered for interviews. Other programs have no threshold score.

Should I do a subinternship in internal medicine?

During a subinternship rotation, the medical student is a "subintern," and assumes the roles and responsibilities of an intern. Nearly all U.S. medical schools offer internal medicine subinternships, and some schools require all students to complete one before graduation.[8]

While few residency programs require students to complete an IM subinternship, most program directors recommend that students complete a subinternship in the specialty they have chosen.[9] This offers students benefits beyond enhancement of the residency application. In a survey of senior medical students at the Boston University School of Medicine, the subinternship was found to "be effective in preparing students for many of the challenges they will face as an intern and beyond."[10]

Tip # 2

Dr. Jeffrey Wiese, associate chairman of medicine and internal medicine program director at Tulane University, offers this tip for medical students. "There is a lot going on during fourth year, but do not let it interfere with your sub-I. You must perform well here; this is your chance to show how well you function as an intern. To do so, you must focus 100% of your efforts on the sub-I."[11]

Did you know...

Unlike the junior medicine clerkship, the internal medicine subinternship grade is often solely based on attending or resident evaluations. One fourth or less of medical schools use objective measures such as written examinations.[8] In a survey of clerkship directors, subinternship grade inflation was found to be quite common. "Half of subinternship students receive Honors and one third receive HighPass."[12]

When should I do an internal medicine subinternship?

Aim to schedule your subinternship in the early part of your fourth year. Doing so offers a number of advantages. First, the rotation will allow you to confirm your specialty choice. If you decide that internal medicine isn't for you, you have some time to consider other career options. Second, there will be enough time to include your evaluation and rotation grade in your Dean's letter and medical school transcript. Third, a strong clinical performance will help you obtain an additional letter of recommendation. Finally, students who schedule their subinternship in the later months of November, December, or January may have difficulties arranging interviews.

How important are away electives in internal medicine?

In general, it isn't necessary to do an away elective to match at a program. Per the Drexel University College of Medicine: "Internal Medicine programs do not expect students to do rotations at their site in order to match at the program." However, some students may not be attractive candidates at certain programs. For these students, a strong performance during an away rotation can improve their odds of receiving an interview invitation.

What fourth year electives are recommended for students pursuing internal medicine as a career?

Based on a survey of 11 internal medicine residency program directors, the following electives were recommended:[13]

- Cardiology
- Infectious disease
- Critical care
- Emergency medicine
- Endocrinology
- Rheumatology
- Nephrology
- Pulmonology
- Radiology
- Medicine subinternship

Other rotations that are commonly recommended include dermatology, office-based orthopedics or sports medicine, neurology, psychiatry, office-based gynecology, anesthesiology, ENT, ophthalmology, and urology.

References

[1]What medical students need to know about the internal medicine rotation. http://www.acponline.org/pressroom/ess_clerk.htm. Accessed January 30, 2011.

[2]Green M, Jones P, Thomas J. Selection criteria for residency: results of a national program directors survey. *Acad Med* 2009; 84(3): 362-7.

[3]University of Washington Medicine Clerkship Website. http://depts.washington.edu/medclerk/drupal/pages/Careers-Internal-Medicine. Accessed January 28, 2011.

[4]National Resident Matching Program. *Results and Data: 2010 Main Residency Match*. 2010. http://www.nrmp.org/data/resultsanddata2010.pdf. Accessed January 30, 2011.

[5]Charting outcomes in the match, 2007. http://www.nrmp.org/data/chartingoutcomes2007.pdf. Accessed January 31, 2011.

[6]Clerkship Directors of Internal Medicine. *Primer to the Internal Medicine Clerkship, Second Edition*. 2008. http://www.im.org/Publications/PhysiciansInTraining/Documents/Primer2ndEd.pdf. Accessed January 14, 2011.

[7]UCSF Career Advisors. http://medschool.ucsf.edu/professional_development/advisors/hauer.aspx. Updated May 17, 2007. Accessed January 27, 2011.

[8]Sidlow R. The structure and content of the medical subinternship: a national survey. *J Gen Int Med* 2001; 16: 550-3.

[9]Lyss-Lerman P, Teherani A, Aagaard E, Loeser H, Cooke M, Harper G. What training is needed in the fourth year of medical school? Views of residency program directors. *Acad Med* 2009; 84(7): 823-9.

[10]Green E, Hershman W, Sarfaty S. The value of the subinternship. *Med Educ Online* 2004; 9: 7.

[11] Wiese J. Planning a 4th year curriculum for your career. http://www.tulanemedicine.com/PDFs/Step%203%20Schedule%20advice.pdf. 2006. Accessed January 27, 2011.

[12]Cacamese S, Elnicki M, Speer A. Grade inflation and the internal medicine subinternship: a national survey of clerkship directors. *Teach Learn Med* 2007; 19(4): 343-6.

[13]Residency Program Directors' Expectations of Incoming Residents. http://www.siumed.edu/oec/Year4/ResidencyProgramSurvey-Generalists-090501.pdf. Accessed January 28, 2011.

Surgery Clerkship

Rule # 4 The surgery clerkship will teach you core surgical principles. These principles are utilized in many fields.

The surgery clerkship provides significant exposure to common surgical problems, and allows you to evaluate the specialty as a potential career choice. Although the bulk of your education will take place on the general surgery service, most rotations provide the opportunity to explore several surgical subspecialties. A surgical clerkship education is very valuable, whether or not you choose to practice in a surgical field. Primary care physicians must be familiar with the evaluation and management of patients in the pre-operative and post-operative settings. An understanding of core surgical principles is important across many fields, including ones such as anesthesiology, dermatology, and emergency medicine. From a personal standpoint, you or a family member is likely to undergo surgery in your lifetime, and you'll find that an understanding of the pre-operative, operative, and post-operative stages will be valuable.

Regardless of your chosen career, your surgery clerkship grade will be a factor used in the residency selection process, due to an emphasis on core clerkship grades in the residency selection process. The University of Colorado Department of Surgery writes that "most surgery programs look very favorably on an 'Honors' grade in your MS3 surgery clerkship rotation and may factor in the grades you received in your Medicine and Ob/Gyn rotations."[1] It's not easy to honor the clerkship. In a survey of medical schools across the country, Takayama found that only 27% of students achieve the highest grade in the surgery clerkship.[2]

Many students approach the surgery clerkship with considerable anxiety. In one study, students were most concerned about fatigue, long hours, workload, insufficient sleep, lack of time to study, mental abuse (getting yelled at or relentless pimping), and poor performance.[3] Unfamiliarity with the operating room environment was also concerning.

In the Surgery Clerkship chapter, we provide tips for operating room success, a checklist for thorough pre-rounding, a step-by-step guide to presenting patients, and time-saving templates for the pre-op, post-op, and op notes. This information will maximize your education as well as your performance. This chapter includes recommendations for those students interested in pursuing general surgery as a career.

About the rotation

The surgery rotation has the reputation of being the most demanding of all 3rd year clerkships. Because it places considerable demands on time and energy, students find the rotation to be challenging and exhausting. Factors contributing to this are the early start, long hours, intensity of the work, and accelerated pace of the work. The surgical hierarchy also contributes, as some feel that it tends to glorify those high on the totem pole while making the junior members of the team feel unimportant.

Having said this, many students, including some who were initially apprehensive and fearful, end up loving their experience. At most places, you spend the bulk of your time on the general surgery service. You may also have the opportunity to rotate through one or more of the surgical subspecialties. Among others, these include trauma, plastic/reconstructive, transplant, vascular, and cardiothoracic surgery.

Typical Day

Here's what a typical day on the surgery clerkship looks like:

5:00 – 6:00 AM	Pre-rounds
6:00 – 8:00 AM	Morning/Work rounds
8:00 – 12:00 NOON	Surgery, clinic, or work time
NOON – 1:00 PM	Noon conference
1:00 – 6:00 PM	Surgery, clinic, or work time
6:00 PM - ?	Afternoon rounds

What should you carry with you?

- Stethoscope
- Penlight
- Tape
- 4 x 4's
- Alcohol swabs
- Steri-strips
- Cotton-tipped applicators
- Staple removal kit
- Bandage scissors

Your Team

The team usually consists of the following individuals:

Attending physician

The attending physician is typically a faculty member at the medical school (clinical or academic) who has been assigned to be the leader of the team. The attending's primary goal is to ensure that the patients assigned to the team receive the best possible care.

   The team's contact with the attending is often limited to the surgery itself. At most places, the attending and chief surgical resident do most of the operating. Just how much the chief surgical resident is allowed to do is based on the type of hospital (private vs. public), nature of the surgery, and complexity of the case. At times, the team may meet with the attending during attending rounds.

Chief surgical resident

Second in charge, the chief surgical resident is responsible for the management of all patients on the team. He or she runs the team on a daily basis. For this reason, it's important that all team members keep the chief surgical resident abreast of all major issues pertaining to the patients. As the most senior resident, chiefs do most of the operating. At many places, it is the chief surgical resident who will complete your evaluation.

Junior and senior surgical resident(s)

The resident physician is a house officer who, at the minimum, has completed an internship. Third and fourth year house officers are considered senior surgical residents. The senior surgical resident is basically the chief's right hand. When the chief isn't conducting work rounds with the team, the senior surgical resident fills in. He or she may also spend quite a bit of time in the OR, assisting the chief and attending.

   Second-year house officers are known as junior residents. The junior resident, along with intern, is responsible for ensuring that all patient care tasks are completed.

Interns

By definition, internship refers to the first year of residency training that follows medical school graduation. Next to medical students, interns are the most junior members of the team. They are responsible for executing the treatment plan that the team has devised. Interns have a lot on their plate, which is why they need to function quickly and efficiently to accomplish the day's activities with regards to patient care.

   You will probably have the most interaction with the intern, since he or she will also follow your assigned patients. When issues arise in the management of your patient's condition(s), you should first discuss the matter with your intern. Although many interns love to teach, this isn't always possible given the demands placed upon them. On a daily basis, some of their responsibilities include scheduling tests and procedures, checking lab test results, entering orders, drawing blood, writing daily progress notes, checking wounds, and changing dressings.

Pre-rounds

During the Surgery Clerkship, your day will typically begin with pre-rounds. During pre-rounds you see your patients alone. The goal is to identify any new events that occurred in your patient's course after you left the hospital on the previous day. This information will be presented to the resident and intern during work rounds, also known as morning walk rounds, which immediately follow pre-rounds.

What to do during pre-rounds

A considerable amount of patient data needs to be gathered during pre-rounds. This information allows you to make an assessment of the patient's condition and decide on the day's plan.

Checklist for pre-rounds

___ Postoperative day # (if applicable)
___ Vital signs (T_{max}, $T_{current}$, RR, BP, P)
___ Ins/Outs (24 hour & morning shift)
___ List of current medications
___ Antibiotic therapy (name and day of therapy)
___ Patient's complaints/concerns
___ Physical examination
___ Events overnight according to nurse
___ New notes in the chart
___ New lab test results
___ New microbiology test results
___ New imaging test results
___ New orders since you last saw the patient

Pre-rounds: 10 Tips for Success

Tip # 1   Set aside enough time. The amount of time needed for pre-rounds depends on your responsibilities, whether you need to write the daily progress note during pre-rounds, the number of patients you're following, and the complexity of your patients' conditions. As you might expect, you'll need extra time at the start of the rotation because of the new environment.

Tip # 2   Use an organized system of data gathering. You'll need easy access to this data during your morning work rounds presentation.

Tip # 3   A review of the chart for any new progress notes is a must. This is one of the keys to getting up to speed on your patient's hospital course. Read all new progress notes, including those left by nurses.

Tip # 4   Always look at the orders. New orders may be written after you leave the hospital. Often, these orders aren't documented in the progress notes.

Tip # 5   Your intern may know things about your patient that you don't. He or she will receive report (sign-out) from the cross-covering intern, who cares for your patient while your team is out of the hospital. Always ask your intern if he or she knows anything about your patient that you don't.

Tip # 6   Perform a heart, lung, abdomen, and lower extremity exam on every patient, irrespective of the reason for hospitalization.

Tip # 7   Always check the computer for the most up-to-date lab test results. Don't rely on the chart, because it often takes some time for the most recent results to make their way to the patient's chart.

Tip # 8   Some lab test results take days to return. Check on pending test results every morning.

Tip # 9   The successful student not only gathers the necessary data, but also sets aside time to organize and process the information before presenting the patient during work rounds.

Tip # 10   Offer to help pre-round on other patients to lighten the load on your resident. Residents may reward such efforts with additional teaching and opportunities to perform procedures.

Work Rounds

During work rounds, also known as morning or resident walk rounds, the team (usually without the attending) travels from room to room, seeing each of the patients on the service. The most junior member of the team (junior medical student, subintern, intern) following the patient is required to update the team on the patient's progress. This update includes any significant events that have occurred overnight, the results of any diagnostic testing, and the current condition of the patient. The information you present will help the team formulate a diagnostic and therapeutic plan.

Because the day's first surgery generally takes place at 8 AM, work rounds in surgery begin early. Rounds, progress notes, orders, test scheduling, and consults often have to be completed before 7:30 AM. Patients need to be properly evaluated and treated before the team goes to the OR for the rest of the day.

7 Questions to Ask Your Resident Before Your First Work Rounds

Question # 1   What time do work rounds start?

Question # 2   Where do work rounds start?

Question # 3   How would you like me to present newly admitted patients?

Question # 4   How would you like me to present established patients?

Question # 5   What information would you like me to include in these presentations?

Question # 6   How much time do I have to present the patient?

Question # 7   Do progress notes need to be completed before work rounds begin?

Step-by-Step Approach to the Work Rounds Presentation

Step 1   Begin with a short summary of the patient to remind the team of his or her problems. Give the patient's name, age, gender, and chief complaint or working diagnosis/reason for hospitalization. For the postoperative patient, also state the postoperative day #, operation, and indication for operation.

This is postoperative day # 2 for Mr. Jones, a 72-year old man s/p left hemicolectomy for colon adenocarcinoma.

Step 2   Present the subjective data, which should include how the patient's symptom(s) have changed, new symptoms, and events that have occurred since yesterday's rounds. For the postoperative patient, also report physical activity, use of incentive spirometer, pain control, and bowel habits.

He has no new complaints. His pain is minimal. He has tolerated sips of clear liquids without difficulty. He said he passed flatus once during the night. He walked around the ward three times yesterday and once earlier this morning.

Step 3   Present the objective data, beginning with the vital signs. Start with the T_{max} (maximum temperature over the past 24 hours) followed by the $T_{current,}$ P, BP, RR, and oxygen saturation (and weight if pertinent). Then report the intake and output information followed by a brief physical examination. The exam should always include the heart, lung, abdomen, and extremity exam. Always report the examination of the surgical site in postoperative patients. Pay special attention to occult arrhythmias, breath sounds, bowel sounds, presence of abdominal distention or tympany, lower extremity edema, and peripheral pulses. Use a Doppler in all vascular patients or if there is a loss of pulse that you felt before.

T_{max} last night 99.5 F, $T_{current}$ is 97.8 F, pulse 66, blood pressure 115/68, respiratory rate 14. His heart has a regular rate and rhythm, and his lungs have crackles at the bases only. His abdomen is soft, nontender, and nondistended. Positive bowel sounds. No lower extremity edema. Positive dorsalis pedis and posterior tibialis pulses. The wound is clean, dry, and intact.

Step 4   Present the results of laboratory and diagnostic tests. Always check just before rounds for new laboratory or microbiology data. Old results may be mentioned if comparison is needed.

The BUN this morning was 30, and the creatinine was 1.6. His white blood cell count was 10.5, his H & H was 10.4 and 31%, and his platelet count was 105.

Step 5   The final step is the assessment and plan. Consider the status of each of the patient's problems and then state the plan. For postoperative patients, consider postoperative recovery as one of the patient's problems or issues to be addressed here, including physical activity (increase activity level?), diet (advance diet?), and postoperative pain control.

Work Rounds: 10 Tips for Success

Tip # 1   Show up for work rounds 5 minutes before they're scheduled to start. All patients need to be seen before going to the OR, and the OR start time is not flexible.

Tip # 2   Repeat after us: Brief and concise. Brief and concise. Patients must not only be seen, but daily progress notes and orders must be written before the first case in the OR begins. Improve team efficiency by delivering brief presentations. Presentations on uncomplicated patients shouldn't take more than 45 to 60 seconds.

Tip # 3   Practice your presentation at the end of pre-rounds. Make sure that you convey the necessary information in an organized manner without exceeding the allotted time.

Tip # 4   Aim to present your patients without relying heavily on your notes.

Tip # 5   There is definitely an order to the work rounds presentation. Students who adhere to the proper order are clearly seen as being more advanced. Use the SOAP format.

Tip # 6   As the day's plan for each patient is defined during work rounds, add each patient-care task to your to-do list. Do not rely on memory.

Tip # 7   Your team would like to hear your own plan for the patient because it reflects your thinking process. Don't defer to the intern for discussion of the assessment and plan.

Tip # 8   Residents may teach during work rounds. They often pass along important pearls of information, which may very well be the answers to your attending's questions later in the day.

Tip # 9   Listen carefully to all patient presentations even if you aren't directly following the patient. These presentations add to your education.

Tip # 10   Demonstrate enthusiasm. Ask questions and make it clear that you want to absorb as much as you can from the rotation experience.

Preoperative Note

You will be expected to write a preoperative note for every patient you are following. You are "following" a patient if you are participating in his or her care. Simply put, the purpose of the preoperative note is to convey to the readers of the chart, especially the surgical team, that the patient is ready for surgery. It answers the question "Have the things that need to be done before surgery actually been done?"

Within the first days of the rotation, you will be asked to write a preoperative note. We provide a template below.

Preoperative Note Template

Title of note
Date and time
Preoperative diagnosis
Procedure planned
Attending surgeon
Anesthesia planned
History and physical
Allergies
Lab test data
    CBC
    Chem 7
    PT/PTT
    Urinalysis
Type & Screen or Crossmatch (# units)
ECG
Chest X-ray
Consent
NPO status/Bowel prep (if necessary)
Name/Signature

Sample Preoperative Note

1/01/11 8PM General Surgery Gold Service Preoperative Note

Preoperative diagnosis:	Acute cholecystitis
Procedure planned:	Laparoscopic cholecystectomy
Attending surgeon:	Dr. Brown
Anesthesia:	General
History and physical:	Written 1/01/11
Allergies:	No known drug allergies (NKDA)
CBC:	Include results here
Chemistry:	Include results here
Urinalysis:	Include results here
Type and screen:	Completed 1/01/11
ECG:	Not indicated
CXR:	No evidence of acute cardiopulmonary disease (film dated 1/01/11)
Consent:	Signed by patient on 1/01/11, witnessed and in chart
	NPO as of midnight

Joe Lister
MS-3

Brief Operative Note

You will be expected to write a brief operative note for every patient you are following. At the end of an operation, the brief operative note should be written in the progress notes section of the chart. The main purpose of the note is to inform chart readers of the events that occurred in the OR.

Brief Operative Note Template

Title of note
Date and time
Pre-op diagnosis
Post-op diagnosis
Procedure and indication
Surgeon (attending)
First assistant (most senior resident)
Second assistant
Student
Anesthesia (GETA, MAC, epidural, spinal)
Input (IV fluids + blood products)[1]
Output (EBL[2] + UO[3] + drains + any other)
Drains (location of placement, type)
Findings
Specimens/cultures
Complications
Disposition (PACU, ICU, floor)
Name/signature

[1]Obtain this information from anesthesiologist
[2]EBL = estimated blood loss
[3]UO = urine output

Sample Brief Operative Note

1/01/11 3 PM General Surgery Gold Service Brief Operative Note

Pre-operative diagnosis:	Colon cancer
Postoperative diagnosis:	Colon cancer
Procedure:	Left hemicolectomy with en-bloc partial bladder resection
Attending surgeon:	Dr. Brown
First assistant:	Dr. Jones
Student:	Harry Cushing MS-3
Anesthesia:	Dr. N. Tubate. General anesthesia endotracheal tube
Input:	3L normal saline + 250 mL albumin + 2U pRBCs
Output:	550 mL EBL + 800 mL UO + 150 mL NG tube
Findings:	Firm mass in left colon with gross invasion of the dome of the bladder; no liver or peritoneal metastases appreciated.
Specimens:	Left colon and bladder sent to pathology for permanent section and staging.
Drains:	Foley draining to gravity; nasogastric tube to low intermittent wall suction (LIWS); Jackson-Pratt drain in left paracolic gutter to bulb suction.
Complications:	No known complications
Disposition:	To post-anesthesia care unit (PACU) in stable condition, extubated

Harry Cushing
MS-3

Postoperative Note

A wide variety of problems can develop in the postoperative patient, some of which are quite serious. It is important to detect these problems early, which is why a member of the team must evaluate the patient postoperatively. The findings of the postoperative evaluation should be included in the postoperative note.

Postoperative Note Template

Title of note
Date and time
Procedure
Subjective
    Level of consciousness/mental status
    Pain control
    Nausea/vomiting
    Ambulation
    Voiding
    PO intake
Vital signs
    Temperature
    Heart rate
    Blood pressure
    Respiratory rate
Input (crystalloids, colloids, blood products)
Output (urine, drain, tube)
Physical examination
Laboratory/radiographic data
Assessment/plan
Name/signature

Sample Postoperative Note

1/01/11 10 PM General Surgery Gold Service Postoperative Note

52-year old man s/p left hemicolectomy and partial bladder resection for locally advanced colon cancer. Reports adequate pain control with patient-controlled anesthesia (PCA). Has not yet ambulated. Denies nausea or vomiting.

Objective:
General:	Awake, alert and oriented. Appears comfortable.
Vitals:	T_{max} = 37.5 C, T_c = 37.6 C, RR = 14, P = 66, BP = 130/80
Output:	200 cc UO; 50 cc per NG tube
Heart:	Regular rate and rhythm
Lungs:	Clear to auscultation; good inspiratory effort
Abdomen:	Non-distended. Absent bowel sounds
Wound:	Dressing in place; minimal blood staining
Extremities:	Ted hose and sequential compression devices in place on both lower extremities

Postoperative labs/imaging: Glucose 156

Asessment/Plan: 52-year old man s/p left hemicolectomy for locally advanced colon cancer

-Will continue PCA for pain control
-Patient encouraged to use incentive spirometry
-Continue intravenous fluids and keep NPO
-Out-of-bed in morning
-Medical oncology service consulted; will see patient in morning regarding adjuvant therapy
-H&H, serum biochemistries pending for AM

Dina Carrel
MS-3

Step-by-Step Approach to Writing the Daily Progress Note

You will be expected to write a daily progress note for every patient you are following. The purpose of the daily progress note is to update readers of the patient's hospital course since the last progress note was written.

Meet with the resident or intern at the beginning of the rotation to discuss how the daily progress note should be written. Even if you know how to write a progress note, recognize that residents often have their own preferences.

Step 1: Follow the proper order. Daily progress notes should be written using the SOAP format. SOAP is an acronym for "subjective, objective, assessment, and plan." Begin your note with the title, date, time, and postoperative day # (POD #), if applicable.

Surgery MS3 Progress Note
1/01/11 6:30 AM
POD # 2

Step 2: In the subjective portion of the note, describe the patient's complaints. Include new complaints or symptoms as well as any change in old complaints or symptoms. In the postoperative patient, don't forget to write about pain (location, severity, duration, quality, effectiveness of analgesic therapy), ambulation/activity, bowel habits (presence/absence, constipation/diarrhea, flatus, bowel movements), appetite, diet (tolerating?), and incentive spirometry use.

Patient does report some peri-incisional pain but states that his pain is fairly well controlled with PCA. No flatus or bowel movements. He is ambulating without difficulty. He has been using the incentive spirometer every few hours.

Step 3: In the objective section of the note, begin with the vital signs. Include the T_{max} (maximum temperature over the past 24 hours and when it occurred), $T_{current}$, pulse, respiratory rate, and blood pressure. For the latter 3 vital signs, also include ranges if there has been significant fluctuation. Oxygen saturation, the amount of supplemental oxygen being administered, and weight should be documented, if pertinent to the patient.

T_{max} – 99.7 F $T_{current}$ – 99.2 F   P – 66   R – 14   BP – 115/68

Step 4: Write down the I/Os over the past 24 hours. The total input includes oral and intravenous fluids. The total output may include urine, stool, emesis, drain, and NG tube output. Each drain output should be recorded separately as well.

24 hour I/O 2300cc/2200cc, urine output 1400cc

Step 5: Document brief physical examination. Comment on general appearance as well as heart, lung, abdominal, and extremity exams. Focus also on the area of interest (why patient was hospitalized). In the postoperative patient, comment on the condition of the incision site/wound (appearance, discharge, tenderness).

General – Awake, alert, and cooperative
Heart – RRR, normal S1 and S2, no murmurs/rubs/gallops
Lungs – CTA bilaterally
Abd – NABS, NT, ND
Ext – No clubbing, cyanosis, or edema, SCDs in place
Incision site – Clean, dry, and intact

Step 6: List any laboratory test results that were done over the past 24 hours which weren't documented in a prior note. You may include previously reported lab test results if trends are important. Don't forget to include the date and time of all lab test results. If results aren't available, write "pending." These can be charted later as an addendum.

Step 7: List the results of any other diagnostic studies (i.e. radiology, cardiology, pathology). Include the date and time of the study.

Step 8: Write the assessment and plan. Start with a short statement of the patient's age, gender, and reason for being in the hospital. For both the preoperative and postoperative patient, discuss the patient's general condition (significant improvement? new concerns?). Then discuss the diagnostic and therapeutic plan.

For the postoperative patient, the plan for the day should also include issues related to:

- pain control: increase/decrease/discontinue/switch from PCA to po?
- diet: advance?
- patient activity: increase activity level?
- incentive spirometry

- antibiotics: discontinue?
- drains: discontinue?
- staples: discontinue?
- intravenous fluids: change or discontinue?
- lines/catheters: discontinue?

Patient is a 72-year old male who is POD # 2 s/p appendectomy
for acute appendicitis.
-Overall doing well
-Encourage continued ambulation
-Encourage continued use of incentive spirometry
-Will switch from PCA to po analgesia
-Continue NPO
-Continue DVT prophylaxis with SCDs

OR Success: 20 Tips

Tip # 1 During orientation to the OR, learn about the principles of aseptic technique and the correct way to scrub, gown, and glove before surgery. This is the first step towards becoming more comfortable in the OR.

Tip # 2 Unless there are no cases scheduled or your help is required on the floors or in the clinics, plan to be in the OR every day. Actively participating in the OR allows you closer interaction with surgical faculty.

Tip # 3 Before leaving for the day, check the OR schedule to see which cases your attending will be performing. In general, you are expected to participate in the surgery of all patients you are following. If your patient(s) are not scheduled for surgery, ask your resident to assign you a case. Having a case assigned the evening before, rather than the morning of surgery, allows you to prepare adequately for the case, thus maximizing your learning.

Tip # 4 Read about the case before the next day's surgery, preferably the night before rather than the morning of surgery. Your morning reading time may be lost if patient issues arise, requiring your attention. This may lead to poor preparation, which is usually obvious to the surgical attending.

Did you know...

In interviews conducted with students and surgeons, Lyon found that surgeons "size up the medical students, interpreting their behavior particularly as it relates to motivation and commitment. These interpretations have an effect on how they, in turn, respond as teachers." One surgeon offered his approach to students:[4]

> "Surgeons are human and if there's somebody there who's full of enthusiasm and obviously gone to the trouble to read something about it in advance, and specifically requests that you show them this or that, you can't help getting stimulated by their interest and responding accordingly. Whereas if you ask a few questions or you make a few forays and the student stands there looking not only ignorant but uninterested then you find yourself not even bothering to talk to them."

Tip # 5 You will be asked questions about the case during surgery. For the patient's condition, be prepared to answer questions about the pathophysiology, symptoms, signs, lab tests, imaging tests, medical management, indications for surgery, timing of surgery, surgical approaches, preoperative evaluation, complications, outcome, prognosis, and postoperative management.

Did you know...

The Department of Surgery at the University of Washington School of Medicine offers the following advice to medical students in the operating room: "If you do not know the answer to a question, it is better to say, 'I don't know, but I will look it up.' Some people suggest stating everything you know about the general topic. In my experience, most people don't have the attention span or patience for this approach. Also, never make up an answer. You will be setting yourself up for heavier interrogation."[5]

Tip # 6   A good way to prepare is to begin by reading the appropriate section in your basic surgical textbook. Also use a "high yield" book such as *Surgical Recall*, which will focus the information you read in your textbook and highlight the major points of the case. A surgical atlas will provide a quick outline of the key maneuvers your surgical team will perform.

Tip # 7   Review the patient's chart before surgery. Familiarize yourself with the patient's clinical presentation and hospital course.

Tip # 8   Eat breakfast before scrubbing. Hunger in the OR can distract you from your focus. It also increases your risk of fainting during surgery.

Tip # 9   While fairly self-explanatory, it bears repeating. Do not consume coffee, tea, soft drinks, or other caffeine-containing products before entering the OR. Cases can run long, and caffeine is a diuretic.

Tip # 10   Once scrubbed in, you won't be able to access your pager. Leave your pager with the circulating nurse before you scrub.

Tip # 11   After entering the OR, introduce yourself to the scrub nurse, circulating nurse, anesthesiologist, and any surgical assistants. The OR team is much more likely to teach and help you if you are polite and respectful.

Did you know...

In interviews with students, Lyon was able to explore the challenges they face in the operating room environment. "Students have to learn to negotiate the physical environment of the operating theatre as a workplace, to learn the protocols, familiarize themselves with the culture, and cope with emotional impact of surgery..." One student described the experience:[6]

"I remember when I went to theatre for the first time, it was quite intimidating. It took several visits to theatre before I was comfortable with the environment, i.e. getting changed, turning up in the right gear to the right place, having some idea of who's who and then knowing where to position myself in theatre without desterilizing everything."

Tip # 12 Before surgery starts, offer to help your resident, circulating nurse, and scrub nurse with any tasks that need to be completed. You may be able to assist in the transfer of the patient to the surgical table, placement of the Foley catheter, and preparation of the skin.

Tip # 13 When first asked to scrub, it's common for students to be unsure of the protocol, even after an orientation. Correct technique can impact patient outcomes, so ask your resident for help if you need to.

Tip # 14 All operating room personnel, including scrubbed and nonscrubbed team members, are expected to maintain the sterile field. You must make every effort to avoid contaminating your surgical gloves. Gloves can become contaminated when you inadvertently touch your hand to your face or any other part of your body or clothing that isn't sterile. Dropping one or both of your gloved hands below the level of the waist is also considered contamination.

Tip # 15 Questions are encouraged, but only at the appropriate time. Before asking a question, always ask the surgeon if it's a good time to do so.

Tip # 16 Retracting is an important job in the OR. Proper exposure of the field of interest is paramount to a successful surgery, and armed with a retractor, this is your mission. The attending will most likely choose the correct retractor for you and put it in the correct place with appropriate tension. Mimic this exactly and hold it steady, but be aware of what's going on and try to adjust accordingly with the surgeon's permission.

Tip # 17 If you are given the opportunity to cut sutures, the correct length of a suture is whatever the attending prefers. Always ask how long the ends of a suture should be the first time you cut.

Tip # 18 If you do feel faint during surgery, notify the other sterile team members as soon as possible. Students have fainted forward, contaminating the sterile field. Let the team know, ask to step back, and scrub out.

Did you know...

In a survey of 630 students, 77 reported having at least one near or actual syncopal event in the operating room. Eighty-eight percent were female students.[7] The most prevalent contributing factors were hot temperature, prolonged standing, wearing a surgical mask, and the smell of diathermy. Eating and drinking prior to entering the operating room were found to be helpful in prevention, as was moving the legs while standing.

Tip # 19 Always help transfer the patient to the gurney after the case and accompany the team to the PACU. Participate in your patient's care there.

Tip # 20 Practice tying knots outside the OR. If you're ever given the opportunity to tie knots or place sutures in the OR, you'll be prepared.

Did you know...

In a survey of medical students at the end of the surgery clerkship, a significant number had driven the camera during laparoscopic procedures (87.9%), made an incision (43.1%), or dissected tissues (30.2%).[8]

Rule # 5   **If you're interested in a surgical field, the process of strengthening your application should start now.**

During or following a clerkship in surgery, some students decide to pursue a career in general surgery. In the 2010 NRMP Match, 895 U.S. seniors matched into a general surgery residency program.[9]

How hard is it to secure a position in a general surgery residency program?

In the 2010 NRMP Match, 1,077 positions were available in categorical general surgery residency programs. 150 U.S. senior medical students went unmatched, making general surgery a competitive specialty. Osteopathic students may apply for positions in both the NRMP and AOA Match. Only 20 osteopathic students secured a position in an allopathic general surgery residency.

Of U.S. senior applicants who matched in 2007, the mean USMLE Step 1 score was 222.[10]

Of U.S. senior applicants who matched in 2007, 12.1% were members of the honor organization AOA.[10]

When should I ask for a letter of recommendation?

If your surgery attending has been impressed with the quality of your work, ask for a strong letter of recommendation at the end of your clerkship. You don't need to wait until the fourth year of medical school when it's time to submit applications. Asking early often leads to a stronger letter of recommendation. Per the words of the Drexel University College of Medicine: "They will have your performance fresh in their mind and can write a stronger LOR."[11]

Tip # 3
If possible, find ways to work closely with well-known surgery faculty members, such as the chairman, program director, clerkship director, and senior attending physicians. Strong letters written by these faculty members will carry more weight.

How can I strengthen my application for residency?

The process begins with an accurate and objective analysis of your background, accomplishments, and credentials. We're usually not the best judges of the strength of our own candidacy, so it's preferable to seek the opinion of faculty involved in the residency selection process. The chairman, program director, or clerkship director at your school would be ideal faculty members to approach in this regard.

Your academic record will be a major factor used in the residency selection process. In the document "So, you want to be a surgeon," the American College of Surgeons offers the following advice:[12]

> *If your record places you in the lower half of your class or if you scored below the mean on the USMLE, you may not get many invitations to interview relative to the number of places you apply. Placement in the second quartile of your class or at least a mean score on the USMLE tests will make you competitive for many good independent medical center-based programs and some university-based programs. If you are in the top quartile of your class, have scores well above the mean on the USMLE examinations, and have some honors on your clinical clerkships, there are quite a few university-based programs you can consider. If you have been elected Alpha Omega Alpha and have many major clinical honors, you should be competitive for any program in the country.*

Tip # 4

If your USMLE Step 1 score is low, plan on taking the USMLE Step 2 CK exam before submitting applications. A high score on this exam can strengthen your application, and alleviate any concerns that programs may have with your Step 1 performance.

While important, academic credentials only tell part of your story. Programs are interested in assessing your non-cognitive skills: commitment, passion, dedication, motivation to excel, and professionalism, among others. Other components of your application, including your letters of recommendation, extracurricular activities, leadership positions, and volunteerism, will be used in this regard. Following analysis of your strengths and weaknesses, determine ways to strengthen your candidacy and follow through with those strategies.

Did you know...

In a survey of over 140 surgery residency program directors, negatives in an application included failing a course or the boards, poor academic performance, extended period of unexplained absence from medical school, professionalism or ethics concerns, and strong grades and scores but otherwise blank application.[13]

How can I identify a mentor or advisor?

If you're considering a career in surgery, developing a relationship with a mentor is very important. Before beginning the surgery clerkship, few students have a surgical mentor. In a survey of UCSF medical students, only 10% reported having one before starting the rotation.[14] As you progress through your clerkship, your interactions with surgery faculty may help you identify a mentor who is best suited for your particular needs. If you can't identify a mentor through your clerkship interactions, you should schedule a meeting with the clerkship director, program director, or chairman to express your interest in pursuing surgery as a career.

Tip # 5

Select a surgery faculty member as an advisor or mentor. The person you choose should have a strong understanding of the application and residency match process.

Tip # 6

During your surgery clerkship, you will work most closely with residents. Having gone through the residency application process relatively recently, residents can be a rich source of information. Cultivate relationships with your residents, and keep in touch after the clerkship ends.

Should I do a subinternship in surgery?

During a subinternship rotation, the medical student is a "subintern," and assumes the roles and responsibilities of an intern. Many schools require all students to complete a subinternship before graduation, and you may be able to fulfill this requirement through a surgery subinternship. Although few residency programs require a surgery subinternship, most program directors recommend that students complete a subinternship in the specialty they have chosen to pursue as a career.[15] The subinternship offers students benefits beyond enhancement of the residency application. In a survey of senior medical students at the Boston University School of Medicine, the subinternship was found to "be effective in preparing students for many of the challenges they will face as an intern and beyond."[16]

When should I do a surgery subinternship?

Aim to schedule your surgery subinternship in the early part of your fourth year. Doing so offers a number of advantages. First, the rotation will allow you to confirm your specialty choice. If you decide that surgery isn't for you, you have some time to consider other career options. Second, there will be enough time to include the evaluation of your performance and rotation grade in your Dean's letter and medical school transcript. Third, a strong clinical performance will help you obtain an additional letter of recommendation. Finally, an earlier subinternship avoids conflicts in scheduling residency interviews.

How important are away electives in general surgery?

In general, it isn't necessary to do an away elective to match at a program. Fabri found that, while away rotations increased the likelihood of receiving an interview, they had no effect on the probability of matching.[17] However, some students may not be attractive candidates at certain programs based on their paper record alone. For these students, a strong performance during an away rotation can improve the odds.

What fourth year electives are recommended for students pursuing general surgery as a career?

Suggested electives include:

- Radiology
- Anesthesiology
- Critical care
- Emergency medicine
- Surgical pathology
- Gastroenterology
- Infectious disease

References

[1]Univeristy of Colorado Department of Surgery. http://www.ucdenver.edu/academics/colleges/medicalschool/education/studentaffairs/studentgroups/SurgicalSociety/Pages/FAQ.aspx. Accessed January 30, 2011.

[2]Takayama H, Grinsell R, Brock D, Foy H, Pellegrini C, Horvath K. Is it appropriate to use core clerkship grades in the selection of residents? *Curr Surg* 2006; 63(6): 391-6.

[3]Pettitt B. Medical student concerns and fears before their third-year surgical clerkship. *Am J Surg* 2005; 189(4): 492-6.

[4]Lyon P. A model of teaching and learning in the operating theatre. *Med Educ* 2004; 38(12): 1278-87.

[5]Farjah F. Primer For Third Year Surgical Clerkship. http://depts.washington.edu/surgstus/CLERKSHIP/TIPS.html. Updated November 15, 2007. Accessed January 18, 2011.

[6]Lyon P. Making the most of learning in the operating theatre: student strategies and curricular initiatives. *Med Educ* 2003; 37(8): 680-8.

[7]Jamjoom A, Nikkar-Esfahani A, Fitzgerald J. Operating theatre related syncope in medical students: a cross sectional study. *BMC Med Educ* 2009; 9: 14.

[8]Berman L, Rosenthal M, Curry L, Evans L, Gusberg R. Attracting surgical clerks to surgical careers: role models, mentoring, and engagement in the operating room. *J Am Coll Surg* 2008; 207(6): 793-800.

[9]National Resident Matching Program. *Results and Data: 2010 Main Residency Match.* 2010. http://www.nrmp.org/data/resultsanddata2010.pdf. Accessed January 30, 2011.

[10]Charting outcomes in the match, 2007. http://www.nrmp.org/data/chartingoutcomes2007.pdf. Accessed January 31, 2011.

[11]Requesting letters of recommendation. http://webcampus.drexelmed.edu/cdc/medRecomInfo.asp. Accessed January 21, 2011.

[12]American College of Surgeons. *So, You Want To Be A Surgeon.* http://www.facs.org/residencysearch/. Accessed January 22, 2011.

[13]Gutnick L. Essentials of Matching in General Surgery http://www.amsa.org/AMSA/Libraries/Committee_Docs/Essentials_of_a_ Getting_into_a_ Surgical_Residency.sflb.ashx. Accessed January 23, 2011.

[14]Cloyd J, Holtzman D, O'Sullivan P, Sammann A, Tendick F, Ascher N. Operating room assist: surgical mentorship and operating room experience for preclerkship medical students. *J Surg Educ* 2008; 65(4): 275-82.

[15]Lyss-Lerman P, Teherani A, Aagaard E, Loeser H, Cooke M, Harper G. What training is needed in the fourth year of medical school? Views of residency program directors. *Acad Med* 2009; 84(7): 823-9.

[16]Green E, Hershman W, Sarfaty S. The value of the subinternship. *Med Educ Online* 2004; 9: 7.

[17]Fabri P, Powell D, Cupps N. Is there value in audition extramurals? *Am J Surg* 1995; 169(3): 338-40.

Chapter 4

Pediatrics Clerkship

Rule # 6   The care of pediatric patients poses unique challenges.

During the pediatrics clerkship, students gain experience and skills in the evaluation and management of common medical problems in infants, children, and adolescents. The Department of Pediatrics at the University of South Alabama writes that "there are few areas in medicine where knowledge of pediatrics will not be necessary."[1] In pediatrics, there is an emphasis on family-centered care. Learning how pediatricians deliver family-centered care will be of benefit, regardless of your medical specialty choice. The Institute for Patient- and Family-Centered Care writes that families "are essential to patients' health and well-being and are allies for quality and safety."[2]

As a core clerkship grade, your performance in Pediatrics is important to residency programs in other specialties. In a survey of over 1,200 residency program directors across 21 medical specialties, grades in required clerkships were ranked as the # 1 factor used in the selection process.[3] In a survey of medical schools across the country, Takayama found that only 29% of students achieve the highest grade in the pediatrics clerkship.[4]

Dr. Andrew Bremer, a pediatric endocrinologist and assistant professor in the Department of Pediatrics at Vanderbilt University, is the author of the *Pediatrics Clerkship: 101 Biggest Mistakes And How To Avoid Them.* He writes that "the pediatrics clerkship is different in many respects from other core clerkships and students are often uncertain of how best to navigate the transition from adult to pediatric care. The challenges of learning how to interact with pediatric patients, take and perform the pediatric history and physical exam, and present patients during rounds presents a steep learning curve for students in the first few weeks of the clerkship."[5]

In the Pediatrics Clerkship chapter, you'll find templates and outlines to help you fulfill your daily responsibilities and tasks. You'll learn how to effectively pre-round, succinctly and accurately present new and established patients, and develop comprehensive write-ups using our checklist. Do you know what elements to include in the neonatal, growth, and developmental histories? This chapter details those elements. For those students interested in pediatrics as a career, this chapter provides insight into the pediatric residency selection process.

About the rotation

The pediatric clerkship is usually two months in duration, and includes inpatient, outpatient, emergency room, and nursery experiences. As pediatrics is mostly an outpatient specialty, the pediatric clerkship will often incorporate several hours of clinic per week – even during inpatient months. Although often considered less rigorous than the general medicine and surgery clerkships, the pediatrics clerkship will introduce you to all facets of pediatric medicine, ranging from the care of pre-term neonates with bronchopulmonary dysplasia to the care of adolescents with eating disorders. The clerkship is multidisciplinary in that it incorporates many of the skills learned from the internal medicine, surgery, OB/Gyn, and psychiatry clerkships, and tailors those skills towards the care of children.

Typical day

Here's what a typical day on the pediatrics rotation looks like:

7:00 – 8:00 AM	Pre-rounds
8:00 – 9:00 AM	Work rounds
9:00 – 10:00 AM	Morning report or work time
10:00 – 12:00 Noon	Attending rounds
Noon – 1:00 PM	Noon conference
1:00 - ?	Work time (± student conferences)

What should you carry with you?

- Stethoscope, with pediatric bell and diaphragm, if available
- Ophthalmoscope for evaluating the red reflex
- Otoscope with pneumatic attachment for viewing and evaluating the mobility of the tympanic membrane
- Calculator, as most pediatric medications are dosed in mg/kg
- Reflex hammer
- Measuring tape for measuring head circumference, other
- Tongue blades
- Penlight
- Pens
- Toy for distracting apprehensive children
- Books, electronic and/or printed

Your team

During your pediatrics inpatient time, you will usually be part of a team responsible for the care of patients on the general medical floor or in the nursery. The team usually consists of the following individuals:

Attending physician

The attending physician is typically a faculty member at the medical school (clinical or academic) who has been assigned to be the leader of the team. The attending's primary goal is to ensure that the patients assigned to the team receive the best possible medical care. Providing a solid educational experience for residents, interns, and medical students is also an important role. The attending is also responsible for evaluating all the team members. The team's contact with the attending is usually limited to attending rounds, a period of time during the day in which the entire team meets.

During your pediatrics outpatient time, you may either work with an individual community pediatrician or an academic pediatrician with a hospital-affiliated clinic. This time is generally more one-on-one, with you working directly with an established pediatrician. Depending on the physician, he or she may want you to see patients by yourself, and then report back to them on the history and physical exam. Alternatively, the pediatrician may request that you shadow him or her as you see patients together. If you see patients by yourself, then the pediatrician will generally see the patient with you in the room again after the two of you have discussed the case.

Residents

The resident physician is the house officer who, at a minimum, has completed an internship. The resident is responsible for overseeing the care of all the patients on the service. The resident supervises the work of the interns and medical students, and ensures that the treatment plans for the individual patients are implemented. The resident is also responsible for teaching the junior members of the team. Resident teaching may include didactic lectures, demonstration of procedures, or pimp questions.

Interns

By definition, internship refers to the first year of residency training that follows medical school graduation. Next to the medical students, interns are the most junior members of the team. The interns are responsible for executing the treatment plan on their patients and for writing the medical orders and daily progress notes. They are also responsible for communicating daily with the family on the condition of their child.

You will probably have the most interaction with the interns, since they will also be following patients assigned to you by the resident. The intern will probably expect you to write the daily progress note on your patients, which they will addend and cosign before it's entered into the permanent medical record. Some institutions permit medical students to write orders, which then need to be cosigned by a physician before the order is executed. Other institutions will only permit orders written by physicians. When issues arise in the management of your patient's condition(s), you should always notify the intern immediately. If the intern isn't available, notify the resident. Although interns love to teach, this isn't always possible given the demands placed upon them. On a daily basis, some of their responsibilities include scheduling tests and procedures, drawing blood or performing other procedures, checking lab test results, entering orders, writing daily progress notes, and communicating with their patients' families.

Pre-rounds

Your day will begin with pre-rounds. Pre-rounds refers to the period of time before work rounds begin. During pre-rounds, you will see your patients individually (or sometimes with the intern). The goal of pre-rounds is to identify any new events that have occurred in your patient's course since you left the hospital the previous day. This information will be presented to the resident and intern during work rounds, which immediately follow pre-rounds.

What to do during pre-rounds

Successful pre-rounding requires that you do all of the following:

- Review the chart for any new progress notes that may have been placed since you left the hospital.

- Review the patient's orders. Look for new orders, since sometimes changes that occur in the patient's course are not documented in the progress notes.

- Speak with the intern (cross-covering intern) who was taking care of your patient while your team was out of the hospital to see if any new events occurred. If this isn't possible, touch base with your intern who will get sign-out from the cross-covering intern.

- Speak with the nurse who was involved in your patient's care to see if they have any concerns about the patient. In pediatrics, the nurses are an important source of information, particularly if the patient's family isn't available.

- Speak with the patient's family to see if they have any concerns or questions regarding the care of the patient. In pediatrics, the patient's parents are often the only ones who know how the child is feeling. You should try to ascertain the following:

  - Has the patient's overall condition improved, stayed the same, or worsened?
  - Does the patient still have the same symptoms? If so, have the symptoms improved, stayed the same, or worsened?
  - Does the patient have any new symptoms?
  - Does the patient have any new concerns?

- If the patient can talk to you, talk with him or her. Although most children are exceedingly shy around strangers, particularly physicians, sometimes the child will tell you something they didn't even tell their parents. Ask the child the same questions you asked the parents.

- Examine the patient. You should do the following:
    - Write down vital signs (including weight).
    - Pay particular attention to I/O's.
    I's = everything the patient has taken by mouth/IV/NG.
    O's = everything the patient has put out in urine/stool/emesis/NG tube/other tubes or drains.
    - Perform brief physical exam
    - Examine the area of interest; for example, if the patient has foot cellulitis, take a look at the foot. At the minimum, you should perform a HEENT (head, eyes, ears, nose, and throat), heart, lung, abdominal, and extremity exam, irrespective of the complaint which led to the hospitalization.

- Check to see if lab or diagnostic test results have returned: labs, cultures, ECG, radiographs, other.

- Gather your thoughts and formulate your assessment and plan for each problem.

- Get ready to present this information during work rounds.

Pre-rounds: 10 Tips for Success

Tip # 1 As a general rule, give yourself about twenty minutes to pre-round on each patient. That way, you'll have enough time to complete the data-gathering tasks and formulate a coherent assessment and plan.

Tip # 2 Have a toy handy – in the pocket of your laboratory coat or near the equipment you'll be using – tso distract apprehensive children.

Tip # 3 Have fun stickers in your pocket so you can give patients a sticker after you examine them or perform a procedure.

Tip # 4 Respect the nurses taking care of your patients and treat them with the same courtesy that you expect for yourself. This respect and courtesy can go a long way toward building trust with your fellow caregivers.

Tip # 5 If your patient and one or more parents are sleeping, gently awaken the parents first and inform them that you are going to examine their child. Then proceed to awaken the child and complete the physical examination. By alerting the parents first, you avoid the possibility of their being awakened abruptly by the cry of their child during the physical examination.

Tip # 6 Inform the older pediatric patient of what you will do during the physical examination before you do it.

Tip # 7 For patients who are old enough to understand, ask how they feel they're doing while you're performing the physical examination. That way, if they feel something isn't going well, you can address it then and there while you are physically present.

Tip # 8 In addition to performing a general physical examination, specifically examine any part of the body for which the patient is being hospitalized. If the patient is hospitalized for an infected decubitus ulcer on the back, examine the ulcer every morning.

Tip # 9 Touch base with the cross-covering intern to ask if any significant events occurred with your patients while you were out of the hospital. If this isn't possible, speak with your intern.

Tip #10 Organize the information gathered from pre-rounds in such a way that it can be easily accessed and conveyed to the team during work rounds.

Work Rounds

During work rounds, the entire team (except the attending) will either do "sit-down rounds" – during which the team will usually sit around a table and discuss each patient individually - or do "walk-rounds" – during which the team will walk from one patient's room to another, discussing each patient along the way. Whether a resident does "sit-down rounds" or "walk-rounds" is often determined by the number of patients on the service. Either way, the resident will expect the most junior member of the team following the patient to present. After the presentation, the team will discuss the patient's progress and any new events that have occurred, and then formulate a treatment plan.

The key to giving a solid presentation on work rounds is to do a great job pre-rounding. The work rounds presentation should be brief; ask your resident how long it should be. It should include information the resident wishes to hear, and since every resident is different, always ask about specific expectations and preferences. As in most other clerkships, the good work rounds presentation includes all the pertinent information in its most concise form.

5 Questions To Ask Your Resident Before Your First Work Rounds

Question # 1   What time do work rounds begin?

Question # 2   Where do work rounds start?

Question # 3   How would you like me to present newly admitted patients?

Question # 4   How would you like me to present established patients?

Question # 5   How much time do I have to present patients during rounds?

Step-By-Step Approach to the Work Rounds Presentation

Step 1: Present the patient to the team by giving the patient's name, age (post-gestational age, if appropriate), ethnicity, gender, and working diagnosis or reason for admission to the hospital.

Amber Smith is a 10-day old, 40 2/7 week post-gestational age white female admitted to the hospital for a fever of unknown origin with a temperature of 101.2° F and dehydration.

Step 2: Present the subjective data, which should include the patient's current status and any events or complaints that have occurred or developed since the previous day's rounds.

No new events occurred overnight. The parents state that the patient is now eating better and that her fussiness has decreased.

Step 3: Present the objective data, beginning with the vital signs.

Over the past 24 hours, the Tmax (maximum temperature) was 99.8° F. Current pulse is 125, respiratory rate 40, and blood pressure 85/45. Weight today is 3800 grams – an increase of 20 grams from yesterday and an increase of ~5 ½ % from her birthweight of 3600 grams. In's were 100cc/kg/day via IV fluids with D5 ¼ NS + KCl 2mEql/100cc plus breastfeeding PO ad lib. Urinary output was 3cc/kg/hour, and the patient had 3 formed stools.

Step 4: Present the physical exam findings from your most recent exam. Always include the HEENT, heart, lung, abdominal, and extremity exam. Also include findings pertinent to the patient's reason for admission. Present both pertinent positives and pertinent negatives.

Physical exam is notable for clear tympanic membranes bilaterally, clear oropharynx, moist mucus membranes, clear chest, soft abdomen, no skin rashes, and well-perfused extremities.

Step 5: Present the laboratory test results. Include only new lab test results. Old results may be presented if needed as a reference point.

All lab results this morning were normal. The serum bicarbonate was 24, as compared to 18 on admission 24 hours ago. All CSF, blood, and urine cultures have been negative for 24 hours.

Step 6: Present the results of any diagnostic studies or imaging tests.

Chest x-ray performed yesterday revealed no infiltrates, effusions, or cardiomegaly. The radiologist reported the film as normal for age.

Step 7: Discuss the problems and treatment plan. The problems should be discussed in order of decreasing importance. Provide an assessment for each problem followed by the management plan.

> *Problem #1 is fever of unknown origin. The patient has been receiving IV ampicillin and IV gentamicin since admission, and will continue to receive these IV antibiotics for at least 48 hours pending the results of her CSF, blood, and urine cultures. If the cultures come back positive, we will continue IV antibiotic therapy based on the identification and sensitivities of the pathogenic organism. If we continue IV gentamicin beyond 48 hours, we will also check serum levels to confirm appropriate dosing. If the cultures come back negative after 48 hours, we will discontinue the IV antibiotic therapy.*

> *Problem #2 is dehydration. The patient has been breastfeeding well per her mother's report since admission and has also been receiving maintenance IV fluids. This morning, her serum bicarbonate is normal. The plan will be to decrease her IV fluid rate and strictly monitor her I/O's and daily weight. If the patient can breastfeed well enough to gain weight and maintain adequate hydration, we will discontinue her IV fluids.*

At the end of your presentation, the resident may agree or disagree with your assessment and plan. Don't be upset if the resident disagrees with you. At this point in your career, you aren't expected to be proficient at formulating the assessment and plan. What is more important is that you demonstrate that you've thought about your patient's examination, and have tried to formulate a plan based on your findings.

Checklist for Pediatrics Write-Up, also known as History and Physical or Admit Note

The written case presentation, or "write-up," is a detailed formal account of the patient's clinical presentation and illness. Although many students consider this task to be a bit tedious, developing the skills needed to document a patient's clinical course appropriately and comprehensively is essential in modern-day medicine. Effective written communication is a learned skill, and the ability to efficiently and succinctly document a patient's case is vital for communication between physicians and essential for delivering high quality patient care. Write-ups are often reviewed and graded by attending physicians and clerkship directors.

Chief Complaint (CC)

___ Chief complaint is included (use words of patient or parent if possible).
___ Source of the history is included (child, parent, guardian).

History of Present Illness (HPI)

___ First sentence includes the necessary and relevant information: age, gender, ethnicity, chief complaint, duration of chief complaint, relevant PMH.
___ HPI is presented in a chronological fashion beginning with when patient was at baseline or usual state of health.
___ Chief complaint is defined properly: location, quality or character, frequency, onset, course, duration, severity, radiation [of pain], precipitating factors, alleviating factors, associated symptoms.
___ Pertinent positives and negatives are included.
___ Information about evaluations performed by other physicians prior to hospitalization, including results of diagnostic testing and response to treatment, is included.
___ Elements of the PMH, social history, and family history relevant to the HPI are incorporated.
___ Information from the review of systems pertinent to the chief complaint is included.

Past medical history (PMH)/Past surgical history (PSH)

___ Complete with sufficient detail for diagnoses, including date of diagnosis, how the diagnosis was made, past studies done for evaluation, dates of any surgeries or hospitalizations, therapy previously received, current therapy, and current status of the problem.
___ PMH includes prenatal, birth, neonatal, feeding, growth, and developmental history. See following table.

What to include

	What to include
Prenatal history	Number of previous pregnancies and their results Duration of maternal pregnancy Any maternal illnesses or complications during pregnancy Amount of maternal weight gain during pregnancy Any unusual maternal exposures during pregnancy: radiation, chemicals, drugs, other Any medications (prescription or non-prescription) taken during pregnancy Duration and adequacy of maternal prenatal care Results of tests performed during pregnancy, time and type of movements fetus made in utero
Birth history	Date, place, weight, height, head circumference Type of presentation: cephalic, breech, other Duration of labor Complications of labor (e.g., failure to progress) Type of delivery: normal spontaneous vaginal delivery, Cesarean section, vacuum-assisted, forceps-assisted, other Anesthetics used during labor
Neonatal history	APGAR scores Birth weight Any perinatal complications: resuscitation at birth, cyanosis, parenteral nutrition, oxygen requirements, incubator stay, jaundice, rashes, infection, other Age at discharge Results of neonatal screening tests: hearing screen, vision screen, newborn metabolic screen, other
Feeding history	How well baby took the first feeding If breast fed: partially, entirely, for how long? If formula fed: partially, entirely, amount/24 hours, type, need for any formula change, for how long? Age at weaning Typical feeding schedule When solids were introduced, and how they were tolerated Any vitamin supplementation: type, amount, date started, duration Present diet: amount of cereal, vegetables, fruit, dairy, meat Any potential feeding problems (e.g., aspiration with thin liquids)
Growth history	History of height, weight, head circumference, and BMI with respect to national standards. In order to do this properly, you need access to age- and gender-appropriate growth charts.
Develop-mental history	Ages at which the patient attained neurodevelopmental milestones, including smiling, maintaining a sitting position without support, walking without support, first words, first sentence, and bowel/bladder continence Ages at which any attained milestones were lost, if applicable How the patient is doing in school The patient's activities outside of school The patient's personality, behavior, and habits

Immunizations

___ List all immunizations the patient has received, including date of administration, boosters, and complications

___ If immunization history is not up to date, those that are lacking are included.

___ Reasons why the patient is not up to date on immunizations are documented.

Medications

___ Include dose, route, and frequency of each medication

___ Include over the counter and herbal preparations

___ Medications being given for the same condition are grouped together

___ If patient is not compliant with a medication, include a notation

Allergies

___ Include nature of adverse reaction

Social History

Include the following:

___ Primary caregivers

___ Other caregivers

___ Education level of primary caregivers

___ Socioeconomic status of the patient's parents

___ Religious affiliation of the patient's parents

___ Marital status of parents

___ Major or traumatic life events (deaths, accidents, divorce)

___ Where the patient lives

___ Type and condition of living environment and year built

___ Attends day care or school or at home

___ Any sick contacts prior to hospitalization

___ Pets at home

___ Use of alcohol, tobacco, or any other drugs

___ Sexually active if applicable (sexual orientation, history of sexually transmitted disease)

___ Performance in school, including attendance, relationship with other students, relationship with teachers

___ Working and if so, where and type

Family History

Include a family tree when possible with following information:

___ State of health of parents, siblings, children

___ Age of family members at time of diagnosis with important conditions

___ Family history of CAD, DM, HTN, and cancer beyond first degree relatives

Review of systems (ROS)

___ All systems are included.

___ Each system is explored in sufficient depth.

___ ROS does not include information already given in HPI.

See page 97 for complete ROS

Physical examination

___ Description of patient's general appearance is included.
___ Includes vital signs, O_2 saturation, and orthostatics, if pertinent
___ Includes height, weight, head circumference (up to the age of 2 years), and percentiles for each from growth chart
___ Physical examination does not include any judgments or interpretations (e.g. wheezing consistent with asthma)
___ Complete, including the following commonly omitted parts of the exam:

- Skin examination
- Thyroid examination
- Lymph node survey beyond just "neck nodes"
- Neck veins
- Distal pulses
- Liver span
- Mental status
- Cranial nerves
- Strength/sensation
- Cerebellar function
- Reflexes

See page 98 for complete physical exam.

Laboratory and other studies

___ All lab and diagnostic test results are reported.
___ Basic lab test results are reported first.

Problem list

___ All active medical problems are included.
___ All abnormalities in the physical exam are included.
___ All abnormal lab test results are included.

Assessment & Plan

___ Begins with summary statement that reviews key history, physical exam, and lab data.
___ Assessment & Plan is problem-based rather than systems or organ-based.
___ Problems are listed in descending order of importance.
___ Assessment is provided for every problem.
___ Differential diagnosis is offered for major problems.
___ Differential diagnosis includes potentially life-threatening causes of the patient's symptoms.
___ Provide information that supports your working or most likely diagnosis
___ Provide information to explain why other conditions in the differential diagnosis are less likely
___ Diagnostic and therapeutic plan is presented for every problem, along with rationale
___ Specifics of plan are included: medication dosages and routes of administration, IV rates/volumes/solutions, etc.

General

___ Write-up is legible
___ Write-up is free from spelling and grammatical errors
___ Medical abbreviations used are recognized as appropriate
___ References are included

Review of Systems for Pediatrics Write-Up

General:
Overall health, growth, and development including change in weight, appetite, activity level, and fatigue

Head:
Headache, dizziness

Eyes:
History of strabismus, glasses, eye infection, discharge, redness, visual problems, change in vision

Ears:
Hearing problems, vertigo, tinnitus, discharge, ear pain

Nose:
Discharge, epistaxis, sinus problems

Mouth & throat:
Sore throat, dental abnormalities, hoarseness, choking with feeds

Respiratory:
Cough (productive vs. nonproductive), shortness of breath, wheezing, hemoptysis

Cardiovascular:
Palpitations, cyanosis, fatigue, chest pain, shortness of breath, orthopnea, paroxysmal nocturnal dyspnea, syncope, murmur, edema

Gastrointestinal:
Dysphagia, abdominal pain, colic, nausea, vomiting, diarrhea, constipation, melena, hematochezia, jaundice

Genitourinary:
History of urinary tract infection, hematuria, enuresis, dysuria, frequency, polyuria, hesitancy, vaginal discharge

Gynecologic:
Number of pregnancies, number of children, abortions, age of menarche, last menstrual period, vaginal bleeding, breast mass

Endocrine:
Heat or cold intolerance, polydipsia, polyuria

Musculoskeletal:
History of joint abnormalities or arthritis, joint pain, joint swelling, muscle pain, weakness, limb-length inequalities, gait abnormalities

Skin:
Rash, hives, discoloration, unusual skin pigmentation, swelling, change in skin color, problems with hair

Neurologic:
History of convulsions, tics, weakness, headache, dizziness, mental status changes, disorientation, numbness, tingling, memory change

Psychiatric:
Depression, change in personality, unusual behaviors

Physical Examination for Pediatrics Write-Up

General: Patient's general appearance: well-nourished, mildly dehydrated, cachectic, other

Vital signs: Temperature, heart rate, respiratory rate, blood pressure, and, if applicable, pulse oximetry and orthostatic vital signs

Measurements: Weight, height, head circumference (up to 2 years of age), and BMI. Also include the patient's percentile with respect to height, weight, head circumference, and BMI

Head: Shape, size, fontanelles, sutures, presence of lesions, trauma, TMJ

Eyes: Pupil size, pupil shape, pupil reactivity, appearance of eyes, visual fields, visual acuity, palpebral fissures, function of the extraocular muscles, red reflexes for newborns, fundal papilledema

Ears: Configuration of the ears, gross auditory acuity, external ear, tympanic membranes, discharge

Nose: Nasal septum, turbinates, mucous membranes, discharge, sense of smell, symmetry, frontal and maxillary sinus tenderness

Mouth & throat: Lips, gums, tongue, teeth, oropharynx, palate, tonsils, uvula

Neck: Presence of any masses, webbing, thryomegaly, cervical lesions (sinus tracts), lymphadenopathy, range of motion, torticollis, rigidity, carotid bruits, tracheal deviation, range of motion, shoulder shrug

Chest: Symmetry, expansion, lesions, gynecomastia, Tanner stage in females

Respiratory: Lung sounds (wheezes, crackles, rhonchi, egophony), inspiratory/expiratory chest movement, use of any accessory muscles of respiration, clubbing, cyanosis, percussion, tactile fremitus, diaphragmatic excursion

Cardiovascular: Point of maximum impulse, heart sounds, rubs, gallops, murmurs, heaves, thrills, jugular venous distention, edema, pulses (carotid, femoral, popliteal, dorsalis pedis, posterior tibial)

Gastrointestinal:	Surgical scars, abdominal tenderness, distention, bowel sounds, liver span, bruits, spleen size, ascites, masses, rebound tenderness, guarding (voluntary, involuntary), costovertebral angle tenderness
Genitourinary:	Tanner stage of the genitalia. For males, comment on the location of the testicles and whether they are both descended into the scrotal sac, circumcision, hydrocele, hernia, and phimosis. For females, comment on the appearance of the genitalia, vaginal orifice (intact hymen), and clitoral enlargement
Musculoskeletal:	Range of motion, atrophy, weakness, instability, joint tenderness, joint swelling, joint redness, spinal deviation, gait abnormalities, limb-length inequality
Neurologic:	Mental status, cranial nerve function, motor function, sensory function, deep tendon reflexes, cerebellar function, spasticity, tremor, rigidity, clonus
Lymphatic:	Lymphadenopathy: cervical, supraclavicular, axillary, trochlear, inguinal
Skin:	Rash, lesions, discoloration, pigmentation

Oral Case Presentation: Newly admitted patients

The day after you evaluate and admit a new patient is the post-call day. On post-call days, the attending will expect formal presentations on newly admitted patients. You will be responsible for presenting the patients assigned to you by the resident. Before presenting a newly admitted patient, you should be aware of your attending's preferences and expectations. Here we describe a step-by-step method of presenting newly admitted patients.

Step 1: Identify patient. Provide full name, room number, and medical record number.

Step 2: Chief complaint and source of information

Step 3: History of Present Illness

	Recommendations
Do...	Start the HPI with an introductory statement that includes the patient's age, gender, ethnicity, relevant PMH, and chief complaint, including duration
	Present the story of the patient's illness in chronological order
	Describe the patient's symptoms fully: onset, precipitating and palliative factors, quality, radiation and region, severity, temporal aspects
	Include pertinent positives and negatives from the review of systems
	Inform your listeners of how the illness has affected the patient's and family's lifestyle
	End the story with a brief description of the patient's visit to their physician or emergency room that prompted hospital admission
Don't...	Use days of the week (Monday, Tuesday, etc.) but rather days prior to admission
	Forget to offer information about any sick contacts prior to the hospitalization
	Forget to report any associated symptoms

Step 4: Past medical history

Step 5: Past surgical history

Step 6: Immunization history

	Recommendations
Do...	Provide the relevant immunization history
	State that "all immunizations are up to date" if applicable to your patient
	Report any missed immunizations and why
Don't...	Report all immunizations the patient has received unless your listeners ask you to do so

Step 7: Medications

	Recommendations
Do...	Report all prescription and non-prescription medications the patient is receiving
	Group medications being given for the same condition together
Don't...	Report the indication for each medication unless asked to do so
	Report the dosage, frequency, and route of administration of each medication unless asked to do so
	Report medications that you and your team started after the patient was hospitalized

Step 8: Allergies

Step 9: Family history

Step 10: Social history

	Recommendations
Do...	Report social history relevant to the patient's current illness
	Provide information about whom the patient lives with, and where
Don't...	Provide a detailed social history unless it has bearing on the patient's current illness

Step 11: Review of systems

Step 12: Physical examination

	Recommendations
Do...	Begin the reporting of the physical examination with a comment about the patient's general appearance
	Report the actual vital signs: temperature, pulse, respiratory rate, blood pressure
	Follow a standard order when presenting the physical examination (from head down)
	Report the patient's height, weight, head circumference (for patients < 2 yrs of age), and BMI along with their percentiles
Don't...	Forget to describe the patient's general appearance (which students commonly do)
	Just say "the patient is afebrile and vital signs are stable"
	Forget to pass along orthostatic vital signs, when applicable
	Make any judgments about physical examination findings (just report the findings)
	Show ambiguity when reporting the information with comments such as "I think I heard a murmur"

Step 13: Laboratory and other diagnostic test data

	Recommendations
Do...	Present basic data before more specialized tests
	Report all abnormal lab test results
	Bring the ECG with you to rounds for the team to review
	Bring any imaging studies with you to rounds for the team to review.
Don't...	Skip around. Keep elements of a given laboratory test panel (CBC, Chem-10) together
	Feel compelled to mention every normal test result
	Forget to bring an old ECG with you for comparison
	Forget to bring old radiographs with you for comparison
	Forget to report a normal test result if it's an important piece of information that will help your listeners exclude a condition in the differential diagnosis

Step 14:   Assessment and plan

Give a brief summary of the patient and his or her problems. Following this, discuss each problem in descending order of importance. Offer an assessment and plan for each problem.

Oral Case Presentation: Outpatient

A step-by-step approach to presenting the outpatient to your preceptor follows:

Step 1: State the patient's name, age (post-gestational age, if appropriate), ethnicity, and gender. Also, if appropriate, state the patient's percentile with respect to height, weight, head circumference, and body mass index (BMI)

Step 2: State the last time the patient was seen at the clinic if the patient is a returning patient. Otherwise, make sure the attending knows that the patient has never been seen in the clinic before.

Step 3: State the chief complaint or reason for the clinic visit. Noting that this appointment is for a routine well child examination is appropriate.

Step 4: State the HPI in chronological order. If the patient is being seen for a sick visit, focus the HPI on the pertinent positives and negatives relevant to the chief complaint. If the patient is being seen for a well child visit, focus the HPI on acquired milestones or any significant events or interval illnesses in the patient's life since the last clinic visit. If the patient is living with a chronic disease, give an interval history on the status of the underlying disease.

Step 5: For a sick visit, provide any pertinent past medical history relevant to the chief complaint.

Step 6: Provide the immunization history.

Step 7: Report all medications the patient is receiving, including all herbal, over-the-counter medications, or supplements. Note the amount, amount per kilogram per day or amount per kilogram per dose, frequency, and route.

Step 8: Report allergies to medications, along with the specific reaction observed.

Step 9: Provide the social history, including the child's caretakers. This section shouldn't receive much attention if the patient is well known to the clinic attending and there haven't been any significant alterations in the social history. Note whether the child attends school or day care.

Step 10: For a sick visit, provide any family history relevant to the chief complaint.

Step 11: Provide the complete review of systems. Inquire about how the child is eating, voiding (urination and stooling), and whether or not the child has lost or gained any weight. If the child has presented for a sick visit, much of this data may have already been presented in the HPI and need not be repeated here. You should supply information regarding how the child is progressing along his or her growth curves with respect to height, weight, head circumference (for those patients less than two years of age), and BMI.

Step 12: Provide the physical examination. Start with general appearance and vital signs. You should perform a complete physical examination. In the clinic setting, it's only acceptable to perform a focused physical exam if the attending directs you to do so.

Step 13: Provide additional data that is important and available, including laboratory results and the findings of other diagnostic procedures such as diagnostic imaging, ECG, and echocardiogram. Such data will typically be available only in follow-up cases. The acute or new patient will generally not yet have laboratory data available in the clinic.

Step 14: Provide the assessment and plan. Begin with a concise summary of the patient and his or her problems. Next, prioritize the patient's clinical problems. For each new problem, formulate a differential diagnosis ranked in order of likelihood. Finally, discuss a clinical plan of care to address each problem.

Pediatric Daily Progress Note (SOAP note)

Title of note/date/time

Subjective: Include presenting symptoms (better, worse, or same?), new symptoms, any concerns or problems, and significant events over the past 24 hours. Also include diet, sleep, pain, voiding, bowel movements, and ambulation. Make inquiries with patient, family, and nurse.

Objective:
Vital signs: Tmax, current temperature, HR, RR, BP
For HR, RR, and BP, provide range over 24 hours
If on O_2, indicate oxygen saturation and FiO_2
Daily weight, if applicable
24-hour I/O (in/out)
In = break down by po and IV (indicate type of intravenous fluids and amount)
Out = urine output (in cc/kg/hour), number of stools
8-hour I/O

Physical exam: include general appearance, HEENT, neck, lung, cardiovascular, abdomen, extremities, and neuro as well as other areas relevant to patient's symptoms

Medication list: include name, dosage, route, frequency, and # of days patient has been on antibiotic(s) if applicable

Lab test results: begin with basic tests and include culture results

Other studies: ECG, imaging tests, other

Assessment / Plan:

Begin with very brief summary and overall impression of patient with age, gender, and reason for hospitalization or diagnosis. Include hospital day # or postoperative day #.

Provide assessment, followed by plan, for each of the patient's problems, beginning with the most important problem first.

Signature

Printed name/pager #

Rule # 7   **If you're interested in the field of pediatrics, advance planning will help your residency application.**

During or following a clerkship in pediatrics, some students decide to pursue a career in the field. In the 2010 NRMP Match, 1,711 medical students matched into the field.[6]

Of U.S. senior applicants who matched in 2007, the mean USMLE Step 1 score was 217.[7]

Of U.S. senior applicants who matched in 2007, 11.6% were members of the honor organization AOA.[7]

How hard is it to secure a position in a pediatrics residency program?

There are 8,124 total residents training in nearly 196 ACGME-accredited pediatrics training programs.[8] Of these, 67.0% are graduates of U.S. allopathic medical schools, 24.2% are international medical graduates, and 8.5% are osteopathic graduates. In recent years, approximately 2,400 positions have been available each year in the NRMP Match. Assuming there are no major red flags in the application, U.S. medical students are readily able to match in the field. However, it can be very difficult to secure positions in top tier pediatrics residency programs.

When should I ask for a letter of recommendation?

If your pediatrics attending has been impressed with the quality of your work, ask for a strong letter of recommendation at the end of your clerkship. There is no need to wait until the fourth year of medical school when it's time to submit applications. Asking early often leads to a stronger letter of recommendation.

Tip # 7

If possible, find ways to work closely with well-known pediatric faculty members, such as the chairman, program director, clerkship director, or senior attending physicians. Strong letters written by these faculty members carry more weight.

Did you know...

If you have performed at a high level during an away or audition elective, you should consider asking your attending for a strong letter of recommendation. A strong letter written by a program's own faculty member often carries greater weight than letters written by other physicians.

How can I strengthen my residency application?

The process begins with an accurate and objective analysis of your background, accomplishments, and credentials. Since we are often not the best judges of the strength of our candidacy, it's preferable to seek the opinion of faculty involved in the residency selection process. The chairman, program director, or clerkship director at your school would be ideal faculty members to approach in this regard.

Dr. Su-Ting Li, program director of the pediatrics residency program at the University of California – Davis School of Medicine, offers the following advice:[9]

> *In order for a student's advisor to be most helpful, the student needs to be honest with the advisor – students should give their advisor their curriculum vitae, personal statement, USMLE scores, transcript, and clerkship comments in advance of a personal meeting with the advisor. They should come to the meeting prepared to discuss (1) any difficulties they had during medical school, (2) what they are looking for in a program (if they know), and (3) how they can improve their CV and personal statement.*

Did you know...

Low USMLE scores are a red flag for program directors. The concern is that the applicant might have difficulty passing future standardized exams, including the USMLE Step 3 exam and the pediatric board exam. Failing the latter reflects poorly on the program, since board passage rates are used by applicants in assessing the quality of a training program. A score < 200 is generally considered low, and applicants with low scores are encouraged to take the USMLE Step 2 earlier in their fourth year. For students who passed the Step 1 after a failed attempt, the Step 2 score carries even more weight.

Following analysis of your strengths and weaknesses by your advisor, determine ways to strengthen your candidacy and follow through.

How can I identify a mentor or advisor?

If you're considering a career in pediatrics, developing a relationship with a mentor is important. As you progress through your clerkship, your interactions with faculty will help you identify the mentor best suited for your particular needs. If you're unable to identify a mentor through your clerkship interactions, schedule a meeting with the clerkship director, program director, or chairman to express your interest in pursuing pediatrics as a career.

> **Did you know...**
>
> Dr. Li offers the following advice to guide students seeking a mentor.[9]
> "Students who have decided to apply to pediatric residency should find an
> advisor who can (1) offer general advice on the application process, (2)
> optimize their application, and (3) help them develop their list of programs.
> The ideal advisor would be someone who is knowledgeable about
> pediatrics and the pediatrics residency application process, and is
> invested in the success of the student."

Should I perform research in the field?

Participating in research to strengthen your application during your third
or fourth year is not a requirement. In fact, one large survey showed that
published medical school research was ranked last in importance among
a group of 16 residency selection criteria.[3] However, if you're interested in
top tier residency programs, research provides a way to distinguish your
application and demonstrate your potential for academic accomplishments in the field.

> **Did you know...**
>
> Many programs value extracurricular activities, especially if applicants
> have shown commitment and have served in leadership capacities. Dr.
> Tim Kelly, Vice Chair for Education in the UCSF Department of Pediatrics,
> writes that extracurricular and volunteer activities are "very important,
> especially activities that are in service of children or activities that
> emphasize a leadership or development role (as opposed to just
> participation)."[10]

How important are away or audition electives in pediatrics?

In general, it is not necessary to do an away elective to match at a program. However, some students may not be attractive candidates at certain programs based on their paper record alone. For these students, a
strong performance during an away rotation can improve the odds. Dr. Li
offers the following advice:[9]

*An away elective is an opportunity for the applicant to (1)
impress the residency program and (2) decide whether the program is the best match for them...Away electives can either help
or hurt an applicant's application. Rotating at a new site requires
learning a new system. Some students quickly adapt to new systems and perform well on day 1. Students who take longer to
adapt to new systems will have more difficulty excelling, and an
away rotation would likely not be in their best interests. Appli-*

cants who are superstars on paper often will be highly ranked even without an away elective, and a less-than-stellar away elective may hurt their application. Applicants who are superstars on paper and clinical superstars from day 1 of their rotation, can use away electives to decide whether the program is the best match for them. Applicants with average paper applications, but who are clinical superstars, may be able to impress programs during their elective, and are most likely to benefit from an away elective.

What fourth year electives are recommended for students pursuing pediatrics as a career?

If you're considering pediatrics, but are not completely sure if it's the right specialty for you, taking a pediatric elective early in your fourth year will allow you to make a more informed decision. Rotations may include an outpatient rotation, subinternship, or a pediatrics subspecialty elective. In addition, a strong performance will lead to an additional letter of recommendation. There will also be enough time to include the evaluation of your performance and rotation grade in your Dean's letter and medical school transcript.

As you might expect with such a broad specialty, there are differences of thought in how the fourth year should be structured for students interested in pediatrics. The University of Washington recommends the following:[11]

- Dermatology
- ENT
- ICU (medicine or surgery)
- Ophthalmology
- Orthopedics
- Pediatric psychiatry
- Pulmonary

Other rotations often recommended by pediatric educators include allergy, anesthesiology, radiology, and neurology. The Medical College of Wisconsin recommends that students "take advantage of the opportunity to take an interesting elective before residency when there is little time to do so. This might include a research elective or elective in another country. Third world experiences are particularly valuable."[12]The University of California Davis School of Medicine feels that students should "avoid spending more than 12 weeks total doing pediatric rotations."[13]

References

[1]Univeristy of South Alabama Pediatrics Clerkship Handbook. http://www.usouthal.edu/peds/reshome/documents/PEDIATRICCLERKSHIPHANDBOOK4.10.pdf. Accessed January 30, 2011.

[2]Institute for Patient- and Family-Centered Care. http://www.ipfcc.org/advance/topics/primary-care.html. Accessed January 30, 2011.

[3]Green M, Jones P, Thomas J. Selection criteria for residency: results of a national program directors survey. *Acad Med* 2009; 84(3): 362-7.

[4]Takayama H, Grinsell R, Brock D, Foy H, Pellegrini C, Horvath K. Is it appropriate to use core clerkship grades in the selection of residents? *Curr Surg* 2006; 63(6): 391-6.

[5]Bremer A, Goldstein B, Nirken M, Desai S. *Pediatrics Clerkship: 101 Biggest Mistakes And How To Avoid Them.* Houston; MD2B: 2005.

[6]National Resident Matching Program. *Results and Data: 2010 Main Residency Match.* 2010. http://www.nrmp.org/data/resultsanddata2010.pdf. Accessed January 30, 2011.

[7]Charting outcomes in the match, 2007. http://www.nrmp.org/data/chartingoutcomes2007.pdf. Accessed January 31, 2011.

[8]Brotherton S, Etzel S. Graduate medical education, 2009-2010. *JAMA* 2010; 304(11): 1255-70.

[9]Desai S, Katta R. The Successful Match: Getting into Pediatrics. Submitted to www.studentdoctor.net for publication.

[10]UCSF Career Advisors. http://www.medschool.ucsf.edu/professional_development/advisors/kelly.aspx. Updated May 17, 2007. Accessed January 27, 2011.

[11]The University of Washington 2009 Top 10 Elective Clerkship Recommendations. http://staff.washington.edu/spomerin/Catalogue/TOP%2010%202008.pdf. Accessed January 25, 2011.

[12]Medical College of Wisconsin Career Guides. http://www.mcw.edu/FileLibrary/User/pconfer/registrarpdf/20102011/CareerGuides.pdf. Accessed January 15, 2011.

[13]University of California Davis Specific Residency Advice. http://www.ucdmc.ucdavis.edu/mdprogram/.../Specific-Residency-Advice-2008.doc. Accessed December 14, 2010.

Chapter 5

Psychiatry Clerkship

Rule # 8   **Many psychiatric patients present initially to other specialties, making knowledge of psychiatric disease important to all physicians.**

Psychiatric disease is highly prevalent, and physicians in all specialties need to be familiar with a variety of psychiatric diseases. The skills learned in this core clerkship are essential for all students, irrespective of specialty choice. All physicians must ensure that patients with psychiatric disease are recognized, diagnosed, and treated correctly. In fact, most patients with psychiatric illness initially present to primary care physicians and specialists, not psychiatrists. "It is known that among outpatients attending specialist clinics, about 15% of those given a diagnosis have an associated psychiatric disorder, and an average of 20 – 30% of those given no medical diagnosis have a psychiatric disorder."[1]

While less than 5% of U.S. medical school graduates match into the field, your psychiatry clerkship grade will be used as a factor in the residency selection process for all fields, as all place considerable value on core clerkship grades. In a survey of medical schools across the country, Takayama found that only 35% of students achieve the highest grade in the psychiatry clerkship.[2]

Even for students who've completed a number of clerkships, the psychiatry clerkship poses unique challenges, and can be anxiety-provoking. Dr. Kimberly McLaren is an assistant professor of psychiatry at the University of Washington and the author of the book, *Psychiatry Clerkship: 150 Biggest Mistakes And How To Avoid Them*. She states that a variety of factors contribute to this apprehension, including the need to learn a new psychiatric "language," as well as the need to learn how to interact with psychiatric patients.[3] In this field, students must leave the comfort zone of the medical-style interview and examination. "Medical students rotating through psychiatry often feel like tourists in a strange country. A new language and new customs confront them at every turn," writes Dr. Glen Gabbard, professor of psychiatry at the Baylor College of Medicine.[3]

In the Psychiatry Clerkship chapter, you'll learn how to present patients and complete write-ups. You may already be knowledgeable about these tasks, but presentations and write-ups in psychiatry are completely different from those in other specialties. In one study, major problem areas identified in medical student psychiatry write-ups included inadequate gathering of developmental histories, omission of sexual histories, brief mental status descriptions, and no attempts at developing a biopsychosocial formulation.[4] In this chapter, you'll find outlines and templates to guide you through the unique facets of psychiatric examinations and documentation. Checklists for the mental status exam highlight unique specifics, such as psychomotor activation, affect, perception, and sensorium. Other outlines help in the creation of a biopsychosocial formulation, as well as the multi-axial DSM diagnosis.

About the rotation

The psychiatry clerkship is usually of two months' duration and may consist of inpatient, outpatient, consult/liaison, or psychiatric emergency center experiences. Students generally find this an interesting rotation with clinical experiences not found elsewhere in medical school. This clerkship should introduce you to the diagnosis and treatment of mental illness, as well as provide a framework for relating to patients in all areas of medicine. You will also learn about subspecialties of psychiatry, including child and adolescent, geriatric, forensic and substance addiction psychiatry.

Typical Day

A typical day on the psychiatry clerkship will vary according to your assignment. The workday on the clerkship is generally 8 AM to 5 PM. If you're working on an inpatient unit or consult-liaison team, you will need to pre-round on the patients assigned to you before attending rounds. Following attending rounds, you will have time to speak with your patients more, discuss treatment plans, follow up on any labs or studies ordered, and contact families. If you have a patient who is involuntarily committed, you should try to attend the commitment hearing if possible. In a psychiatry emergency center or outpatient rotation, you will typically begin seeing new patients when you arrive and may discuss the patients with the resident or attending as they are seen.

What should you carry with you?

In psychiatry, your most important instrument will be yourself. You need to be prepared to listen for what a patient is saying and for what they are not saying, and determine if it makes sense. You also need to pay attention to how you feel in interacting with a particular patient, as this is often an important clue to what is going on with the patient diagnostically. You will need to perform a mental status exam for each patient. You may also be responsible for performing physical exams on patients, focusing especially on the neurologic exam, and therefore may need the following equipment:

- Stethoscope
- Penlight
- Reflex hammer
- Tuning fork

Your team

During your psychiatry clerkship, the members of your team may vary according to which service you are assigned. In general, though, you will be part of a multidisciplinary team responsible for the care of patients assigned to your team. The team usually consists of the following individuals:

Attending physician

The attending physician is typically a faculty member at the medical school (clinical or academic) who has been assigned to be the leader of the team. The attending's primary goal is to ensure that the patients assigned to the team receive the best possible care. Providing a solid educational experience for residents, interns, and medical students is also an important goal. The attending is responsible for evaluating all team members. The team's contact with the attending varies according to the type of service to which you are assigned. On an inpatient unit, contact with the attending may be limited to attending rounds, a period of time during the day in which the entire team meets. In a clinic, consult/liaison or emergency center setting, you may have ongoing contact with the attending as each new patient is seen.

Residents and interns

The resident physician is a house officer who, at the minimum, has completed an internship. By definition, internship refers to the first year of residency training that follows medical school graduation. Your team may have only a resident, only an intern, or both a resident and an intern. The residents and interns are responsible for executing the treatment plan that the team has devised. You will probably have the most interaction with the intern or resident, since he or she will also follow patients assigned to you. When issues arise in the management of your patient, you should first discuss the matter with the resident or intern. Your team may also have an upper-level resident, who may be responsible for teaching medical students. This may consist of didactic lectures or pimp questions.

Psychiatric nurses

The nurses on a psychiatric unit have the most contact with patients and are an invaluable source of information about the patients. They usually report on each patient during multidisciplinary rounds, and can be helpful in determining the consistency with which a patient may be exhibiting symptoms. They also provide informal therapy with patients throughout the day (and night). Nurses in the psychiatric emergency center also have significant contact with patients and can provide important diagnostic information.

Social worker

On an inpatient unit, the social worker will perform the psychosocial assessment and may gain important information from the patient and family that will help the team formulate the treatment plan. The social worker may also facilitate group therapy and work with patients individually. They will be especially helpful in discharge planning during multidisciplinary rounds. In the psychiatric emergency center, social workers can also provide useful information from a brief psychosocial assessment, and may also help facilitate involuntary commitment of patients.

Occupational therapist

The occupational therapist on an inpatient unit works with patients, in groups and individually, on skills such as grooming and hygiene, leisure activities, and psychiatric education. They will also report on patients during multidisciplinary rounds. Because of the time that they spend with patients during the day, they are often helpful in providing information on improvement of symptomatology and ability to reintegrate into society.

Psychiatric techs

Psych techs work on inpatient units and in the psychiatric emergency center. They have been specially trained in dealing with acutely agitated patients and maintaining the safety of the unit, both for patients and for staff. They have ongoing contact with patients throughout their shift and can be useful sources of information about how patients are doing. The techs will also be available to you when evaluating or examining patients. You should ask them to accompany you to see patients until you know the patient well and don't feel that the patient is a threat.

Patient and family

On a psychiatry service, the patient is an important part of the team. A treatment plan should be completed at admission and updated periodically, and the plan should be reviewed with the patient. Because the psychiatry clerkship usually does not entail many procedures or checking on test results, you will spend most of your time talking with the patient and family. You should spend time talking with your patients daily, especially with those who may be depressed or whose thought disorder is improving, as these patients will be the most verbal. Those patients who are more acutely ill may be able to engage in playing games, such as ping-pong or dominoes, or craft projects. This time with the patient will allow you to better understand the patient's symptomatology.

The family, when available, is also an integral part of the team. However, except in the case of an emergency, you must have the patient's permission to talk with anyone about their admission or care. Confidentiality is paramount in psychiatry, and you should not acknowledge to anyone that a patient is under psychiatric care without the express consent of the patient. If the patient provides consent, part of your job will be to gather information from the family, schedule and attend family meetings, and make sure that the family is aware of the treatment plan, particularly concerning discharge planning. The family will often need education about their loved one's illness and how they can help minimize relapses. The family burden of psychiatric illness can be quite overwhelming, and simply listening to the family's frustrations can be very helpful. You can also refer them to support networks, such as the National Alliance for the Mentally Ill (NAMI), which is a nationwide support and advocacy organization of consumers, families, and friends of people with severe mental illnesses. Information can be obtained from their website at www.nami.org.

Checklist for Psychiatry Write-Up

____ Chief complaint is included.
____ Source of the history is included.

History of Present Illness (HPI)

____ Identifies time of symptom onset
____ Includes duration of symptoms
____ Traces development of symptoms from onset to the current time (chronological order)
____ Addresses why the patient has sought medical/psychiatric attention now
____ Precipitants of the patient's symptom(s) are included such as death or illness in family, marital problems, relationship problems [family, significant other, friend], medical illness, work difficulties, stressful events at school, financial difficulties, legal problem, anniversary of negative event, medication noncompliance, substance abuse, other stresses or changes
____ Includes factors that alleviate the patient's symptoms
____ Pertinent features of the past psychiatric history
____ Pertinent features of the past medical or surgical history such as current illness or previous surgery that is contributing or accounting for the patient's symptoms
____ Pertinent features of the family history are included
____ Pertinent features of the sexual history are included
____ Review of systems that is pertinent to the chief complaint is included
____ Patient's concerns, fears, and thoughts about what may be accounting for his or her symptoms
____ Degree to which the psychiatric illness is affecting the patient's functioning. Specify baseline and current functioning with regards to relationships with family/significant other/friends, occupation, school, and leisure activities

Past psychiatric history

____ Names and contact information of current clinicians: psychiatrist, therapist, psychopharmacologist, social worker, group therapist, primary care physician
____ Dates of last and next appointments with current clinicians
____ Prior hospitalizations (psychiatric or chemical dependency), including age at first hospitalization, total number, reasons for hospitalization, location, voluntary/involuntary status, and date of last hospitalization
____ Suicide attempt history, including number of attempts, methods, and medical lethality of the act
____ Self-mutilation history, including why the patient mutilates and the effect
____ Psychiatric medications taken by patient in the past, including indications for each medication, response, any adverse reactions, maximum dosages reached, and duration of treatment

Past medical history (PMH) / Past surgical history (PSH)

____ All current and past medical problems, including current treatments and
     status of illness (active, well-controlled, remission)
____ Presence or absence of head trauma (include loss of consciousness,
     need for hospitalization, resultant deficits),seizure disorders, liver
     disease, thyroid disease, diabetes mellitus
____ Surgical history and obstetric/gynecologic history
____ Significant childhood illnesses

Medications

____ Names of all prescribed medications the patient is taking, along with
     dosage and route of administration
____ Names of all over-the-counter medications the patient is taking, along
     with dosage and route of administration
____ Names of all herbal supplements the patient is taking, along with dosage
     and route of administration
____ Recently discontinued medications followed by the notation "recently
     discontinued" in parentheses

Allergies

____ Includes nature of adverse reaction

Social History

____ Where the patient was born and raised
____ Performance in school and extent of education
____ Occupation and employment status. If not currently employed, has
     patient ever been employed?
____ Disability status
____ Legal history, including incarcerations, arrests, probation/parole status
____ History of physical, emotional, sexual abuse
____ Sexual history
____ Relationships with parents, siblings, spouse/partner, children, friends

Family History

____ Any history of psychiatric illness in biological relatives, including
     diagnoses, treatment (and whether it was effective), hospitalizations,
     suicide attempts, and completions (include suicide attempts in non-
     biological relatives as well)
____ Medical history in biological relatives, focusing on illnesses with
     psychiatric manifestations, such as thyroid disease, neurological
     disease, other, and those that might dictate treatment, including cardiac
     disease, hepatic disease, renal disease, diabetes mellitus, and other
     conditions.

Review of systems (ROS)

___ All systems are included.
___ Each system is explored in sufficient depth.
___ ROS does not include information already given in HPI.

Mental status examination

___ Appearance: grooming, hygiene, age, weight, oddities
___ Eye contact
___ Behavior: cooperation, attitude
___ Psychomotor activity: decreased, increased, agitated
___ Speech: rate, volume, tone, paucity
___ Mood: in the patient's words
___ Affect: your observation; note congruence with mood and thought content
___ Thought processes: logical, goal-directed, circumstantial, tangential, flight of ideas, loose associations, disorganized
___ Thought content: delusions, obsessions, suicidal/homicidal ideations
___ Perception: illusions, hallucinations
___ Sensorium: level of alertness, orientation, attention/concentration, memory
___ Abstraction
___ Insight
___ Judgment

Physical examination

Patients admitted to an inpatient psychiatry unit should have documentation of a physical examination. Additionally, any patient with psychiatric symptoms that you suspect are secondary to a general medical condition should have a complete physical exam. Every patient presenting to an emergency or admissions department should have vital signs taken and documented. The vital signs may be the first indication that a patient is intoxicated or withdrawing from a substance, or that the patient has an unstable general medical condition. Since there is significant overlap between psychiatric and neurologic illnesses, your neurological examination must be thoroughly documented.

Laboratory and other studies

___ Laboratory data: toxicology screen, alcohol level, pregnancy test, serum drug levels, metabolic panel, complete blood count
___ Other diagnostic test data: CT scan, MRI, EEG, ECG, other radiographs

Biopsychosocial formulation

The biopsychosocial formulation serves to summarize the salient features of your write-up. It takes into consideration the biological, psychological, and social factors that may be contributing to your patient's current presentation. It should include:

____ Biological factors contributing to illness: personal and family history of psychiatric illness, medical illness with psychiatric symptoms, psychoactive medications, drugs, alcohol
____ Psychological factors contributing to illness: coping strategies, defense mechanisms, relationships, abuse, other
____ Social factors contributing to illness: occupational or financial problems, relationships, support system
____ Spiritual factors contributing to illness

Multiaxial DSM Diagnosis

Your diagnosis section is complete if you have included the following:

____ Differential diagnosis: discuss major categories of Axis I disorders and Axis II personality disorders
____ Multiaxial DSM Diagnoses

>   Axis I: Clinical Psychiatric Disorders
>   Axis II: Personality Disorders
>   Mental Retardation
>   Developmental Disorders
>   Axis III: General Medical Conditions
>   Axis IV: Psychosocial and Environmental Stressors
>   Axis V: Global Assessment of Functioning

Treatment Plan

____ Biological treatments: hospital admission, medications, diagnostic tests, treatment of underlying medical conditions, discontinuing medications or illicit drugs that may be contributing to illness
____ Psychosocial treatments (psychotherapy)
____ Social interventions: social services consult to help with any outstanding social needs, referral to support groups
____ Spiritual interventions: pastoral consult or counseling

General

____ Write-up is legible
____ Write-up is free from spelling and grammatical errors
____ Medical abbreviations used are recognized as appropriate
____ References are included

Daily Progress Note

1/14/11 9 A.M. Psychiatry Service MS III Note

Subjective: Patient-reported complaints, relevant social developments, clinical symptoms you are following including sleep, appetite, mood, anxiety, suicidal/homicidal ideation, hallucinations, delusions, others, as described by the patient.

Objective:
VS: T   BP   HR   RR
MSE:

Gen – 58-year old WM in hospital attire, well-groomed, appearing his stated age, lying in bed in NAD, reading newspaper
Sensorium – alert and fully oriented
Attitude – pleasant and cooperative with interview
Psychomotor – no significant agitation or retardation
Speech – normal rate/tone/volume
Mood – fine
Affect – full range and congruent
Thought content – appropriate, no delusional content, no paranoia, no SI/HI
Thought processes – logical and goal-directed, no evidence of thought disorder
Perceptual – no AVH
Insight – good
Judgment – good

Meds: Sertraline 50 mg po qd
Clonazepam 0.5 mg po tid
Trazodone 50 mg po qhs prn
Propanolol 20 mg po tid
Isordil 20 mg po tid
Albuterol 2 puffs q6 hours
Atrovent 2 puffs q6 hours

Labs: Relevant labs (esp. drug levels)

Studies: MRI, CT, EEG, ECG, others

A/P: Patient is a 58-year old WM with major depressive disorder, PTSD, HTN, CAD, COPD, doing well with stable mood on sertraline; clonazepam covering anxiety; trazodone effective for insomnia.

• Continue sertraline 50 mg po qd for depression, PTSD
• Continue clonazepam 0.5 mg po tid for anxiety
• Continue trazodone prn for insomnia.
• Will provide supportive psychotherapy as needed

Joe Medstudent, MS III

Step-by-Step Approach to Presenting Established Patients

The key to giving solid patient presentations is to do a great job pre-rounding. The updates on previously admitted patients should be brief (ask your attending how long they should be) and should include the information the attending wishes to hear. Every attending is different, so always ask the attending what his or her preference is. Below is a step-by-step method to present a previously admitted patient.

Step 1: Present patient to the team by providing the patient's name, age, gender, and chief complaint or working diagnosis/reason for being in hospital

Ms. Jones is a 33-year old AA female who presented with suicidal ideations and is diagnosed with Major Depressive Disorder.

Step 2: Present the subjective data, which should include the patient's current status and any events or complaints that have occurred or developed since yesterday's rounds.

She reports that she is still feeling depressed but is starting to enjoy some of the group activities on the unit. Her appetite and sleep are improving. She has not had any suicidal ideations since yesterday and has not tried to harm herself since admission. In the family meeting yesterday, she expressed some of her concerns about failure to her parents and they seemed supportive. She said she felt better after the meeting.

Step 3: Present the objective data, beginning with the vital signs.

Vital signs are within normal limits.

Step 4: Present the findings from your most recent mental status exam. Your attending may want to hear either a complete mental status exam or just the pertinent findings.

On mental status exam, Ms. Jones was showered, dressed, and eating her breakfast in the day area. Speech was normal in volume and tone. Mood was "still down." Affect was constricted, but with slightly increased range. Thought processes were logical and goal-directed. Thought content was negative for suicidality or delusions. No hallucinations. Judgment and insight are intact.

Step 5: Present the laboratory test results. Include only new lab test results. Old results may be presented if needed as a reference point.

All laboratory test results are normal except for the TSH, which is high at 7.8.

Step 6: Present the results of any diagnostic studies or imaging tests.

MRI of the brain was negative.

Step 7: Discuss the treatment plan for each issue, providing an assessment followed by the management plan.

Ms. Jones's depression seems to be improving with her current treatment of fluoxetine 20 mg daily. The plan is to continue at this dose and follow her depressive symptoms. We will order complete thyroid function tests to further investigate her hypothyroidism, and may request an endocrine consult. If she continues to deny suicidality, we will plan to discharge her in one to two days, following another family meeting.

The rest of the team, including nursing, social work, and occupational therapy may present their reports and findings prior to the discussion of the treatment plan. When it's time to present your treatment plan, you may need to modify it based upon the reports of the rest of the team. Don't be upset if other team members disagree with you. At this point in your career, you aren't expected to be proficient at formulating the assessment and plan. It's more important that you demonstrate that you've thought through your patient's findings and diagnosis, and that you've tried to formulate an appropriate plan.

Writing Admit Orders

Psychiatric Admission Orders	
Element	**What to write**
Admit to	Psychiatry unit, team, attending
Status	Voluntary or involuntary
Diagnosis	Axis I, II, and III diagnoses
Condition	Good/fair/satisfactory
Vital signs	q day is usually sufficient for most patients on psychiatry units, unless the patient has medical issues or withdrawal symptoms that require more frequent monitoring
Allergies	List drug allergies here; if there are no drug allergies, write NKDA, which stands for no known drug allergy
Activity	Unit restriction, precautions and checks for suicidality, agitation, elopement, other. Also indicate if the patient is allowed to smoke per unit protocol
Nursing	Instructions for nursing care may include fingerstick glucose measurements, wound care, dressing changes, other
Diet	Regular, renal diet, ADA diet for DM, low-sodium, low-protein, lactose-restricted
Consults	Social Work and Occupational Therapy for evaluation and therapy
Medications	Specify the medication as well as the dosage, frequency, and route of administration. Include PRN medications for agitation if indicated
Labs	Specify when and what type of laboratory tests should be ordered
Special	Include anything else here that you haven't listed above

Rule # 9   If you're planning a career in psychiatry, recognize that advance planning can strengthen your application.

During or following a clerkship in psychiatry, some students decide to pursue a career in the field. In the 2010 NRMP Match, nearly 800 allopathic and osteopathic medical students matched into the field.[5]

How hard is it to secure a position in a psychiatry residency program?

There are 4,745 total residents training in nearly 182 ACGME-accredited psychiatry training programs.[6] Of these, 57.6% are graduates of U.S. allopathic medical schools, 33.5% are international medical graduates, and 8.7% are osteopathic graduates. In recent years, approximately 1,100 positions have been available in the NRMP Match. Assuming that there are no major red flags in the application, U.S. medical students are readily able to match in the field. However, it can be difficult to secure positions in top tier psychiatry residency programs. According to Dr. Lowell Tong, director of UCSF medical student education, the "top six or so programs nationally are supercompetitive."[7]

When should I ask for a letter of recommendation?

If your psychiatry attending has been impressed with the quality of your work, ask for a strong letter of recommendation at the end of your clerkship. There's no need to wait until the fourth year of medical school when it's time to submit applications. Asking early often leads to a stronger letter of recommendation.

Tip # 8

If possible, find ways to work closely with well-known psychiatry faculty members, such as the chairman, program director, clerkship director, or senior attending physicians. Strong letters written by these faculty members will carry more weight.

> **Did you know...**
>
> Not all of your letters need to be written by psychiatry faculty members. Most educators recommend submitting two letters from psychiatrists. Of note, some programs mandate that one letter be written by a non-psychiatrist.

How can I strengthen my application for my residency?

The process begins with an accurate and objective analysis of your background, accomplishments, and credentials. Since we're often not the best judges of the strength of our own candidacy, it's preferable to seek the opinion of faculty involved in the residency selection process. The chairman, program director, or clerkship director at your school would be ideal faculty members to approach.

> **Did you know...**
>
> According to Dr. Mina Bak, "while top USMLE scores are helpful, they are probably less crucial in psychiatry, compared to other subspecialties, since evaluation of the whole person is emphasized. USMLE is of practical importance because passing is required for licensure..."[8]

Following analysis of your strengths and weaknesses by your advisor, determine ways to strengthen your candidacy.

How can I identify a mentor or advisor?

As you progress through your clerkship, your interactions with faculty will help you identify an appropriate mentor. If you're unable to identify a mentor through your clerkship interactions, schedule a meeting with the clerkship director, program director, or chairman to express your interest in pursuing psychiatry as a career. Dr. Adam Brenner, director of medical student education in the Department of Psychiatry at University of Texas Southwestern, writes that "most schools have Directors of Medical Student Education in psychiatry, and these people are often the designated counselors for students interested in considering or pursuing a psychiatric career."[9]

Did you know...

Dr. Mendez-Tadel, a practicing psychiatrist and graduate of the psychiatry residency program at the University of Pennsylvania School of Medicine, offers the following advice to students seeking a mentor.[10] "As with any other area of interest, it is essential to develop a good relationship with a resident or an attending who can help you define your career goals...It is also important to get to know your local psychiatry department. Whether you want to remain at the same institution for residency or you want to go elsewhere, the head of the department, the program director or a well regarded attending can be a great ally."

Should I perform research in the field?

Performing research to strengthen your application during your third or fourth year is not a requirement. In fact, one large survey showed that published medical school research was ranked eleventh in importance among a group of 16 residency selection criteria.[11] However, it may be an important differentiating factor if you are applying to highly competitive programs.

How important are away or audition electives in psychiatry?

In general, it's not necessary to do an away elective to match at a program. However, an away elective will provide the student with more accurate information about a program.

What fourth year electives are recommended for students pursuing psychiatry as a career?

If you're considering psychiatry, but aren't completely sure if it's the right specialty for you, taking a psychiatry elective early in your fourth year (outpatient rotation, subinternship, psychiatry subspecialty elective) will allow you to make a more informed decision regarding career choice. In addition, a strong performance will lead to an additional letter of recommendation. There will also be enough time to include the evaluation of your performance and rotation grade in your Dean's letter and medical school transcript.

Did you know...

According to Dr. Mina Bak, "receiving the top grade (e.g., honors) in the core psychiatry rotation is not essential for matching, but it is noticed by selection committees. In many medical schools, the top grade in the core psychiatry rotation has stricter criteria than the top grade in an elective or advanced psychiatry rotation and is therefore of special note. Students not receiving honors in a core psychiatry clerkship may augment their transcript by exceptional performance in subsequent advanced psychiatry rotations."[8]

The University of Washington recommends the following electives:[12]

- Subinternship in Medicine (if interested in adult psychiatry)
- Subinternship in Pediatrics (if interested in child psychiatry)
- Dermatology
- Endocrinology
- Neuroradiology
- Psychiatry electives: consult/liaison psychiatry, addiction psychiatry, emergency psychiatry, outpatient psychiatry

References

[1]World Psychiatric Association. http://www.wpanet.org/detail.php?section_id=8&content_id=109. Accessed January 30, 2011.

[2]Takayama H, Grinsell R, Brock D, Foy H, Pellegrini C, Horvath K. Is it appropriate to use core clerkship grades in the selection of residents? *Curr Surg* 2006; 63(6): 391-6.

[3]McLaren K, Martin C, Hebig P. *Psychiatry Clerkship: 150 Biggest Mistakes And How To Avoid Them*. Houston: MD2B; 2005.

[4]Roman B, Trevino J. An approach to address grade inflation in a psychiatry clerkship. *Acad Psychiatry* 2006; 30(2): 110-5.

[5]National Resident Matching Program. *Results and Data: 2010 Main Residency Match*. 2010. http://www.nrmp.org/data/resultsanddata2010.pdf. Accessed January 30, 2011.

[6]Brotherton S, Etzel S. Graduate medical education, 2008 – 2009. *JAMA* 2009; 302(12): 1357-72.

[7]UCSF Career Advisors. http://medschool.ucsf.edu/professional_development/advisors/tong.aspx. Updated May 17, 2007. Accessed January 27, 2011.

[8]Bak M, Louie A, Tong L, Roberts L. Applying to psychiatry residency programs. *Acad Psychiatry* 2006; 30(3): 239-47.

[9]University of Texas Southwestern Psychiatry as a Career. http://www.utsouthwestern.edu/utsw/cda/dept28657/files/81862.html. Accessed January 17, 2011.

[10]AMA Residency Programs: An Inside Look. http://www.ama-assn.org/ama/pub/about-ama/our-people/member-groups-sections/minority-affairs-consortium/transitioning-residency/residency-programs-an-inside-look.shtml. Accessed January 20, 2011.

[11]Green M, Jones P, Thomas J. Selection criteria for residency: results of a national program directors survey. *Acad Med* 2009; 84(3): 362-7.

[12]The University of Washington 2009 Top 10 Elective Clerkship Recommendations. http://staff.washington.edu/spomerin/Catalogue/TOP%2010%202008.pdf. Accessed January 25, 2011.

Chapter 6

Obstetrics & Gynecology Clerkship

Rule # 10   A knowledge of women's health is required in all fields.

All medical students benefit from an increased knowledge of women's health. The Department of Obstetrics and Gynecology at Yale University writes that "physicians of all specialties will care for female patients who present with reproductive health issues, whether it is a teen seeking contraception, a young athlete with amenorrhea, a pregnant woman with an autoimmune disease, a patient with type II diabetes and abnormal uterine bleeding, or a post-menopausal woman with breast cancer and symptoms of hypoestrogenemia."[1]

Although only 5% of U.S. medical school graduates enter the specialty, the obstetrics and gynecology clerkship is a core clerkship, and therefore this grade will be utilized in the residency selection process of any field. According to the Department of Obstetrics and Gynecology at University of California Davis, "USMLE scores and clerkship grades (especially in ob/gyn, surgery, and internal medicine) are considered factual data and ranked high."[2] However, honoring the rotation is challenging. "Obstetrics and gynecology is a difficult field, and it takes a truly outstanding student to earn an Honors grade in the clerkship," writes Dr. Yasuko Yamamura, clerkship director of the University of Minnesota obstetrics and gynecology rotation.[3] In a survey of medical schools across the country, Takayama found that only 29% of students achieve the highest grade in the obstetrics and gynecology clerkship.[4]

In the Obstetrics and Gynecology chapter, you'll find outlines and templates that will enable you to complete the daily responsibilities unique to the field, including templates for the delivery note, obstetric admission history and physical exam, and postpartum notes following vaginal delivery and Cesarean section. Do you know what LOP, TOA, or IUGR stand for? This chapter reviews the commonly used abbreviations in obstetrics and gynecology. The chapter ends with recommendations for students who wish to pursue obstetrics and gynecology as a career.

About the rotation

The obstetrics and gynecology clerkship is usually six to eight weeks in duration, and provides exposure to women's health issues in both the inpatient and outpatient setting. While clerkship structure varies from school to school, often students rotate through inpatient obstetrics, inpatient gynecology, and outpatient clinics in both obstetrics and gynecology.

Typical Day

A typical day on the obstetrics and gynecology clerkship will vary according to your assignment or service. If you have rotated through general surgery, you'll find that a typical day on the inpatient gynecology service is structured similarly. Your day will start early with pre-rounds. During pre-rounds, you'll see the preoperative and postoperative patients you are following and write daily progress notes. Following this, you will present your patients to the team during work rounds. All of these activities need to be completed by 7:30 or 8:00 AM so that the team can prepare for the first surgical case. Here's what a typical day on the inpatient gynecology service looks like:

5:30 – 6:30 AM	Pre-rounds
6:30 – 7:30 AM	Work rounds
7:30 – Noon	Operating room
Noon – 1:00 PM	Noon conference
1:00 – 5:00 PM	Operating room or student conferences
5:00 - ?	Follow-up of postoperative patients

On obstetrics, you will primarily be in the labor and delivery (L&D) suite. You will pre-round on postpartum patients and present these patients to the team during work rounds. As new patients are admitted, you will be involved in their initial evaluation ("admission history and physical"). With your team, you will follow the progress of laboring patients, participate in delivery, and write progress and delivery notes. Here's what a typical day on the inpatient obstetrics service looks like:

5:30 – 6:30 AM	Pre-rounds
6:30 – 7:30 AM	Work rounds
7:30 – Noon	L&D suite
Noon – 1:00 PM	Noon conference
1:00 – 5:00 PM	L&D suite or student conferences
5:00 - ?	Follow-up of postpartum patients

Students often take call with the team. Residents on call may spend their time on the labor floor, in the operating room, or in the emergency department. Being an active participant on call allows you to evaluate newly admitted patients, write notes and orders, and perform other tasks required for patient care.

In the outpatient setting, you should be prepared to evaluate common problems.

Commonly encountered problems in outpatient obstetrics and gynecology	
Outpatient clinic	Common problems encountered
Gynecology	Annual exam Abnormal Pap smear Vaginal discharge Abdominal/pelvic pain Abdominal/pelvic mass Difficulty conceiving Contraceptive counseling
Obstetrics	Contractions Abdominal pain Bleeding Leaking fluid Baby not moving

What should you carry with you?

- Stethoscope
- Pregnancy wheel
- Penlight

Your team

During your obstetrics & gynecology clerkship, the members of your team may vary according to which service you are assigned. The team usually consists of the following individuals:

Attending physician

The attending physician is typically a faculty member at the medical school (clinical or academic) who has been assigned to be the leader of the team. The attending's primary goal is to ensure that the patients assigned to the team receive the best possible care. Providing a solid educational experience for residents, interns, and medical students is also an important goal. The attending is responsible for evaluating all team members. The team's contact with the attending varies according to the type of service assigned. On an inpatient unit, contact may be limited to attending rounds, a period of time during the day in which the entire team meets with the attending, or in the operating room. In a clinic, you may have ongoing contact as each new patient is seen.

Residents and interns

The resident physician is a house officer who, at the minimum, has completed an internship. By definition, internship refers to the first year of residency training that follows medical school graduation. The typical team has a senior resident, junior resident, and intern. The residents and interns are responsible for evaluating patients and executing the treatment plan that the team has devised. You will probably have the most interaction with the intern, since he or she will also follow patients assigned to you. When issues arise in the management of your patient, you should first discuss the matter with the resident or intern.

Other team members

Students frequently work with other team members. These include nurses, midwives, and anesthetists, all of whom can teach you important skills.

Commonly Used Abbreviations

AB	Abortion
AFP	Alpha fetoprotein
AFI	Amniotic fluid index
AMA	Advanced maternal age
AROM	Artificial rupture of membranes
ASCUS	Atypical squamous cells of unknown significance
BMD	Bone mineral density
BPD	Biparietal diameter
BPP	Biophysical profile
BTL	Bilateral tubal ligation
CIN	Cervical intraepithelial neoplasia
CS	Cesarean section
CST	Contraction stress test
CTX	Contractions
CVS	Chorionic villus sampling
CX	Cervix
D & C	Dilatation and curettage
DUB	Dysfunctional uterine bleeding
EAB	Elective abortion
EDC	Estimated date of confinement
EDD	Estimated date of delivery
EGA	Estimated gestational age
FAVD	Forceps assisted vaginal delivery
FH	Fundal height
FHR	Fetal heart rate
FHT	Fetal heart tones
FL	Femur length
FM	Fetal movement
GBS	Group B streptococcus
GC	Gonorrhea
GDM	Gestational diabetes mellitus
GTT	Glucose tolerance test
HELLP	Hemolysis, elevated liver enzymes, low platelets
HGSIL	High-grade squamous intraepithelial lesion
HPV	Human papilloma virus
HSG	Hysterosalpingogram
IUD	Intrauterine device
IUFD	Intrauterine fetal demise
IUGR	Intrauterine growth retardation
IUP	Intrauterine pregnancy
L & D	Labor and delivery
LAVH	Laparoscopic assisted vaginal hysterectomy

LGSIL	Low grade squamous intraepithelial lesion
LMP	Last menstrual period
LOA	Left occiput anterior
LOT	Left occiput transverse
LOP	Left occiput posterior
LOF	Leak of fluid
LTCS	Low transverse Cesarean section
LTV	Long term variability
MAB	Missed abortion
MAC	Maternal age considerations
MSAFP	Maternal serum alpha-fetoprotein
NSVD	Normal spontaneous vaginal delivery
PID	Pelvic inflammatory disease
PIH	Pregnancy-induced hypertension
PMP	Postmenopausal bleeding
PPD	Postpartum day
PPH	Postpartum hemorrhage
PPROM	Preterm premature rupture of membranes
PROM	Premature rupture of membranes
PTL	Preterm labor
ROA	Right occiput anterior
ROT	Right occiput transverse
ROP	Right occiput posterior
SAB	Spontaneous abortion
SGA	Small for gestational age
SROM	Spontaneous rupture of membranes
SSE	Sterile speculum exam
STV	Short term variability
SVD	Spontaneous vaginal delivery
TAB	Therapeutic abortion
TAH/BSO	Total abdominal hysterectomy/Bilateral salpingo-oophorectomy
TL	Tubal ligation
TOA	Tubo-ovarian abscess
TVH	Total vaginal hysterectomy
VAVD	Vacuum-assisted vaginal delivery
VB	Vaginal bleeding
VBAC	Vaginal birth after C-section
VTX	Vertex

Obstetrics Admission History and Physical

Date and time

Identification: 28 y/o G3P2 (**G**ravidity = how many times woman has been pregnant; **P**arity = how many times woman has given birth)

EGA[1]:   38 3/7 weeks

LMP[2]:   Date of the first day of the last menstrual period

EDC[3]:   Specify due date and method of determination (LMP or by US at __ weeks)

CC: Painful contractions, which started at 0900, and now occurring every 9 min.

HPI: Patient is a 28 y/o G3P2 at 38 3/7 EGA, dated by ultrasound at 12 weeks, presenting with painful contractions, which started at 0900, and are now occurring every 9 minutes. She reports good fetal movement, intact membranes, and no vaginal bleeding.

                Following this, provide prenatal data, including number of visits, first visit, last visit, weight gain, BP range, lab test results (AFP, glucose tolerance test, blood type, hemoglobin/hematocrit, rubella status, Pap, RPR, GC, Chlamydia, HIV, group B streptococcus, hepatitis B surface antigen, urinalysis, PPD, and amniocentesis), and ultrasound results.

Past OB Hx: For each pregnancy, list year, spontaneous vaginal delivery (SVD) versus Cesarean section (C/S), age at term, gender, weight, length of labor, complications, and developmental problems in child. Provide information about abortions, if pertinent.

Past Gyn Hx: Include menarche, menses, history of STDs, abnormal Pap test results

PMH:

PSH:

Meds:

Allergies:

Family history:

Social history: List any use of tobacco, alcohol, or drugs

ROS:

PE: Include general appearance, vital signs, HEENT, neck, heart, lungs, breast, abdomen, and extremities

              For vaginal exam, document cervical dilation, effacement, station, and position. Also document presenting part and status of membranes.

              Provide fundal height in cm and estimated fetal weight by Leopold's maneuver

              Include fetal heart rate on monitor

Lab tests: List prenatal and current test results

Other tests: Provide ultrasound results, if done

Assessment: 28 y/o G3P2 at term in early active labor, reassuring fetal heart rate tracing
              Intrauterine pregnancy at 38 3/7 weeks
              History of UTI treated at 28 weeks
              Current urinalysis with no findings c/w UTI

Plan: Admit to L&D
              NPO except for ice chips
              IV – D5LR at 125 mL/hour
              Hemoglobin/hematocrit
              Continuous fetal monitoring
              Anticipate NSVD

[1] EGA = estimated gestational age
[2] LMP = last menstrual period
[3] EDC = estimated date of confinement

Sample Delivery Note

Date and time

This is a 28-year old G____ now P____ who was admitted for _____ (active labor, post-term induction, other). With progression of labor that was _____ (spontaneous, aided by pitocin), she delivered a _____ (viable, nonviable) _____ (male, female) infant weighing _____ grams at _____ (time). Nose and oropharynx were bulb suctioned at the perineum. Amniotic fluid was _____ (clear, meconium stained). Apgar scores were _____ and _____. Delivered _____ (LOA, ROA, LOP, etc.) over _____ (intact perineum, midline episiotomy). A nuchal chord _____ (x # was identified, was not identified) and _____ (if identified, clamped and cut or reduced). Placenta was delivered _____ (spontaneously, by manual extraction) _____ (intact, fragmented) with a _____ (2 or 3 vessel cord). The uterine fundus was _____ (firm, atonic) with _____ (no bleeding, minimal bleeding, or bleeding requiring intervention). The episiotomy lacerations were repaired with _____ (type of suture). The perineum, vagina, and cervix were inspected - _____ (no lacerations, # and degree of lacerations repaired with type of suture under local versus spinal anesthesia). Infant was taken to _____ in _____ condition. EBL = _____. Ms. _____ was taken to _____ in _____ condition. Placenta and umbilical artery blood gas _____ (were sent, were not sent). Doctors _____ and _____.

Sample Postpartum Note (vaginal delivery)

Date and time
MS3 Note

S: Include information about patient's ambulation, diet, voiding, lochia (vaginal bleeding), pain control, breastfeeding, and contraception plan along with any other complaints.

O: Vitals (Tmax, Tcurrent, BP with ranges if preeclampsia, P, R)
CV – RRR, no m/r/g
Resp – CTA bilaterally
Breasts – engorged versus non-engorged, tender versus nontender
Abdomen – bowel sounds? soft? Include location of fundus (___ cm below umbilicus) and whether firm or tender
Perineum – assess for lochia (scant, minimum, moderate), visual inspection for hematoma/edema/sutures
Ext – assess for edema or tenderness

Labs – Postpartum hemoglobin 10.2 (pre-delivery 11.3)

A: S/P NSVD, postpartum day # 1 – doing well, afebrile, and tolerating diet.

P: Continue postpartum care. (Can address issues related to pain control, breastfeeding, contraception, vaccines, and discharge/follow-up).

Sample Operative Note for Cesarean Section

1/10/11   3 PM

Preoperative diagnosis:	Intrauterine pregnancy at term with arrest of descent
Postoperative diagnosis:	Same
Procedure:	Low Transverse Cesarean Section
Attending surgeon:	Dr. Smith
Resident:	Dr. Jones
Student:	Harry Cushing, MS3
Anesthesia:	(Spinal, epidural, general)
EBL:	850 mL
Output:	800 mL UO
Findings:	Live 3,452 gram female infant with Apgars of 9 and 9, clear amniotic fluid, normal uterus, ovaries, and tubes
Complications:	No known complications
Drains:	If any
Path:	If sent
Disposition:	To Recovery Room

Harry Cushing
MS-3

Sample Obstetrics C-section Postoperative Note

MS3 Ob/Gyn Progress Note
Date and time

S: Patient is a 33 y/o G2P2 who delivered by C-section at 37 3/7 weeks, and is now POD # 1. Prenatal course was uncomplicated. She did well overnight with no complaints. She is tolerating a regular diet with no difficulty. No nausea or vomiting. She is not passing gas and has had no bowel movements. She is urinating without difficulty. Her pain is under excellent control with medication. She has been ambulating from the bed to the bathroom. Baby is doing well with breastfeeding.

O: Tmax – 99.4   Tcurrent – 98.8   R – 14   P – 84   Ins/Outs
CV -
Resp -
Breast – engorged? Tender?
Abd – soft? Bowel sounds? Include location of uterine
     fundus (___ cm below umbilicus) and whether it is firm
     or tender
Incision – Clean, dry, intact?
Perineum – visual inspection for hematoma/edema/sutures
Ext – edema or tenderness?

Labs - Postpartum hemoglobin 9.8

A/P: 33 y/o G2P2 POD # 1 s/p C/S for failure to progress – doing well

For the postoperative patient, the plan for the day should include issues related to:
     - pain control: increase/decrease/discontinue/switch
        from PCA to po
     - diet: advance?
     - patient activity: increase activity level?
     - incentive spirometry
     - antibiotics: discontinue?
     - drains: discontinue?
     - staples: discontinue?
     - intravenous fluids: change or discontinue?
     - lines/catheters: discontinue?
     - contraception plans

Harry Cushing
MS3

Sample Gynecology Preoperative Note

Same as Surgery Preoperative Note. See page 66.

Sample Gynecology Operative Note

Same as Surgery Operative Note. See page 68.

Sample Gynecology Postoperative Note

Same as Surgery Postoperative Note. See page 70.

Sample Gynecologic History and Physical

Title/name/date
Chief complaint
HPI: Include age, gravidity, parity, and chief complaint in the first line
Past medical history
Past surgical history
Past gynecologic history: Include information listed in the following table.

Elements of the past gynecologic history	
Element	**What to include**
Menstrual history	Last menstrual period Menarche Menstrual frequency, cycle duration, heaviness Intermenstrual bleeding or spotting Dysmenorrhea Menopausal symptoms (if pertinent) History of current or past hormone replacement therapy
Pap history	Last Pap exam History of abnormal Pap test results, colposcopy, cryotherapy, laser, cone biopsy, LEEP, hysterectomy
Sexual history	Orientation Number of partners in lifetime Age of first coitus History of physical or sexual abuse
Contraception method	
Sexually transmitted infections	Include episodes of pelvic inflammatory disease
Breast health	Include whether patient knows how to perform breast self-examination Frequency of breast self-examination Last mammogram History of abnormal mammogram

Past obstetric history: Include date and type of delivery, gender, weight at birth, gestational age, and complications during or following pregnancy

Family history
Medications
Allergies
Social history
Review of systems
Physical exam
Lab tests
Assessment and plan

Rule # 11   If you're interested in the field of Obstetrics and Gynecology, begin planning your application now.

During or following a clerkship in obstetrics and gynecology, some students decide to pursue a career in the field.

How hard is it to secure a position in an obstetrics and gynecology residency program?

There are 4,815 total residents training in nearly 250 ACGME-accredited obstetrics and gynecology training programs.[5] Of these, 71.8% are graduates of U.S. allopathic medical schools, 19.9% are international medical graduates, and 8.1% are osteopathic graduates. In recent years, over 1,100 categorical positions have been available in the NRMP Match. In the 2010 Match, 84 U.S. seniors went unmatched.[6] The specialty can be considered a moderately competitive specialty.

When should I ask for a letter of recommendation?

If your obstetrics and gynecology attending physician has been impressed with the quality of your work, ask for a strong letter of recommendation at the end of your clerkship. There's no need to wait until the fourth year of medical school when it's time to submit applications. Asking early often leads to stronger letters of recommendation. Most programs require three letters of recommendation, and generally prefer that two are written by obstetrics and gynecology faculty members.

Tip # 9

If possible, find ways to work closely with well-known obstetrics and gynecology faculty members, such as the chairman, program director, clerkship director, and senior attending physicians. Strong letters written by these faculty members typically carry more weight.

Did you know...

Some residency programs request that one letter of recommendation come from the chairman. However, many students don't have opportunities to work closely with the chairman. Dr. Eugene Toy is Vice Chair of Academic Affairs and residency program director in the Department of Obstetrics and Gynecology at The Methodist Hospital in Houston. He writes that students shouldn't worry if they find themselves in this position. "Even if the student doesn't have a chance to work clinically with these people, a student can set up one or two meetings. For instance, I have written plenty of letters of recommendation on the basis of meeting with students, learning about their interests and passions, and reading their evaluations."[7]

How can I strengthen my application for residency?

The process begins with an accurate and objective analysis of your background, accomplishments, and credentials. We're often not the best judges of the strength of our own applications, and therefore it's preferable to seek the opinion of faculty involved in the residency selection process. The chairman, program director, or clerkship director at your school would be ideal faculty members to approach in this regard. In advice given to University of Washington medical students, Dr. Vicki Mendiratta, clerkship director of the obstetrics and gynecology rotation writes that the "3rd year is an excellent time to review your credentials to date" and to "make reasonable recommendations regarding your residency options."[8]

Tip # 10

If your USMLE Step 1 score is low, consider taking the USMLE Step 2 CK exam before submitting applications. A high score on this exam can strengthen your application and alleviate any concerns programs may have with your Step 1 performance. In a recent study of residents in eight obstetrics and gynecology programs, researchers found a significant correlation between USMLE Step 1 scores and the Council on Resident Education in Obstetrics and Gynecology (CREOG) in-training examination. The latter is an examination taken during residency, and is used by programs to identify residents "who are likely to pass the American Board of Obstetrics and Gynecology written examination."[9]

Following analysis of your strengths and weaknesses by your advisor, determine ways to strengthen your candidacy and follow through.

How can I identify a mentor or advisor?

If you're considering a career in obstetrics and gynecology, developing a relationship with a mentor is very important. As you progress through your clerkship, your interactions with faculty will help you identify a mentor best suited for your particular needs. If you're unable to identify a mentor through your clerkship interactions, you may schedule a meeting with the clerkship director, program director, or chairman to express your interest in pursuing obstetrics and gynecology as a career.

Tip # 11

Select an obstetrics and gynecology faculty member as an advisor. The person you choose should have a strong understanding of the application and residency match process. Dr. Toy writes that "the two most important factors are availability/interest of the faculty member, and experience/ expertise of the faculty member to give good advice. Sometimes a faculty member will be well qualified but have little time for students due to their busy schedule. In these circumstances, a student should not feel badly about gaining advice from another faculty. Other factors include honesty and integrity, confidentiality, and the mentor's placing the students' interests as higher than one's own or the institution's.[7]

Should I perform research in the field?

Performing research to strengthen your application during your third or fourth year is not a requirement, according to the Department of Obstetrics and Gynecology at the University of Virginia. "Short research experiences may not enhance your residency selection potential as it will not likely lead to a publication or even substantial results to discuss in an interview."[10] Dr. Toy writes that other criteria are more important in the residency selection process. "For instance, clinical performance on medical school rotations, commitment to the specialty, attitude and ability to work with people, performance on standardized tests, and work ethic are more important."[7] He advises students to "work on addressing their weakest area based on what matters most to residency programs. For example, if the student's USMLE step 1 score was average or slightly below average, then spending time studying for the USMLE Step 2 examination would be more important than research."

Did you know...

Many programs value extracurricular activities, especially if applicants have shown commitment and have served in leadership capacities. Dr. Elena Gates, chief of the division of general gynecology in the UCSF Department of Obstetrics, Gynecology, and Reproductive Sciences, comments on the subject. She writes that "commitment and leadership in a few" activities is far better than "superficial participation in a large number."[11] Extracurricular activities, particularly those "showing commitment to women's health" are even better, according to Dr. Mindy Goldman, director of the UCSF Women's Health Cancer Care Program.[12]

How important are away or audition electives in obstetrics and gynecology?

In general, it's not necessary to do an away elective to match at a program. However, some students may not be attractive candidates at certain programs based on their paper record alone. For these students, a strong performance during an away rotation can improve the odds. Dr. Carol Major, program director of the University of California Irvine obstetrics and gynecology residency program, recommends that "students in the middle of their class definitely should do an externship at competitive programs that they are interested in. An externship will allow a competitive program an opportunity to better evaluate a student who happens to fall in the middle of their class. A good job on an externship may also result in another good letter of recommendation, which can help support a student's application."[13] Dr. Toy writes that he always advises "a student doing an audition elective to be prepared to work harder than any other student in the history of the hospital, to put off any leisure during that month until after the rotation is over, and to do more research, read more, arrive earlier, and stay later than any other resident."[7]

What fourth year electives are recommended for students pursuing obstetrics and gynecology as a career?

Scheduling an advanced clinical elective in obstetrics and gynecology early in the fourth year will allow those students considering the field to confirm their interest. In addition, a strong performance will lead to an additional letter of recommendation. There will also be enough time to include the evaluation of your performance and rotation grade in your Dean's letter and medical school transcript.

Among the advanced clinical elective choices offered at most U.S. medical schools are maternal-fetal medicine and gynecologic oncology. The Department of Obstetrics and Gynecology at Northwestern University writes that these rotations can "better prepare the student for advanced graduate training."[14]

The University of Virginia Department of Obstetrics and Gynecology recommends that students consider the following electives if interested in pursuing a career in obstetrics and gynecology:[10]

- Urology
- Radiology
- Dermatology
- Ambulatory medicine elective
- Surgery
- Medical/surgical intensive care unit
- Medical Spanish

The Department reminds students that "these are suggestions and not meant to limit you. Look for areas you always wanted to know more about or think may provide unique learning opportunities." Other electives that are often recommended include infectious disease, medical genetics, emergency medicine, obstetric anesthesia, and adolescent medicine.

References

[1]Yale University Department of Obstetrics and Gynecology. http://medicine.yale.edu/obgyn/education/medstudents/index.aspx. Accessed January 30, 2011.

[2]University of California Davis Department of Obstetrics and Gynecology. www.ucdmc.ucdavis.edu/gme/ppts/residency_advice_1.pps. Accessed January 30, 2011.

[3]University of Minnesota Department of Obstetrics and Gynecology. http://www.obgyn.umn.edu/education/medstudent/clerkship/home.html. Accessed January 30, 2011.

[4]Takayama H, Grinsell R, Brock D, Foy H, Pellegrini C, Horvath K. Is it appropriate to use core clerkship grades in the selection of residents? *Curr Surg* 2006; 63(6): 391-6.

[5]Brotherton S, Etzel S. Graduate medical education, 2008 – 2009. *JAMA* 2009; 302(12): 1357-72.

[6]National Resident Matching Program. *Results and Data: 2010 Main Residency Match*. 2010. http://www.nrmp.org/data/resultsanddata2010.pdf. Accessed January 30, 2011.

[7]Desai S, Katta R. The Successful Match: Getting into Obstetrics and Gynecology. May 30, 2010. http://www.studentdoctor.net/2010/05/the-successful-match-getting-into-obstetrics-and-gynecology/. Accessed January 30, 2011.

[8]University of Washington Department of Obstetrics and Gynecology. http://depts.washington.edu/obgyn/clerkship/electives.html. Accessed January 30, 2011.

[9]Armstrong A, Alvero R, Nielsen P, Deering S, Robinson R, Frattarelli J, Sarber K, Duff, P, Ernest J. Do U.S. medical licensure examination step 1 scores correlate with council on resident education in obstetrics and gynecology in-training examination scores and American board of obstetrics and gynecology written examination performance? *Mil Med* 2007; 172(6): 640-3.

[10]University of Virginia. www.healthsystem.virginia.edu/internet/obgyn/.../medstudentquestions.pdf. Accessed January 30, 2011.

[11]UCSF Career Advisors. http://medschool.ucsf.edu/professional_development/advisors/gates.aspx. Updated May 17, 2007. Accessed January 27, 2011.

[12]UCSF Career Advisors. http://medschool.ucsf.edu/professional_development/advisors/goldman.aspx. Updated May 17, 2007. Accessed January 27, 2011.

[13]University of California Irvine Career Guidance Handbook: Obstetrics and Gynecology. http://www.meded.uci.edu/education/residencyselection/obgyn.html. Accessed January 30, 2011.

[14]Northwestern Department of Obstetrics and Gynecology. http://www.meded.uci.edu/education/residencyselection/obgyn.html. Accessed January 30, 2011.

Chapter 7

Family Medicine Clerkship

Rule # 12   **The family medicine clerkship provides exposure to a wide-ranging spectrum of wellness and disease in the outpatient setting.**

According to the Society of Teachers of Family Medicine, the family medicine clerkship provides "essential patient care knowledge and skills necessary for generic medical school development, regardless of ultimate career choice."[1] The family medicine clerkship teaches students the role of the family physician in the delivery of primary care in the United States. You will learn how to evaluate and manage patients with a wide variety of acute and chronic medical problems.

The experiences in the family medicine clerkship are important to your growth as a physician, regardless of specialty. Physicians in most specialties care for patients in the outpatient setting. Since family medicine clerkships are largely outpatient rotations, you will see medicine as it's practiced in the ambulatory setting. The clerkship will show you how family physicians "identify, prioritize, and manage the multiple medical problems of many patients in time limited visits," writes Dr. Robert Taylor, professor of family medicine at the Oregon Health & Science University.[2]

Through this clerkship, you will hone your skills in interviewing, examination, and clinical problem-solving. These skills are important ones for all physicians, even if you ultimately decide to enter anesthesiology, urology, or another field.

The family medicine clerkship is a core rotation, and your clerkship grade will be a factor in the residency selection process, regardless of your specialty choice. In a survey of medical schools across the country, Takayama found that only 34% of students achieve the highest grade in the family medicine clerkship.[3]

About the rotation

The family medicine clerkship is usually of 4 to 8 weeks' duration, and provides exposure to acute and chronic medical problems commonly encountered in the field. Family medicine clerkships generally take place in an outpatient family medicine clinic in or near the main medical school campus. Rural rotations are also offered at many schools. Although largely an outpatient experience, you may also be asked to accompany your preceptor to the hospital for rounds.

Typical Day

A typical day on the family medicine clerkship will be based on your preceptor's office schedule. While some preceptors have regular office hours, an increasing number of family physicians have extended hours. If your preceptor has patients in the hospital, you may have attending rounds before clinic.

7:00 – 8:00 AM	Hospital rounds (if preceptor has patients in the hospital)
8:00 – Noon	Morning clinic
Noon – 1:00 PM	Noon conference or lunch
1:00 – 5:00 PM	Afternoon clinic

What should you carry with you?

- Stethoscope
- Penlight
- Reflex hammer
- Tongue blades

Your team

The team usually consists of the following individuals:

Attending physician

The attending physician is typically a faculty member at the medical school (clinical or academic) who has been assigned to be your faculty preceptor. Family physicians practice in a variety of settings, and you may find yourself working in a solo practice, group practice, rural clinic, or academic center. The attending's primary goal is to ensure that clinic patients receive the best possible care. Providing a solid educational experience for you is also an important goal. In the clinic, you will have ongoing contact with the attending as each new patient is seen. You may shadow your preceptor, or you may be asked to evaluate patients on your own. If so, after performing the history and physical exam, you will present the patient to your preceptor and discuss the assessment and plan. You will then see the patient together to conclude the visit.

Residents and interns

If your family medicine clerkship takes place at an institution that has a residency training program, you may work closely with residents in both the inpatient and outpatient setting. The resident physician is a house officer who, at the minimum, has completed an internship. By definition, internship refers to the first year of residency training that follows medical school graduation.

For more information about evaluating patients in the family medicine clinic, turn to Chapter 16 on the Outpatient Setting.

References

[1]The Family Medicine Clerkship Curriculum. http://www.stfm.org/documents/fmcurriculum(v3).pdf. Accessed January 30, 2011.

[2]Taylor R. *Fundamentals of Family Medicine: The Family Medicine Clerkship Textbook*. New York; Springer-Verlag: 2003.

[3]Takayama H, Grinsell R, Brock D, Foy H, Pellegrini C, Horvath K. Is it appropriate to use core clerkship grades in the selection of residents? *Curr Surg* 2006; 63(6): 391-6.

Chapter 8

Patients

Why did you become a doctor? There may be a number of reasons, but the most important one is the same across the board: to take care of patients. Everything that you learn, and everything that you practice, throughout four years of medical school, is all in the service of one mission. You are here to make each and every individual patient better.

It is an amazing privilege and responsibility to take care of patients. You can read about a disease all that you want, but to be able to speak to and examine a patient with that disease is an unsurpassed learning experience. It is an incredible responsibility as well. You will be asking patients the most intimate and intrusive types of questions. You will be asking patients to offer their arm for a needle and to disrobe for an exam. In return, you have a responsibility to heal the sick, and protect your patients from harm.

A respected surgeon recently published a startling account of his own commission of a major medical error: wrong-site surgery.[1] Dr. Ring, in the *New England Journal of Medicine,* stated "I realized I had performed the wrong procedure...I hope that none of you ever have to go through what my patient and I went through." The article breaks down the pathogenesis of this major error, and the conclusion is startling as well: small errors in the care of patients can lead to major consequences.

From ancient times onwards, medical practice has posed dangers to patients. In modern times, those dangers are shockingly common. Medical error is thought to be the <u>third</u> leading cause of death in the US.[2] Those errors include the unbelievable: one report described an average of 27 cases in one year, per New York hospital, of invasive procedures performed on the <u>wrong</u> patient.[3] Those errors also include the shockingly common. Nosocomial infections have now become so commonplace that we consider them routine. When a patient develops a hospital-related infection, we document it as a nosocomial infection and treat the infection without questioning why it occurred. However, many of those infections are preventable, and should never have occurred at all.

Protecting patients is critical. Caring for patients is just as important. With all of the amazing advances in modern medicine, it's easy to overlook one basic fact: the best medical care involves caring for the patient, not just the illness. In 1927, Dr. Francis Peabody published his now-famous essay "The Care of the Patient."[4] He reminds us that our patients are not cases. They are individuals.

When a patient enters a hospital, one of the first things that commonly happens to him is that he loses his personal identity. He is generally referred to, not as Henry Jones, but as "that case of mitral stenosis in the second bed on the left." ...

The disease is treated, but Henry Jones, lying awake nights while he worries about his wife and children, represents a problem that is much more complex than the pathologic physiology of mitral stenosis...

In this chapter, our focus is on the patient. You are the team's expert on your own patients. From protecting your patients to healing them, medical students have great power to improve medical care. You will learn the steps that students can take, even at their level, to protect their patients from physical harm. You will also learn a number of strategies that you, as a student, can utilize to improve patient care and outcomes.

Rule # 13   "First, do no harm."
—Hippocrates

Medical error is thought to be the third leading cause of death in the U.S.[2] Ask any practicing physician. The longer a patient stays in the hospital, the higher the chances of complications. Sometimes these complications are due to mistakes.

A report by the Institute of Medicine, widely described in the mainstream media, found that as many as 98,000 deaths occur yearly because of medical errors.[3] Numbers like that are hard to fully comprehend, but other studies have found that medical errors are shockingly common. In response to the Institute of Medicine study, researchers surveyed practicing physicians and members of the public. They found that 35% of physicians and 42% of members of the public reported errors in their own or a family member's care.[5]

Medical care has great potential to harm patients, and the numbers support this fact. Patients have been alerted by the media to this fact. Dr. Richard Klein wrote a book directed to patients, in which the title itself is very striking: *Surviving your doctors: why the medical system is dangerous to your health and how to get through it alive.*[6]

Even as a medical student, you can do great harm to your patients. You can directly harm your patient in many ways. You may transmit a nosocomial infection. You may write an illegible order that is misunderstood by the nursing staff. Your patient may then suffer a potentially fatal overdose. You may make a prescribing error, inadvertently substituting one medication for another that sounds similar, such as Toprol for Topamax (an antihypertensive for a migraine medication). You may fail to document your patient's medication allergy, thus bypassing all of the pharmacy's computerized safeguards.

You are the team's expert on your own patients, and therefore you have the ability to prevent and catch medical errors. Prevention begins with a thorough history and physical exam, a comprehensive problem list, a complete medication list, and an accurate list of drug allergies. These items alone can prevent many medical errors. Sound too obvious? Researchers at the University of Illinois looked at drug allergy documentation by physicians, nurses, and medical students, and found that 20% of individuals failed to document drug allergies in their admission notes.[7]

Recognize that your interns are inexperienced, overworked, and fatigued, and may not be able to catch all of your mistakes. Although you don't have ultimate responsibility for patient care decisions, you are on the front lines of patient care and therefore play a critical role in the prevention of medical errors.

Rule # 14   You will probably witness a medical error.

A newspaper report described a patient safety course taught by Dr. Sax, professor of surgery at Brown University. He asked a group of second-year students, about to begin clinical clerkships, the question "How many of you are scared to death that you're going to hurt or kill someone?" "Every hand in the room went up."[8]

As increasing attention is focused on medical errors, research is underway on prevention at all levels of training, including that of medical students. According to one study, 76% of medical students had observed a medical error.[9] However, only about 50% of these students reported the error to the resident or attending physician.

Although you are likely to witness a medical error, you may or may not receive any official training in how to handle this situation. In recent years, a number of organizations have called upon medical schools to increase patient safety training during medical education. In a 2006 survey of internal medicine clerkship directors in the U.S. and Canada, researchers sought to determine the patient safety curricula in medical schools. Only 25% of schools had explicit patient safety curricula.[10] However, some strides are being made in the education of medical students on topics of patient safety.

In his required course at Brown, Dr. Sax highlighted what medicine can learn from the aviation industry's strides in safety: "an emphasis on good communication, careful record-keeping, diligent use of checklists and, especially, an environment in which everyone feels free to speak up about any doubts and report their own errors without fear of retaliation."[8]

We outline in this chapter further measures that students can take to prevent or catch medical errors.

Rule # 15   Medical students have the power to protect patients.

The issue of medical errors is so vast and complex that it may appear insurmountable. However, every individual in health care has the power to protect patients. One inspiring success story is that of Dr. Ellison Pierce, and his contributions to anesthesia safety. In the book *Complications: A Surgeon's Notes on an Imperfect Science*, Dr. Atul Gawande presents this story. Dr. Pierce was committed to reducing errors in anesthesia, and was able to mobilize the American Society of Anesthesiology, as well as others, to attack the issue. He helped to increase research funding and brought in the expertise of many individuals, including engineers and anesthesia machine designers. In one decade, overall anesthesia death rates dropped to less than a twentieth of what they had been.[11]

As a student, you may feel that your lack of clinical knowledge, relative inexperience, and lack of confidence would prevent you from identifying and preventing errors. However, because you have relatively fewer patients to follow, you may be able to devote extra time and greater attention to your patients, thus allowing you to pick up on errors that others on the team may miss. In a recent study, four real case histories of how students prevented or could have prevented harm were described.[12] Two are summarized below:

Case scenario # 1

An elderly patient with end stage Alzheimer's disease was admitted for placement of a percutaneous endoscopic gastrostomy tube. The patient's code status was "Do Not Resuscitate" (DNR). Following insertion of the tube, the patient went into cardiac arrest while in the PACU. A code was called. After resuscitation efforts commenced, the third year medical student following the patient arrived on the scene. The student knew that the patient was DNR but wasn't sure what to do, since resuscitation efforts had already started. The student didn't know that such efforts could be stopped. After several minutes had passed, the student decided there was no harm in reminding everyone of the patient's DNR status. After he spoke up, resuscitation efforts were ceased.

Event description	Contributing factors or problems	Role of medical student	Lessons learned
DNR order not followed	No system for alerting DNR orders to team. Student hesitant to communicate knowledge of DNR order	Communicated DNR order to team	Students encouraged to communicate with team members when there are questions about proper procedures
Seiden S, Galvan C, Lamm R. Role of medical students in preventing patient harm and enhancing patient safety. *Qual Saf Health Care* 2006; 15(4): 272-6.			

Case scenario # 2

During the first clerkship of her third year of medical school, a student was asked to follow a 21-year old male with ulcerative colitis. The patient was admitted for total abdominal colectomy. The first three postoperative days were uneventful. However, on day # 4 of the hospitalization, the patient developed vomiting and appeared quite ill. A plain abdominal x-ray showed free air under the diaphragm, raising concern for the possibility of perforation. The student's review of the patient chart revealed that the ordered postoperative famotidine (Pepcid) was not being administered to the patient because the order had never been transcribed to the medication administration record. Subsequent abdominal imaging showed no findings of perforation, and the free air was deemed to be residual from the surgery. Following nasogastric tube drainage and institution of famotidine therapy, the patient improved.

Event description	Contributing factors or problems	Role of medical student	Lessons learned
Drugs ordered but not administered	Drug order system requires transcription from hand written order to computer based medication administration record. No formal practice of confirming that ordered drugs are administered.	Drug administration was not confirmed	Students are in a position to follow the practice of confirming that orders are carried out and medications administered.

Seiden S, Galvan C, Lamm R. Role of medical students in preventing patient harm and enhancing patient safety. *Qual Saf Health Care* 2006; 15(4): 272-6.

As these cases indicate, students have the power to prevent or recognize medical errors. In the first scenario, the student initially hesitated to speak up, a common occurrence. As the authors state: "Our experience and that of others shows that students may feel hesitant and delay communicating a known error because of their junior or outsider status and the intimidation they feel from the medical hierarchy."

Medical errors may be committed by any member of the health care team, including the attending physician. As a medical professional, it is your duty to speak up if you believe you have information that is critical to safe patient care. When speaking up, avoid confrontational statements or accusatory stances. You can just state your thoughts directly. "I was thinking about Mr. Burton's indwelling catheter and I wondered if..." You can also phrase your comments in the form of a question, or use defusing phrases such as "I may be mistaken but..." or "This might be a crazy question..."

Rule # 16   Use every technique possible to protect your patients.

A young mother, a pillar of the community, died last year following a routine outpatient surgery. She was a teacher, a Girl Scout leader, and a mother of two young children, and she had undergone a routine orthopedic procedure. The night of her procedure, she woke up at home with shortness of breath, and then died of a pulmonary embolism.

As you progress in your training, you will sadly witness outcomes like this. In some cases, these tragedies are preventable.

In 2009, the National Quality Forum published a set of 34 safe practices to reduce the risk of patient errors. Some of these practices are listed on the next page, including ways in which medical students can make an impact.

Ways in which medical students can enhance patient safety	
What you can do?	**Why**
Do your part to create a healthcare culture of safety	As a member of the healthcare team, you have the opportunity and obligation to "contribute to the quality and safety of patient care."[9]
Use only standardized abbreviations	While medical abbreviations are time savers for busy clinicians, research has demonstrated that certain abbreviations frequently contribute to errors in patient care. In 2004, the Joint Commission on Accreditation of Healthcare Organizations (JCAHO) issued its National Patient Safety Goals. Among the new requirements were recommendations to standardize abbreviations and acronyms and creation of a list of abbreviations not to be used. As you rotate through your school's affiliated healthcare institutions, obtain their list of acceptable abbreviations, and adhere to these guidelines.
Stay up to date with vaccinations	All healthcare workers are at risk for exposure to influenza, and can be vectors in the transmission of influenza to patients. In one survey of physicians and nurses at a major teaching hospital, the overall influenza vaccination rate was only 73%.[13]
Wash hands before and after each patient encounter.	Decontaminate hands with either a hygienic hand rub or by washing with a disinfectant soap prior to and after direct contact with the patient or objects immediately around the patient.
Ensure patients that need venous thromboembolism (VTE) prophylaxis receive it.	In one study of nearly 200,000 discharges from over 200 hospitals, the appropriate VTE prophylaxis rate was only 33.9%, highlighting the low rate of prophylaxis in U.S. acute care hospitals.[14] With every newly admitted patient, assess the need for VTE prophylaxis, and ensure that all eligible patients receive appropriate prophylaxis.
Ensure that written documentation of the patient's preference for life-sustaining treatments is prominently displayed in his or her chart.	In a recent survey of nursing executive members representing academic health centers, researchers learned of how institutions identified DNR orders: • 56% only use paper documentation • 16% use electronic health records • 25% use color-coded wristband in addition to either paper or electronic documentation. Of note, over 70% reported "situations when confusion around a DNR order led to problems in patient care."[15]

Evaluate your patient upon admission and regularly thereafter for the risk of developing pressure ulcers. This evaluation should be repeated at regular intervals during care.	The incidence of pressure ulcers in hospitalized patients is approximately 10%, with most ulcers occurring early in the hospitalization period. A commonly used scale to determine pressure ulcer risk is the Braden scale.[16] Once patients at risk are identified, institute measures to prevent pressure ulcer development. These measures include repositioning the patient at regular intervals, use of pressure reduction devices, and maintaining head of the bed at the lowest degree of elevation possible.
Communicate changes in patient status and new diagnostic information to team in a timely and clearly understandable manner	Ineffective communication can lead to suboptimal patient care and medical errors. In an observational study of nearly 50 surgeries, communication failures were common, occurring in approximately 30% of exchanges.[17]
Collaborate with pharmacist colleagues	Physicians often underutilize pharmacist colleagues. Pharmacists are able to actively participate in the medication-use process, including being available for consultation with prescribers on medication ordering, review of medication orders, preparation of medications, dispensing of medications, and administration and monitoring of medications.

Some information above adapted from The National Quality Forum Safe Practices for Better Healthcare: a consensus report. 2009 update. Report available at www.qualityforum.org.

Rule # 17   Identify patients who are at risk for the hazards of hospitalization.

The elderly Mr. K was admitted to the hospital with pneumonia. As many elderly individuals do, he often had trouble sleeping, and hospitalization, with its beeping machines and vitals in the middle of the night, only worsened his sleep deprivation. The next day, sleep-deprived, he was shaky on his feet and fell.

Patients are admitted to hospitals to get better. Unfortunately, many patients develop iatrogenic complications that are unrelated to their primary diagnosis. They come in with one problem, and then they develop a new one. These complications, which are sometimes referred to as "hazards of hospitalization," include malnutrition, depression, delirium, pressure ulcers, urinary incontinence, falls, restraint use, infection, adverse drug events, and functional decline.[18] Older patients are at particular risk for the development of these problems, and they make up over 1/3 of all new hospital admissions in the U.S. The following table shows some of the risk factors for these problems.

Hospital-acquired risk factor	Hazards
Sleep impairment	Delirium, falls, physical restraints, mortality
Hearing impairment	Delirium
Vision impairment	Delirium, falls, functional decline
Balance, gait, or mobility impairment	Falls, physical restraints, urinary incontinence, pressure ulcers, functional decline
Depression	Delirium, functional decline,mortality
Pain	Delirium, adverse drug events
Cognitive impairment	Delirium, functional decline, falls, pressure ulcers, urinary incontinence, physical restraints, mortality
Malnutrition	Mortality
Urinary or fecal incontinence	Infection, pressure ulcers, functional decline
Bladder or catheter use	Falls, physical restraints
Pressure ulcers	Infection
Physical restraint use	Falls, mortality
Medications	Adverse drug events, delirium, falls, urinary incontinence, physical restraints
Lack of medical continuity	Adverse drug events

Fernandez H, Callahan K, Likourezos A, Leipzig R. House staff member awareness of older inpatients' risks for hazards of hospitalization. *Arch Intern Med* 2008; 168(4): 390-6.

As a student, you can work closely with your medical team to identify risk factors in your patients. The literature has shown that, for some hazards, treatment of risk factors or institution of preventive measures can reduce the incidence of these hazards.

Currently, this facet of patient care is suboptimal. Medical professionals often just don't think about these risk factors, and they certainly don't institute preventive measures as often as required. One example is the use of indwelling urethral catheters, which places patients at an increased risk for infection. In one study of physicians and medical students caring for patients at four university-affiliated hospitals, researchers presented participants with a list of patients they were following. For each patient, the provider was asked, "As of yesterday afternoon, did this patient have an indwelling urethral catheter?" Answers were compared to the findings on examination of the patient. The unawareness rate for medical students was 21%, 22% for interns, and 27% for residents. Even more problematic, catheter use was found to be inappropriate in 31% of the 117 patients with a catheter.[19]

Did you know...

An excellent guide to medical errors and patient safety was published by the Department of Family Medicine at the New York Medical College. It is available at http://www.nymc.edu/fammed/medicalerrors.pdf.

Rule # 18   Prevent medication errors.

Actor Dennis Quaid publicized his family's experience with an entirely preventable medical error that almost killed his twin babies. The babies were supposed to receive Hep-Lock to flush the IV; instead they were given heparin, "the same medication but a thousand times stronger."[20]

They received this overdose twice, and therefore almost hemorrhaged to death, due to events that the hospital later explained were a series of preventable errors.

This type of error has been reported by other hospitals, and in fact many had called for the replacement of Hep-lock IV flushes with saline flushes. Many other types of medication errors occur regularly. The medical team may administer the wrong medication, or the wrong dose. They may administer the right medication to the wrong patient, or the right medication in the wrong way.

In a chapter entitled "Don't let a hospital kill you," author Elizabeth Cohen reports what the actor now teaches patients to ask: is this medication for the right patient, is it the right drug, is it the right dose, is it the right route, and is it the right time.[20] These are the same questions that all medical professionals should routinely ask.

Rule # 19   Don't transmit a nosocomial infection.

According to the CDC, 1.7 million people developed nosocomial infections in 2002, leading to the deaths of nearly 100,000. How are antibiotic-resistant pathogens most frequently spread from one patient to another in healthcare settings? <u>Via the contaminated hands of clinical staff.</u> That means you.[21]

Hand hygiene is described as "the simplest, most effective measure for preventing nosocomial infections", and yet a review of studies that looked at average compliance rates found that most studies estimated compliance rates to be less than 50%.[22] The title of a *Washington Post* article summarized this sad statistic well: "Medicine's dirty little secret: hospitals promote doctors to wash their hands."[23] There are numerous studies that examine how best to encourage compliance among health care professionals, and can be summarized by saying that no one method is uniformly successful.

Hand hygiene is probably the one area in medicine in which I encourage you to teach yourself. Many medical students learn their practices by observing their interns, residents, and attendings. Unfortunately, as studies have demonstrated, these physicians may or may not be compliant with the best practices to avoid nosocomial infections. Lankford and colleagues found that "health-care workers in a room with a senior (e.g. higher ranking) medical staff person or peer who did not wash hands were significantly less likely to wash their own hands."[24]

Your mission is to protect your patients. Cleanse hands between every single patient encounter, even if you were wearing gloves, even if you only shook hands for a second, and even if no one else does so. Hand hygiene may include handwashing with soap and water, hand disinfection with disinfectants and water, or the use of alcohol-based hand rubs.

When I was an intern, my infectious disease attending watched me as I washed my hands, and then turned off the water using my bare hands. He drilled in me the lesson that once your hands are clean, you don't touch anything that could re-contaminate them. If you wash your hands, use your paper towel to turn off the faucet and open the door.

Patients can and do die from nosocomial infections. Recognize that effective prevention of transmission begins with your own personal commitment.

Rule # 20   Your clothing may transmit infections. Change it or wash it.

To investigate if white coats may be a vector for transmission of nosocomial pathogens, University of Maryland researchers cultured the lapels, pockets, and cuffs of medical and surgical grand rounds attendees. Twenty-three percent of the attendees' white coats were contaminated with *S. aureus*. Eighteen percent of the *S. aureus* contaminated coats were methicillin-resistant (MRSA). Prevalence of contamination was greater in those working in inpatient settings, and those who saw an inpatient that day.[25]

In a separate study of the white coats of medical students, researchers found that certain parts of the white coat, including the sleeves and pocket, were more likely to be contaminated. The authors also found that "the cleanliness of the coat as perceived by the student was correlated with bacteriological contamination, yet despite this, a significant proportion of students only laundered their coats occasionally."[26]

Like white coats, neckties have been found to be contaminated with a variety of bacteria, including methicillin-resistant *S. aureus*.[27] Unlike white coats, however, which are laundered, neckties are rarely cleaned.

This has led some infectious disease specialists to recommend forgoing the necktie when a clinician is involved in direct patient care.[28] One suggestion to reduce the risk of bacterial contamination is to clip the necktie to the shirt.

In 2007, after reviewing the literature in this area, the British National Health System implemented a hospital dress code described as "bare below the elbow."[29] The clothing and accessory items that were banned include the white coat, long sleeves, neckties, and hand and wrist jewelry. In the U.S., the American Medical Association is considering adoption of Resolution 720.[30] The resolution, introduced in 2009 by the organization's Medical Student Section (AMA-MSS) and discussed at the 2009 Annual Conference, involves "adoption of hospital guidelines for dress codes that minimize transmission of nosocomial infections." As of yet, no official recommendations have been made.

Rule # 21   You and your accessories and equipment are just one big potential fomite. Disinfect them, change them, or just don't use them.

Stethoscopes, other medical equipment, pagers, artificial nails, computer keyboards, as well as neckties, clothing, and lab coats, are all potential modes of transmission of nosocomial infections.[31, 32, 33] Most medical students recognize this fact. Many don't do enough about this fact.

In 2008, over 1700 medical students having daily patient contact completed a questionnaire about their hygiene practices regarding frequency of white coat replacement and stethoscope disinfection.[34]

Frequency of white coat replacement and stethoscope disinfection (percentage)						
	After every contact	Daily	At least weekly	At least monthly	Less than monthly	Never
White coat	----------	5	63	30	1	0
Stetho-scope	6	13	26	28	15	10

Melenhorst W, Poos H, Meesen N. Medical students need more education on hygiene behavior. *Am J Infect Control* 2009; 37(10): 868-9.

What can you do? Wash or disinfect your hands. Wash or disinfect your stethoscopes. Disinfect your pagers. Wash your hands after handling potential fomites, such as computer keyboards. Wash your clothing.

Don't let patients contact items that aren't typically washed, such as neckties. Don't use artificial nails at all.

In one study, *Staphylococcus aureus* was isolated from 38% of stethoscopes.[35] According to a number of studies, rubbing alcohol pads on stethoscope diaphragms reduces bacterial colonization. In a prospective, randomized, double-blind study of 100 stethoscopes, researchers found that immediate cleaning led to a drop in the rate of contamination from 90% to 28%.[36]

Another strategy is simultaneous cleansing of the hands and stethoscope using an alcohol-based hand foam. In one study, in which stethoscope heads were imprinted onto a chocolate agar plate, bacterial counts were significantly reduced in the post-wash plates.[37]

Rule # 22   The golden rule applies in medicine as well. Treat patients as you would wish to be treated.

What would you seek from your physician if you were the one lying in the hospital bed? In an interesting study done at UCLA, researchers hospitalized nine medical student volunteers who were at the end of their second year of medical school.[38] The goal was to expose students to hospitalization from the viewpoint of a patient. To make the hospitalization experience as realistic as possible, only the Director of Hospital Admissions, the Director of Nursing, and the attending physician on whose service the student was admitted were aware of the student's actual non-patient status. Residents and interns caring for the student patient were kept in the dark. Of the nine student patients, none had ever been hospitalized. Prior to hospitalization, students were coached to present with one of three complaints:

- Severe lower back pain, left lower leg weakness and numbness following a motor vehicle accident
- Dehydration from nausea, vomiting, and diarrhea in an HIV-positive patient
- Loss of consciousness following head trauma secondary to a fall from a ladder

Once admitted, each student patient was evaluated by a house officer team, who performed the history and physical exam. Tests were ordered following the initial evaluation if the team deemed them necessary. Student patients were gowned in typical patient attire, placed in standard hospital beds, given hospital food, and were counseled to follow the team's orders, including "strict bed rest" and "nothing by mouth." Following a one-day hospitalization, students met with faculty members to discuss their experience.

Domain	Representative comments/thoughts
Comfort	Student patients expressed discomfort with having to share a room with another patient and were frequently interrupted from sleep by hospital technology, TVs, noise from hallways, and other patients. Particularly distressing was not knowing what would happen next as well as the slow pace at which things seemed to move.
Interactions	Ratings of nursing staff were highest with students stating that nurses were caring, attentive, and professional. Four of the nine students reported that physicians were distant and cold. One student remarked, "The residents tended to stand far away from me, at the foot of the bed, talk rapidly and walk toward the door even before they finished speaking." Another said "I was ignored by the doctors while the nurses seemed to really care."
Privacy	Several students described feeling awkward when residents came in to round on them. "It felt so intimidating to have them all examining me at once; all trying to feel my abdomen. I felt invaded."
Impact of the experience	One student said that "I think communication is the key. Be compassionate and attentive to possible patient concerns. Patients need to be told what doctors are doing and when delays occur, you need to tell patients why the delays are occurring." Another commented "Communication is important. So is respect. I would tell them when I would drop by and then make sure I keep to that schedule. I would use 'please' and 'may I' a lot more than they do."

Adapted from Wilkes M, Milgrom E, Hoffman J. Towards more empathic medical students: a medical student hospitalization experience. *Med Educ* 2002; 36: 528-33.

Participants felt that the experience of having been a patient would lead them to be far more empathetic than they would have been had they never been hospitalized.

Rule # 23   Introduce yourself correctly.

When meeting a patient for the first time, you must introduce yourself properly. The patient should know exactly who you are as well as your specific role in his care.

Hello, I'm Shawn Patterson. I'm a third year medical student who is part of the team that will be taking care of you while you are here in the hospital. With your permission, I would like to ask you questions related to your medical history.

Did you know...

In the videotaped analysis of histories performed by senior medical students, 30% of all students did not introduce themselves by name.[39] 44% neglected to mention that they were medical students.

Rule # 24   **It is unethical for patients to believe you are a doctor.**

Since you haven't yet received your M.D. degree, you should never introduce yourself as "Doctor."

Did you know...

At the Medical and Public Health Law Site, the LSU Law Center writes that "the practice of introducing a medical student to patients as 'doctor,' 'young doctor,' or a 'student doctor' is fraud. A reasonable person introduced to a doctor in a medical setting assumes that this term denotes a licensed physician with a doctoral degree in medicine."[40]

Not long after you start clerkships, you'll notice that other healthcare professionals will, at times, introduce you as a "student doctor" or "student physician." While these individuals are well-intentioned, this tendency can be deceptive to patients. The danger with attaching the word "doctor" or "physician" to "student" is that the patient may assume that you have the qualifications and responsibilities of a doctor.

Did you know...

In one study of preclinical and clinical students at five Philadelphia area medical schools, researchers found that most preclinical students felt that it was important to introduce themselves as medical students and to request patient's permission before proceeding with the encounter.[41] However, clinical students attached less importance to informing patients of their student status.

If a team member introduces you as a "doctor," clarify your position and role to the patient at the appropriate time. Do so in a way that avoids embarrassment. Even though no harm was meant, patients should have no misunderstandings about the healthcare professionals participating in their care. Once informed, patients are usually receptive to having a medical student involved in their care. For those who aren't, their wishes must be respected.

Making your student status clear preserves the patient's right to refuse your participation in their care. You'll probably find, though, that most patients will readily agree to your participation. Patients often enjoy taking an active role in educating tomorrow's doctors and gain considerable satisfaction through these interactions.

Did you know...

In one study, over 100 adult emergency patients undergoing procedures (sutures, intravenous access, splinting) were surveyed to determine if they would allow first-year medical students to perform the procedure after being told of their relative inexperience.[42] Ninety percent of patients allowed students to perform the procedure.

Rule # 25   **The patient-physician relationship begins with the first words spoken. Greet patients properly in order to establish trust and rapport.**

What do you say to a patient when you meet them for the first time? Are you supposed to shake hands, wave, or just smile? What do patients themselves expect from their doctors?

In a study by Northwestern University researcher Dr. Gregory Makoul, patients reported that healthcare professionals often do not introduce themselves properly or clarify their roles.[43]

Over 400 patients were surveyed regarding preferences for shaking hands and the use of patient and physician names during the initial part of the encounter. Researchers also videotaped patient visits to learn about patterns of greeting behavior demonstrated by physicians.

Patient preferences regarding physician greeting behavior		
	What do patients prefer?	**What do physicians do?**
Handshake	Majority of patients wanted the physician to shake hands with them; only 18% did not.	Only 9 of 19 physicians shook hands with every patient.
Use of patient name	Over half of patients wanted physicians to use their first name, 17% wanted their last name, and 24% wanted both first and last names to be used.	In over 50% of encounters, physicians did not mention patient names at all. When patient names were used, there was a tendency to only use the last name.
Use of physician name	Most patients prefer that physicians introduce themselves using their first and last names. Thirty-three percent expect physicians to only use their last name. Seven percent prefer that physicians use their first name only.	Most physicians use both their first and last names and, when doing so, generally leave out the title "Dr." Thirty percent only used their last name, prefacing it with "Dr." Of note, 11% did not introduce themselves at all.

Data from Makoul G, Zick M, Green M. An evidence-based perspective on greetings in medical encounters. *Arch Intern Med* 2007; 167 (11): 1172-6.

Based upon the study's findings, researchers recommended that physicians shake hands with patients. Remain sensitive to the patient's body language, however, since nearly 20% of patients did not want the physician to shake hands. The authors also suggest using the patient's first and last names initially, along with their own first and last names, when introducing themselves.

Survey participants were also allowed to comment on other aspects of the greeting. Patients preferred that their physicians be smiling, personable, and respectful. Eye contact was important, as was making the patient feel like a priority.

Tip # 12

A successful medical interview requires that you first pay attention to your environment. Make adjustments to the physical arrangements when needed. Turn off the television, close the door, slide the bed curtain for maximum privacy if you are in a two-patient room, and arrange seating to allow for easy and level eye contact. The seated position allows both the physician and patient to be on equal footing. It also reinforces that the physician is ready and able to give their full attention to the patient.

Rule # 26   Your attire can impact your patient's trust and confidence in you as a physician.

On the first day of medical school, Dr. Wilson, dean of the School of Medicine at the University of North Dakota, reminds students that they are junior colleagues of the faculty. "I think it's easy for medical students to see medical school as an extension of their general education, at least for the first couple years. Our students see patients right away, and they learn doctoring skills right away. They need to start behaving like doctors right now…"[44]

For students who will be meeting and examining patients, it is of obvious importance to look like a doctor. Most studies have shown that patients prefer physicians to be well dressed in formal attire. In a study from the Medical University of South Carolina, patients were surveyed to assess whether formal attire influenced the development of trust and confidence in physicians.[45] Patients viewed pictures of physicians in four different dress styles, and were then asked to complete a written survey. These styles were:

- Business attire (suit and neck tie for male physicians, tailored trouser or skirt for female physicians)
- Professional attire (same as business attire but also included white coat)
- Surgical scrubs
- Casual attire (jeans and T-shirt for male physicians, jeans or short skirt for female physicians)

Study participants were asked about their preferences, as well as their trust and confidence in discussing sensitive issues with the physician in each picture. Respondents overwhelmingly favored "physicians in professional attire with a white coat." They were much more likely to share sensitive personal information, including sexual and psychological problems, with professionally dressed physicians.

Rule # 27   Plan your initial interactions with a patient.

In your physical diagnosis course, it was all much more clear-cut. You entered with the attending, he or she introduced you, and then you got started. In rotations, you are typically assigned a patient. You are then expected to locate the patient and get started. There's usually no attending to help you get started or to introduce you. Below is a sample script of how a typical medical student exam might begin:

Beginning the student-patient encounter	
Step	**Script**
Step 1: Ask for permission to enter the patient's room. Confirm the patient's identity.	Good afternoon, are you Mr. Larry Jones? May I come in?
Step 2: Introduce yourself properly, leaving no ambiguity about who you are and what you will be doing.	My name is Katie Litton. I'm a third-year medical student here at ____ and a member of the team that will be taking care of you while you are in the hospital. I believe that Dr. Ran, my resident, informed you that I would be stopping by.
Step 3: Express appreciation for the patient's participation and request permission to proceed.	I really want to thank you for letting me participate in your medical care. Is this a good time for us to talk?
Step 4: Inform the patient that he or she is not obligated to participate.	Mr. Jones, I would like to take your history and then follow that with the physical exam. If there are any parts of the history or physical exam that you would rather not do, please feel free to tell me at any time. Also, if at any point you want to stop, that's perfectly fine too.
Step 5: Inquire about patient's comfort or needs before beginning the interview	Before we start, are there any questions that I can answer for you? Is there anything you need before we start?

Rule # 28   Your patient is not a disease. Do not refer to them as such.

In 1927, Dr. Francis Peabody published his now-famous essay "The Care of the Patient."[46] He reminds us that our patients are not cases. They are individuals. [*JAMA* 88; 1927 The care of the patient Francis Peabody 877-882]

> *When a patient enters a hospital, one of the first things that commonly happens to him is that he loses his personal identity. He is generally referred to, not as Henry Jones, but as "that case of mitral stenosis in the second bed on the left." There are plenty of reasons why this is so, and the point is, in itself, relatively unimportant; but the trouble is that it leads, more or less directly, to*

*the patient being treated as a case of mitral stenosis, and not as
a sick man. The disease is treated, but Henry Jones, lying
awake nights while he worries about his wife and children, represents a problem that is much more complex than the pathologic
physiology of mitral stenosis, and he is apt to improve very
slowly unless a discerning intern happens to discover why it is
that even large doses of digitalis fail to slow his heart rate. Henry
happens to have heart disease, but he is not disturbed so much
by dyspnea as he is by anxiety for the future, and a talk with an
understanding physician who tries to make the situation clear to
him, and then gets the social service worker to find a suitable
occupation, does more to straighten him out than a book full of
drugs and diets. Henry has an excellent example of a certain
type of heart disease, and he is glad that all the staff find him
interesting, for it makes him feel that they will do the best they
can to cure him; but just because he is an interesting case he
does not cease to be a human being with very human hopes and
fears.*

**Rule # 29   The cafeteria, the elevator, the hallway: all
                are public places, and should be treated as
                such.**

Have you noticed the signs in many hospital elevators? "We respect
patient confidentiality." There's a reason these signs have become so
widespread. Physicians and other healthcare professionals used to discuss cases on elevators and in other public locales, as if they were the
only individuals in the vicinity. Obviously, though, you aren't alone in
these locations, and your conversations are frequently overheard.

According to the AMA's Principles of Medical Ethics, medical students and physicians "shall respect the rights of patients including the
right to confidentiality, and shall safeguard patient confidences within the
constraints of the law."[47] While students understand the importance of
maintaining patient confidentiality, adhering to the rules can be challenging and often requires strict vigilance to avoid inadvertent disclosure. In
an article published in the *British Medical Journal*, the authors wrote that
most breaches of confidentiality occur "in settings such as ward rounds in
cubicles with multiple beds and overheard 'discussions management' in
corridors."[48]

Elevators are another hot spot. In a report published in the *American
Journal of Medicine*, researchers described breaches of confidentiality
that occurred in hospital elevators.[49] As the researchers repeatedly went
up and down in elevators, they listened to the conversations of hospital
staff. Analysis of 259 elevator trips revealed that in 14% of trips inappropriate comments were overheard. The most common violations were
breaches of patient confidentiality. In one case, a team of physicians
entered the elevator discussing a patient's test results.

Another study observed medical personnel behavior in a large
emergency department. Observers documented privacy and confidentiality breaches in various patient care areas.[50] Breaches in the triage/wait-

ing area were common, affecting over 53% of patients. Breaches near the physician/nursing station were also frequent, ranging from 3 to 24 per hour. The authors wrote that "all members of the health care team committed confidentiality and privacy breaches."

Some breaches are intentional. In 2008, 25 employees of the UCLA Health System, including six physicians, faced possible disciplinary action for accessing the electronic health record of Britney Spears while she was involuntarily hospitalized.[51]

Confidentiality can also be breached through the Internet. When student affairs deans at U.S. medical schools were asked about their experiences with online posting of unprofessional content by students, 13% of deans reported violations of patient confidentiality.[52] Blogging about a patient encounter with a level of detail that could lead to patient identification was cited as a real life example.

Regardless of whether the breach is inadvertent or intentional, the end result is the same – violation of the patient's privacy and a breach of your ethical responsibility to your patients.

Rule # 30   You are in a position to put your team at risk for a lawsuit. Do not do so.

Why do patients sue their physicians? With so much money at stake, there are numerous studies devoted to answering this question. Why do some patients sue their doctors when there hasn't been a negative outcome? Why would some sue over a tiny scar? Why do some patients, on the other hand, truly experience medical negligence, and then decide not to sue? While physicians may expect that medical errors would be most likely to trigger a lawsuit, several findings point to communication, or rather miscommunication, as the major factor.

For those just starting out in patient care, this can be surprising. Ask any malpractice lawyer. Lawsuits aren't filed due to poor patient care alone. They are filed due to poor patient outcomes and poor communication, even when the medical care provided was entirely within the standard of care. "Poor communication is the leading reason physicians get sued" states Dr. Michota, director of academic affairs for the department of hospital medicine at the Cleveland Clinic.[53]

A number of authors reinforce that communication issues play an important role in a patient's decision to sue. Beckman et al studied depositions made by patients and families who were bringing a malpractice suit.[54] They found that physician relationship issues played a role in 71% of the depositions. They found four themes within the relationship issues. These included perceived desertion of the patient, delivering information poorly, and either failing to understand the patient perspective or devaluing the patient or family views.

These findings underscore the need for students and physicians to always maintain respectful interactions with patients and families. Even if medical science tells you the patient is completely wrong about the cause of his cancer, listen carefully to his point of view and acknowledge his beliefs with respect. Ensure that the patient knows that you are always available to answer questions or respond to concerns. Learn from your attendings and residents how best to deliver bad news. Lastly, even if your team believes that another physician or hospital was medically negligent, it is not your place to discuss this with the patient. Suggestions by another healthcare professional of prior malpractice may also lead to a decision to sue.[54]

Rule # 31   How you speak to a patient can impact your risk of a lawsuit.

In the bestselling book *Blink,* the author Malcolm Gladwell talks about the power of first impressions.[55] In one section, he describes two studies that evaluate a doctor's likelihood of being sued.

In two groups of surgeons, <u>in which there was no difference in the amount or quality of information,</u> communication skills made all the difference. The "better" doctors, who had never been sued, were more likely to exhibit several communication factors:

They were more likely to make "orienting" comments: "I will leave time for your questions."

They were more likely to engage in active listening: "Tell me more about that."

They were more likely to laugh during the visit.

Overall, they spent 18.3 minutes on average with their patients versus 15 minutes.[56]

In a separate study, another researcher, Dr. Ambady, listened to the tapes of these same conversations, and chose 40 seconds of conversation for each doctor.[57] She then changed the frequency of the conversation so that she preserved pitch and rhythm but removed content. Without even knowing what the surgeons were saying to their patients, she was able to predict which surgeons got sued and which didn't. The main difference: one group sounded more dominant, while the other sounded less dominant and more concerned.

In earlier years, we termed these skills "bedside manner". Now we term them "communication skills". There is no doubt that these skills impact patient compliance, patient outcomes, and the risk of lawsuits. As a medical student, and later as a clinician, you will constantly be honing these skills.

Rule # 32   Do what you can to prevent lawsuits.

As you begin rotations, you may be concerned about potential liability. The reality of the situation is that any member of the health care team, including students, can potentially be sued for medical malpractice. However, it is rare for students to be involved in lawsuits.

Your medical school or academic health center will carry liability insurance for you. [There are limits to the policy, and if a judgment is awarded exceeding the limit, a student can be personally liable for the difference.] However, the coverage provided by such policies generally requires that you be engaged in clinical activities that are commensurate to your training level and under the supervision of your medical school's faculty and/or house staff. These policies often include coverage for clinical activities performed during visiting electives at other institutions. In the table below, we offer some general guidelines to help students avoid legal liability while in medical school and, later, as a practicing physician.

Issue	Recommendations
Identification	Your status as a medical student should never be in doubt. Always identify yourself as a student. Always wear identification name tags, and have tags prominently displayed in all patient interactions. All notations made in the patient chart should be signed with a notation indicating your status as a student.
Order writing	Have all orders reviewed and cosigned by your supervisor. Execution of your written order without review, approval, and co-signature of your supervisor exposes you to personal liability should the execution of the order result in harm to the patient.
Performing procedures	When gaining proficiency in basic medical procedures, including placement of intravenous lines, phlebotomy, and catheter insertion, you should be closely and personally supervised by your attending physician or resident. Once you have gained proficiency in a procedure, you must never perform that procedure unless it is ordered by your supervising physician. If you do not feel proficient in a procedure, you must communicate this so that you can be supervised properly. You should never be afraid to say, "I don't know how to do this."
Informed consent	Whenever a proposed treatment or procedure is associated with risk to the patient, informed consent must be obtained. Once the known risks and complications of the procedure have been communicated to the patient, he or she can make an informed decision regarding whether to proceed. While medical students need to learn how to obtain informed consent, it is the attending and resident physician who should ideally obtain informed consent.
Bedside manner	Lawyers will tell you that the best way to shield yourself from a lawsuit is a good bedside manner. When naming physicians in a lawsuit, patients have been known to insist on leaving a particular name out, particularly if the doctor was caring and nice.

Documentation	Thorough and accurate documentation is of obvious importance in delivering high quality patient care. Such documentation is also essential to deterring lawsuits, particularly when there is disagreement later about what was said. Failure to document can lead to a "he said, she said" contest with the patient.
Criticism of other caregivers	Critical comments of another physician's care can trigger a lawsuit. Patients commonly ask healthcare professionals to comment on the care they received elsewhere. In many cases, physicians form opinions based only on the patient's account. According to David Karp, a risk management consultant, this can be problematic. "Too often," he says, "physicians will criticize a colleague's treatment based on the patient's own account of what occurred, without reviewing the case with the previous physician. Such injudicious remarks have triggered many lawsuits, meritorious or not."[58]
Patient's right to confidentiality	Under the Health Information Portability and Accountability Act (HIPAA), private health information cannot be divulged to anyone outside of the medical team without the patient's authorization. This includes the patient's family members and friends. This also includes your spouse, best friend, and classmates.
Disclosure of medical error to patients	As a medical student, you may witness or commit a medical error. You should not disclose such errors to the patient without first discussing it with the senior members of your team. In some cases, what is perceived to be an error is not deemed so after a thorough review of the situation. If an error was made, discussion with risk management is generally recommended before meeting with the patient. In cases of student error, the supervising physician is the appropriate person to disclose the information. Studies have shown that an apology following honest and full disclosure of an error can prevent a lawsuit.

Rule # 33   Excellent patient communication skills translate to better patient care.

It seems painfully obvious that in order to provide the best patient care, you must hone your patient communication skills. However, too many physicians pay lip service to this concept. What does patient communication mean? How does improving your communication skills translate to better patient care and outcomes?

Studies have shown that good communication improves the physician-patient relationship. It also allows more accurate identification of patient problems and enhances compliance with therapy. Overall it leads to greater patient satisfaction with care and results in fewer incidents of malpractice.

The American Academy on Communication in Healthcare has examined this issue in detail.[59] They divide patient-physician communication into three functions: information gathering, relationship building, and education.

Information gathering includes talking to the patient to obtain a correct history of present illness.

Relationship building means using the patient encounter as a means to establish a relationship with the patient, in which the patient believes what you are saying, trusts that you know what you are talking about, and feels confident enough in your abilities to follow through on your recommendations.

Education means learning how to translate evidence-based medicine into easy to understand concepts that your patient can comprehend and internalize.

Did you know...

Considerable research done over the years has demonstrated that physician-patient communication is often suboptimal. In 2004, this led the Institute of Medicine to make the acquisition and development of communication skills a top priority during medical education. That same year, the National Board of Medical Examiners (NBME) began requiring medical students to take a clinical skills examination (USMLE Step 2 CS) as a means to assess competence in communication.

Rule # 34   Information gathering means more than just asking the questions. It includes listening to the patient.

What is the ideal way to gather information from patients? What is the best way to obtain an accurate HPI? Studies have been performed on this issue, because it's an important one. In one observational study of medical interns and residents, trainees often did not allow the patient to tell the story of their illness. "A series of rapidly fired questions often led to disjointed, discontinuous story, or to a series of yes and no answers."[60] With this approach, they found that errors in the medical interview were common.

In an often cited study, Beckman and Frankel found that physicians frequently prevented patients from completing just their opening statements:[61]

- Interruptions occurred after a mean time of just 18 seconds.

- Less than a fourth of patients were actually able to complete their statement.

- Patients who were not interrupted usually completed their statement in less than 60 seconds. No patient took longer than 150 seconds.

In a majority of cases, physicians had interrupted patients after the first complaint, assuming that this was the chief complaint. However, the order in which patients presented their concerns was not related to clinical importance. Therefore, in obtaining the history, the physician may have actually missed the chief complaint.

Published in 1984, this study has received considerable attention and press over the years. To see if it led to a change in physician practice, Marvel repeated the study in 1999 with a group of experienced family physicians.[62] Interruptions were again the norm, with only 28% of patients being allowed to complete their statement. Even more important, once interrupted, the likelihood of the physician allowing the patient to voice other concerns was only 8%.

These deficiencies have considerable potential impact. In some cases, physicians don't even get the chief complaint right. Incomplete information also impacts hypothesis generation and testing, and therefore directly impacts diagnosis and treatment. Such physicians also score lower in patient satisfaction, and many fail to develop the most effective relationships with patients. This impacts compliance, trust, and the risk of lawsuits.

Rule # 35   Incorporate the essential elements of effective information gathering.

In 2001, a group of experts representing medical schools, residency programs, and medical education organizations developed a list of essential elements of physician-patient communication. The resulting Kalamazoo Consensus Statement provides recommendations on gathering information from patients.[63]

● Physicians should use open-ended and closed-ended questions appropriately

Closed-ended questions are those that require patients to answer specifically. An example is a question that asks for a "yes or no" answer. Contrast this with an open-ended question or statement which allows patients to elaborate. "Tell me about your back pain" is an example of an open-ended statement.

There is a role for both types of questions in the physician-patient encounter. It is recommended, however, that physicians begin with open-ended questions, which allows the patient to tell his or her story fully. This can be followed later by closed-ended questions. Unfortunately, physicians sometimes transition too quickly. This "physician-dominated" rather than "patient-centered" approach has been shown to be far less effective.

● Throughout the interview, physicians should structure, clarify, and summarize information. Summarizing information periodically shows the patient that their story has been heard and allows for correction of any misunderstandings.

● The most effective physicians display active listening. This includes nonverbal techniques, such as eye contact and body position, as well as verbal techniques, such as words of encouragement. While we often focus on what is said in the physician-patient encounter, there is no denying the importance of nonverbal communication. The "right" body language can enhance communication. Certain body language indicates that the physician is listening and is interested in what the patient is saying. This includes head nodding, a comfortable degree of eye contact, a forward lean in the chair, and more direct body orientation with uncrossed arms and legs.[64]

Rule # 36   **Communication with patients encompasses more than just talking about their disease. Acknowledge their concerns and feelings, and recognize the impact of the illness on their life.**

Mrs. S was admitted for chemotherapy. In obtaining the history of present illness, the student was doing a thorough job of chronicling the details of the cancer and previous therapies. The patient looked anxious, and finally said "I'm so worried about what will happen to my kids if this chemotherapy doesn't take care of my breast cancer."

Patient communication is much more than just gathering the information related to the illness — although that is obviously critical. It's important to acknowledge the impact that a patient's illness has on every aspect of their life. An illness can create consequences in any or all of multiple realms, including the social, emotional, financial, and professional.

When you're learning how to take a thorough history, it can be hard to incorporate these other concerns. New clerks struggle with this issue, especially since they tend to conduct a medical interview using a script. They worry that they'll miss a critical piece of information if they don't ask every single question on their list. Some students become so focused on the next question that they don't hear the patient, and they don't make eye contact. When you're talking to a patient, it's important not to just ask question after question. Listen to the patient, acknowledge their concerns and feelings, and respond empathically to the patient who expresses concern.

Did you know...

One videotaped analysis of histories performed by senior medical students found that "patients were often forced to repeat key phrases such as 'I was feeling very low' as many as 10 times in order to get students to acknowledge their mood disturbance."[65]

Rule # 37   Patient education is often suboptimal. Begin by discussing the diagnosis and thoroughly reviewing the treatment plan.

Patients want to know their diagnosis, and they want to know the treatment plan. Sounds simple enough. However, studies have shown that patients often desire more information than physicians provide.[66] Physicians in turn often overestimate the time they devote to the task of information giving. In one study of internists, a little more than one minute, on average, was given to this task. However, the internists believed that they had spent approximately nine minutes.[67]

While many patient visits end with a new prescription, research demonstrates that critical elements of medication use are often not communicated to patients. If you're prescribing a new blood pressure medicine, you need to tell the patient about the potential side effects, and you need to tell them how long they need to take the medication. Do they take it forever, until they feel better, or until you tell them otherwise? In one study, adverse effects were addressed for only 35% of new prescriptions, and duration of use information was given for only 34%.[68]

Patient education in a hospitalized setting can be even worse. Forget potential medication side effects. Do patients even know the names of their doctors when they're hospitalized? Northwestern University researchers interviewed 239 hospitalized patients. They were asked the names of their physician and nurse, and the plan of care for the day, including planned tests, procedures, medication changes, and physician services consulted. Only 32% of patients were able to correctly name at least one of the physicians involved in their care.

Just as concerning, almost half of patients did not know what would happen to them in the hospital that day. In 48% of instances, there was no agreement between patients and physicians on the planned tests or procedures for the day.[69]

Rule # 38   As a student, you are in a position to provide high quality patient education.

You will have fewer patients to follow than any other team member. As a result, you will have extra time to spend with your patients. Use this time to educate your patients on their illness. Let them know where things stand, what's in store for them on a particular day, and what they can expect in the long-term. Most patients appreciate patient information brochures. These can be found in your hospital library or online. If provided online, obtain information only from reputable sources. Some patients are actually told to seek out their own information, but a simple Google search may lead to commercial, biased, or even fraudulent sites. Patients may also be interested to hear of local support groups, such as the Scleroderma Foundation or the Arthritis Foundation. Some patients wish to become more involved in their own care, and are not sure how to proceed. The Agency for Healthcare Research and Quality (AHRQ), part of the US Department of Health and Human Services, publishes brochures that patients may find helpful. The website www.ahrq.gov/path/beac-tive.htm includes information on topics such as taking a medication safely, planning for surgery, and helping to prevent medical errors.

Accompany your resident or attending when they visit your patient to discuss discharge instructions. Return to the patient's room later to make sure the patient understood all instructions. You and your team have worked hard to provide the patient with effective treatment. Now, as the patient is being prepared for discharge, you need to ensure that she is ready to assume responsibility for her own care. Make it a point to:

- Speak to the patient in language that she can understand

- Spend the time necessary to educate and counsel the patient. Make sure the patient is familiar with the illness, the names and dosing schedule of all medications, and side effects of therapy

- Determine if the patient actually understands the discharge instructions (verbal and written)

- Allow the patient to ask questions about the diagnosis and treatment plan

---

Did you know ...

In a study involving 47 patients at the time of hospital discharge, researchers sought to determine the level of understanding patients had of their discharge diagnoses and names, purpose, and common side effects of prescribed medications.[70] They found that only 41.9% knew of their diagnosis or diagnoses. Even less were able to list the names (27.9%), purpose (37.2%), and common side effects (14.0%) of their medications.

Rule # 39   Avoid the use of medical jargon.

Some healthcare professionals have a tendency to talk to patients as if they were colleagues. If you haven't witnessed this yet, you will soon. I still remember hearing a liver specialist tell a patient why she had abnormal liver function tests. He was convinced that the patient had hepatic steatosis (fatty liver) and was throwing this word around without defining it. The patient had a perplexed look on her face as he explained to her what the work-up would entail.

Don't use medical terms such as CHF or COPD when explaining to a patient the possible reasons for his difficult breathing, unless the patient clearly understands these terms. Instead, replace these medical terms with language that is easily understood.

In a study of communication between internal medicine residents and standardized patients involving cancer screening, researchers noted the use of a "large number of jargon words and low number of explanations."[71] In another study of physician use of jargon when caring for diabetic patients, 81% of patient encounters involved the use of at least one unclarified jargon term (with a mean of 4 jargon terms/visit). Researchers found low patient comprehension rates.[72]

Rule # 40   Informed consent must be obtained and documented prior to all procedures.

Before a patient agrees to a procedure, they need to know what the procedure involves, including all of the risks and possible outcomes. A patient can only give permission to undergo a procedure if they are fully informed. Informed consent is at the heart of ethical medicine. It is also at the heart of many lawsuits.

Medical students need to learn how to obtain informed consent properly. However, the attending or resident physician should ideally obtain informed consent. Sherman defines informed consent as the "process by which a physician and patient discuss the possibility of the patient deciding to consent to a proposed preventive or therapeutic intervention. The outcome of this process is the patient's decision to receive or forego treatment."[73]

Some physicians delegate this responsibility to other staff members, including nurses. This is not optimal, and some groups consider it wrong. You won't know whether the consent was obtained adequately. You also need to be present for the patient, and be seen as having the time to address and answer any concerns.

You cannot obtain informed consent for a procedure unless you, yourself, have complete knowledge of the risks, benefits, and alternatives of the procedure. You also must be able to answer correctly any questions about that procedure. You must read, ask questions, and be thoroughly educated yourself before you can properly obtain informed consent.

Once consent is obtained, it needs to be well-documented in the patient chart. The documentation should be clear and thorough, including all risks and complications of the procedure discussed with the patient. Consent for the procedure should be signed and dated by the patient, as well as witnessed properly, before being placed in the chart.

Did you know...

In one study, researchers asked first-year surgical residents about the risks, benefits, and alternatives for five surgical procedures, including abdominal aortic aneurysm repair, total thyroidectomy, laparoscopic cholecystectomy, open inguinal hernia repair, and esophagogastrectomy. The authors found that "few residents were able to correctly list all risks, benefits, and alternatives of any of the procedures." Study participants were also asked to answer questions that patients might ask about each procedure. Less than 50% of the questions were answered correctly.[74]

Rule # 41   Family members play a crucial role in patient care. Involve them appropriately.

Physicians often underestimate the influence of family members on patient care, thus overlooking a great resource. Case Western Reserve

University School of Medicine researchers noted that in 32% of all family practice office visits, family members were present.[75] The management of chronic diseases in the outpatient setting often requires the involvement of family members to ensure compliance and successful therapy. Discharge planning and education following hospitalization also requires the input of family members. Clinical trials have shown that significant improvement can be realized in certain patient behaviors when a family member is involved in the treatment. This includes how faithfully patients keep appointments, take their medications as prescribed, and stick to the treatment plan.[76]

Tips for communicating with family members

- Include family members whenever possible when communicating with patients. There are numerous reasons to do so, not the least of which is that it demonstrates respect for the patient and those important to him. Many physicians will walk into a room, look at the patient, and never acknowledge the person who has just spent the night at the bedside. You need to introduce yourself properly and ask about them and their relationship with the patient.

- Before including any family member or loved one in a discussion, ask the patient if he would prefer that you speak to him alone.

- In a family interview, allow each family member to speak. acknowledge, legitimize, and respond to any expressed emotions.

- Avoid taking sides. Siding with a family member can affect the physician-patient relationship. Listen carefully to the family member's concern and then ask the patient to respond to the concern.

- Maintain patient confidentiality. Do not discuss diagnostic or treatment decisions with family members unless you have been given permission to do so. Remember that sensitive personal information such as sexual history or drug abuse may not be accurately conveyed to you in the presence of family members.

- For sensitive issues, an ideal time to ask these questions is during the physical exam when you are likely to be alone with the patient.

- Use what you learn from the interview to create a plan that takes into account the patient's and family's concerns.

- News of certain health conditions, such as diabetes or cancer, can be overwhelming to patients. A family member or close friend may be able to listen better and actually process what you say. They may be the ones to take notes and ask relevant questions.

- If a patient does not speak English, a family member may not be the best translator. Some family members are overwhelmed by bad news and are unable to function well. Children may not have sufficient comprehension of medical issues in order to translate well. Even adult children, particularly those raised in America, may be able to speak their native language at home, but may lack the knowledge to fully translate medical terms. In issues involving personal questions, patients may not be honest if a family member is translating. A patient may not give an accurate sexual history if their child is the translator. Hospitals do have translators available, and many subscribe to telephone translation services for those languages infrequently encountered.

- When planning lifestyle modifications, a spouse or caregiver must be involved. If you recommend a change in diet, in order to be successful the entire family must be involved. Particularly when a spouse does all the grocery shopping and cooking, such information may actually need to be directed primarily at them.

- Interventions such as smoking cessation efforts work best with the support of the family. You can involve them in the discussion and make clear to them how important they are to the patient's success.

- With some chronic diseases, family members become caregivers. The care of a patient with dementia is exhausting, emotionally and physically, and has been shown to affect the health of the caregiver. Some caregivers make Herculean efforts day after day and have no one that recognizes that fact. Do what you can by acknowledging and praising their efforts.

Rule # 42   Utilize professional interpreters.

While family members are often used as interpreters, this practice leads to potential problems. In one study, encounters between physicians and patients were videotaped when either a professional or family interpreter was required. Information transfer was found to be more accurate through a professional interpreter. Family interpreters were found to often speak "as themselves rather than rendering the words of doctor and patient into the other's language."[77]

When interpreters are required, residents may underutilize the service, even when it is readily available. In a study of IM residents at two teaching hospitals with readily available interpreter services, residents indicated that they underused professional interpreters, stating that it was "easier to get by" without doing so. Interpreters were less likely to be used when residents were constrained for time, when family members were available to fulfill the role, or when the resident had some second language communication skills.[78]

Rule # 43   The electronic health record is a technological and medical breakthrough, but it poses unique challenges in patient interactions.

It used to be that you would sit down, with your clipboard ready, and talk to a patient face to face. The electronic medical record (EMR) has changed that. It is definitely a medical breakthrough, but it has introduced different facets to physician patient communication. In a study of third year students in the ambulatory setting, many felt that the EMR affected their ability to establish rapport with patients, and nearly half reported that its use led them to spend less time looking at the patients.[79] Only 21% felt that patients liked them using it.

Researchers at the University of Texas Southwestern Medical School have studied ways to improve EMR-specific communication skills.[80] These involve introducing yourself before turning to the computer, and moving closer to the patient so that they can read the screen. Other strategies involve the patient further, by showing them vital signs, flow-sheets or health trends on the computer screen.

Rule # 44   You cannot take it personally.

Your patients are generally good people. Good people, when faced with the stress of illness, sometimes act in uncharacteristic ways.

Patients lash out at their doctors for many reasons. Being sick enough to be hospitalized is frightening for most people. Patients commonly feel afraid, confused, and powerless. They feel they have no control over what's happening to them. Physical factors, such as acute or chronic pain, may play a role. The realities of living with a life-threatening illness, or dealing with bad news that impacts prognosis or risk of disability, are all severe stressors.

Sometimes the healthcare system itself can be the cause, as in long waiting times for a test, or an intrusive procedure, or denied insurance claims. At other times, the patient-physician relationship will cause a patient to lash out, as when a physician is perceived as arrogant or disrespectful.[81] Understand that there may be a number of factors at play when a patient lashes out at you, and in most cases you should not take it personally.

Rule # 45   You will encounter angry patients. Know what to do.

- Understand why the patient is angry. Generally, patients become angry when we fail to meet their expectations.

- Listen carefully to the patient. Too often, in our hurry to fix the problem, we fail to listen properly.

- Rather than standing over the patient or by the door, ask the patient if you can sit down. Do not sit down on the patient's bed.

- Speak in a normal tone of voice

- Begin by saying, "Mr. Woods, the nurse informed me that you have some concerns regarding your care. Could you fill me in,..?"

- Let the patient speak without interrupting. Avoid the tendency to interrupt the patient to ask a question or offer an explanation. Instead, let the patient speak until he has finished.

- Avoid angry or defensive responses, which only tend to worsen the situation.

- After the patient is finished, summarize what you have heard to make sure you have understood properly. "So Mr. Woods, as I understand it, you expected ..."

- After the patient has expressed his concern, ask him how he feels about the situation. Then acknowledge that feeling. "I can understand how that would make you feel ..."

- Determine what will make the patient feel better. "What can I do to make you feel better about this now?"

- Apologize if appropriate

- Finish your conversation by asking the patient if he is satisfied with your understanding of the situation and your plan to address his concern

---

Tip # 13

Hospitalized patients often feel as if they have no control. This can be extremely distressing. You can diminish this sense by keeping your patients well informed of what will happen next.

Did you know ...

In a survey of second-year medical students at the Kansas University School of Medicine, researchers asked students to report personal characteristics of patients that might evoke a negative personal reaction, interfering with their ability to provide quality clinical care.[82] Comments included:

"Patients who are violent or mean to staff"
"People who treat me with animosity"
"Vulgar, disrespectful, antagonistic patients"
"Drug/alcohol/substance abusers who have horrible, rude, or unpleasant attitudes"
"Chronic complainers who never seem to appreciate care"
"People who don't take responsibility for their actions (everything is everyone else's fault)"

This study raised concerns that students may lose objectivity when caring for patients with certain personal characteristics.

Rule # 46 Know what to do if the angry patient becomes aggressive.

The measures we describe are effective in defusing most situations in which patients express anger. However, despite the use of effective techniques, you won't be able to calm down some patients. In some cases, patients are prone to aggression because of underlying illness, such as alcohol or drug abuse, withdrawal, delirium, or psychiatric conditions such as schizophrenia or bipolar disorder. If a patient's aggression increases or agitation escalates, seek immediate help from others, including hospital security if necessary. Your first priority is your own safety. Patient-initiated assault against health care workers does occur and can affect any member of the team, including students. In a recent study of students at a North American medical school six months following the start of clerkships, six students reported experiencing physical assaults.[83]

Rule # 47   Caretaker fatigue is a real hazard.

During my surgery core clerkship, we were rounding with the team in the county hospital. The patient was the mother of an acquaintance. She was a middle-aged, well-spoken, dignified woman who had just undergone resection of colon cancer. She was in pain, feeling nauseous, and looked frail and uncomfortable. The three burly surgery residents proceeded to stand over her and harangue her to get out of her chair and start walking "because it's for your own good and you can't just sit there." [The dammit was understood from the tone of their voice.]

The sleep deprivation, the angry patients, the toxic colleagues, the constant vigilance due to so many potential mistakes: all are real aspects of our profession. In some cases, these severe stressors can impact students', residents', and clinicians' sense of empathy.

Empathy is one of the most important professional traits. Empathy as it relates to patient care is defined as "a cognitive attribute, which involves an understanding of the inner experiences and perspectives of the patient as a separate individual, combined with a capability to communicate this understanding to the patient."[84]

Did you know ...

In telephone interviews with 192 patients cared for at the Mayo Clinic, researchers identified seven ideal physician behaviors.[85] Patients felt that the ideal physician is confident, humane, empathetic, personal, respectful, forthright, and thorough. Note that technical skills were not one of the seven ideal behaviors. The authors suggested that patients may be inclined to assume that a physician is competent.

You would assume that empathy would grow during medical school. Studies have shown that in fact the opposite occurs for many students, and that as students progress through their medical education, there is frequently a decline in empathy. Educators generally believe that this largely occurs in the clinical years of medical school. Decline in empathy is thought to be, in part, a result of the pressures and stressors of the medical school experience.[86]

Be aware that a decline in empathy can occur during medical school, and look for it and guard against it in yourself. There are no evidence-based guidelines that we can reference on further measures to prevent this, but general guidelines on dealing with stress can help. There are entire books on how to deal with stress and anxiety, and there are a number of effective measures that you can take. Maintain social connections. Utilize physical activity to decrease stress. Take care of your own health. Maintain your own sense of well-being. In short, do whatever it takes so that your stress does not impact the type of care that you provide. The next rule highlights how easy it is for stress to impact professionalism.

Rule # 48   Your own sense of well-being can impact the patient care you provide.

The stressors of patient care are varied and can be severe. This absolutely affects our sense of well-being. In a recent study, residents described well-being "as a balance among multiple parts of their personal and professional lives: family, friends, physical health, mental health, spiritual health, financial security, and professional satisfaction."[87]

When residents have a better sense of well-being, they report having a greater capacity to relate to patients and interact with colleagues. In fact, research has suggested that enhanced personal well-being may lead physicians to deliver more compassionate care to their patients.[88, 89, 90] However, physicians often don't recognize the relationship between personal well-being and care given to patients. In one survey, residents were asked to list attributes associated with professionalism. Among the 28 reported characteristics, "balance between personal and professional life" was listed last among the group.[91]

In one study, interviews with residents highlighted specific areas in which diminished well-being impacted professionalism.

Domain	Effect on professionalism
Relationships with patients	"If you are not feeling well and completely stressed out, you don't have all the tools to deal with patients the way you should…If you are down yourself, it's difficult to give someone else strength, or help somebody to cope…"
Interactions with colleagues	"Somehow my tolerance for [my intern's] mistakes was just much, much lower…And I was very quick to point out things she missed and in a quite harsh way. I feel bad about it because when I kind of lose my balance and don't feel that well, then I just lose perception of how other people feel…"
Performance in patient care	"I think when I'm feeling good and I'm not so stressed out…I'm probably more likely to take the time to get a thorough history, do a more thorough exam, more likely to call the primary care provider, and do those things that are extra but really should be part of what you're always doing."

From Ratanawongsa N, Wright S, Carrese J. Well-being in residency: effects on relationships with patients, interactions with colleagues, performance, and motivation. *Patient Educ* Couns 2008; 72(2): 194-200.

References

[1]Ring D, Herndon J, Meyer G. Case records of The Massachusetts General Hospital: Case 34-2010: a 65-year-old woman with an incorrect operation on the left hand. *N Engl J Med* 2010; 363(20): 1950-7.

[2]Starfield B. Is US health really the best in the world? *JAMA* 2000; 284: 483-5.

[3]Institute of Medicine. *To Err is Human: Building a Safer Health System.* Washington, DC: National Academy Press; 2000.

[4]Peabody F. The care of the patient. *JAMA* 1927; 88: 877-82.

[5]Blendon R, DesRoches C, Brodie M, Benson J, Rosen A, Schneider E, Altman D, Zapert K, Hermann M, Steffenson A. Views of practicing physicians and the public on medical errors. *New Engl J Med* 2002; 347(24): 1933-40.

[6]Klein R. *Surviving your doctors: why the medical system is dangerous to your health and how to get through it alive.* Lanham, Maryland: Rowman and Littlefield Publishers; 2010.

[7]Pau A, Morgan J, Terlingo A. Drug allergy documentation by physicians, nurses, and medical students. *Am J Hosp Pharm* 1989; 46(3): 570-3.

[8]Freyer F. Medical students get lesson in safety. *The Providence Journal*. http://www.projo.com/health/content/PATIENT_SAFETY_COURSE_05-10-10_KEIDSPU_v12.3d1634e.html. Published May 10, 2010. Accessed January 31, 2011.

[9]Madigosky W, Headrick L, Nelson K, et al. Changing and sustaining medical students' knowledge, skills, and attitudes about patient safety and medical fallibility. *Acad Med* 2006; 81: 94-101.

[10]Alper E, Rosenberg E, O'Brien K, Fischer M, Durning S. Patient safety education at U.S. and Canadian medical schools: results from the 2006 Clerkship Directors in Internal Medicine survey. *Acad Med* 2009; 84(12): 1672-6.

[11]Atul Gawande. *Complications: A surgeon's notes on an imperfect science*. New York; Picador: 2002.

[12]Seiden S, Galvan C, Lamm R. Role of medical students in preventing patient harm and enhancing patient safety. *Qual Saf Health Care* 2006; 15(4): 272-6.

[13]Martinello R, Jones L, Topal J. Correlation between healthcare workers' knowledge of influenza vaccine and vaccine receipt. *Infect Control Hosp Epidemiol* 2003; 24(11): 845-7.

[14]Amin A, Stemkowski S, Lin J, Yang G. Thromboprophylaxis rates in US medical centers: success or failure. *J Thromb Haemost* 2007; 5(8): 1610-6.

[15]Sehgal N, Wachter R. Identification of inpatient DNR status: a safety hazard begging for standardization. *J Hosp Med* 2007; 2(6): 366-71.

[16]Prevention Plus, Home of the Braden Scale. http://www.bradenscale.com/products.htm. Accessed January 23, 2011.

[17]Lingard L, Espin S, Whyte S, Regehr G, Baker G, Reznick R, Bohnen J, Orser B, Doran D, Grober E. Communication failures in the operating room: an observational classification of recurrent types and effects. *Qual Saf Health Care* 2004; 13: 330-4.

[18]Fernandez H, Callahan K, Likourezos A, Leipzig R. House staff member awareness of older inpatients' risks for hazards of hospitalization. *Arch Intern Med* 2008; 168(4): 390-6.

[19]Saint S, Wiese J, Amory J, Bernstein M, Patel U, Zemencuk J, Bernstein S, Lipsky B, Hofer T. Are physicians aware of which of their patients have indwelling urinary catheters? *Am J Med* 2000; 109(6): 476-80.

[20]Cohen E. *The empowered patient*. New York: Ballantine Books; 2010.

[21]Institute for Healthcare Improvement. *How-to guide: improving hand hygiene*. http://www.ihi.org/IHI/Topics/CriticalCare/IntensiveCare/Tools/HowtoGuideImprovingHandHygiene.htm. Accessed January 30, 2011.

[22]Pittet D. Improving adherence to hand hygiene practice: a multidisciplinary approach. *Emerg Infect Dis* 2001; 7(2): 234-40.

[23]Medicine's dirty little secret: hospitals promote doctors to wash their hands. *Washington Post*. September 30, 1997.

[24]Lankford M, Zembower T, Trick W, Hacek D, Noskin G, Peterson L. Influence of role models and hospital design on the hand hygiene of healthcare workers. *Emerg Infect Dis* 2003; 9(2): 217-23.

[25]Treakle A, Thom K, Furuno J, Strauss S, Harris A, Perencevich E. Bacterial contamination of health care workers' white coats. *Am J Infect Control* 2009; 37(2); 101-5.

[26]Loh W, Ng V, Holton J. Bacterial flora on the white coats of medical students. *J Hosp Infect* 2000; 45(1): 65-8.

[27]Nurkin S. Is the clinician's necktie a potential fomite for hospital acquired infection? Presented at the 104th General Meeting of the American Society for Microbiology in New Orleans, May 23-27, 2004.

[28]Ditchburn J. Should doctors wear ties? *J Hosp Infect* 2006; 63(2): 227-8.

[29]The Lancet. The traditional white coat: goodbye, or au revoir? *Lancet* 2007; 370: 1102.

[30]AMA Resolution 720. http://www.ama-assn.org/ama1/pub/upload/mm/475/ refcomg.pdf. Accessed January 26, 2011.

[31]Singh D, Kaur H, Gardner W, et al. Bacterial contamination of hospital pagers. *Infect Control Hosp Epidemiol* 2002; 23: 274–6.

[32]Devine J, Cooke R, Wright E. Is methicillin-resistant *Staphylococcus aureus* (MRSA) contamination of ward-based computer terminals a surrogate marker for nosocomial MRSA transmission and handwashing compliance? *J Hosp Infect.* 2001; 48: 72–5.

[33]Gupta A, Della-Latta P, Todd B, San Gabriel P, Haas J, Wu F, Rubenstein D, Saiman L. Outbreak of extended-spectrum beta-lactamase-producing *Klebsiella pneumoniae* in a neonatal intensive care unit linked to artificial nails. *Infect control Hosp Epidemiol* 2004; 25(3): 210-5.

[34]Melenhorst W, Poos H, Meesen N. Medical students need more education on hygiene behavior. *Am J Infect Control* 2009; 37(10): 868-9.

[35]Marinella M. Pierson C, Chenoweth C. The stethoscope. A potential source of nosocomial infection? *Arch Intern Med* 1997; 157(7): 786-90.

[36]Parmar R, Valvi C, Sira P, et al. A prospective, randomized, double-blind study of comparative efficacy of immediate versus daily cleaning of stethoscope using 66% ethyl alcohol. *Indian J Med Sci* 2004; 58: 423-30.

[37]Schroeder A, Schroeder M, D'Amico F. What's growing on your stethoscope? (And what you can do about it). *J Fam Pract* 2009; 58(8): 404-9.

[38]Wilkes M, Milgrom E, Hoffman J. Towards more empathic medical students: a medical student hospitalization experience. *Med Educ* 2002; 36: 528-33.

[39]Rutter D, Maguire G. History-taking for medical students. *Lancet* 1976; 2 (7985): 558-60.

[40]LSU Law Center's Medical and Public Health Law Site. http:// biotech.law.lsu.edu/books/lbb/x477.htm. Accessed January 5, 2011.

[41]Silver-Isenstadt A, Ubel P. Erosion in medical students' attitudes about telling patients they are students. *J Gen Intern Med* 1999; 14(8): 481-7.

[42]Santen S, Hemphill R, Spanier C, Fletcher N. "Sorry, it's my first time!" Will patients consent to medical students learning procedures? *Med Educ* 2005; 39(4): 365-9.

[43]Makoul G, Zick M, Green M. An evidence-based perspective on greetings in medical encounters. *Arch Intern Med* 2007; 167 (11): 1172-6.

[44]UND Medical School students taught professionalism from day one. *Grand Forks Herald*; August 5, 2005. http://www.redorbit.com/news/education/198856/und_medical_school_students_taught_professionalism_from_day_one/. Accessed January 12, 2011.

[45]Rehman S, Nietert P, Cope D, Kikpatrick A. What to wear today? Effect of doctor's attire on the trust and confidence of patients. *Am J Med* 2005; 118: 1279-85.

[46]Peabody F. The care of the patient. *JAMA* 1927; 88: 877-82.

[47]American Medical Association's Principles of Medical Ethics. http://www.ama-assn.org/ama/pub/physician-resources/medical-ethics/code-medical-ethics/principles-medical-ethics.shtml. Accessed January 22, 2011.

[48]Robinson G, Aldington S, Beasley R. From medical student to junior doctor: rules of confidentiality. StudentBMJ 2006; 14: 377-9. http://archive.student.bmj.com/issues/06/10/careers/377.php. Accessed January 27, 2011.

[49]Ubel P, Zell M, Miller D, Fischer G, Peters-Stefani D, Arnold R. Elevator talk: observational study of inappropriate comments in a public space. *Am J Med* 1995; 99(2): 190-4.

[50]Mlinek E, Pierce J. Confidentiality and privacy breaches in a university hospital emergency department. *Acad Emerg Med* 1997; 4(12): 1142-6.

[51]Jones K. Prying in Britney Spears' medical records may cost employees' jobs. *Information Week*. March 17, 2008. http://www.informationweek.com/news/global-cio/compliance/showArticle.jhtml?articleID=206904141. Accessed January 30, 2011.

[52]Chretien KC, Greysen S, Chretien J, Kind T. Online posting of unprofessional content by medical students. *JAMA* 2009; 302 (12): 1309-15.

[53]McNamara D. Awareness of top causes of lawsuits can reduce risk. *Hospitalist News*. April 2009; 12.

[54]Beckman H, Markakis K, Suchman A, Frankel R. The doctor-patient relationship and malpractice. *Arch Intern Med* 1994; 154(12): 1365-70.

[55]Gladwell M. *Blink*. New York; Little Brown and Company: 2005.

[56]Levinson W, Roter D, Mullooly J, Dull V, Frankel R. Physician-patient communication. The relationship with malpractice claims among primary care physicians and surgeons. *JAMA* 1997; 277(7): 553-9.

[57]Ambady N, Laplante D, Nguyen T, Rosenthal R, Chaumeton N, Levinson W. Surgeons' tone of voice: a clue to malpractice history. *Surgery* 2002; 132(1): 5-9.

[58]Rice B. Can you be forced to testify against a colleague? *Med Econ* 2004; 81: 28.

[59]American Academy on Communication in Healthcare. http://www.aachonline.org/. Accessed January 23, 2011.

[60]Wiener S, Nathanson M. Physical examination. Frequently observed errors. *JAMA* 1976; 236: 852-5.

[61]Beckman H, Frankel R. The effect of physician behavior on the collection of data. *Ann Intern Med* 1984; 101(5): 692-6.

[62]Marvel M, Epstein R. Flowers K, Beckman H. Soliciting the patient's agenda: have we improved? *JAMA* 1999; 281(3): 283-7.

[63]Bayer-Fetzer Conference. Essential elements of communication in medical encounters: the Kalamazoo Consensus Statement. *Acad Med* 2001; 76: 390-3.

[64]Beck R, Daughtridge R, Sloane P. Physician-patient communication in the primary care office: a systematic review. *JABFP* 2002; 15(1): 25-38.

[65]Rutter D, Maguire G. History-taking for medical students. *Lancet* 1976; 2(7985): 558-60.

[66]Waitzkin H. Doctor-patient communication: clinical implications of social scientific research. *JAMA* 1984; 252(17): 2441-6.

[67]Waitzkin H. Information giving in medical care. *Journal of Health and Social Behavior* 1985; 26(2): 81-101.

[68]Tarn D, Heritage J, Paterniti D, Hays R, Kravitz R, Wenger N. Physician communication when prescribing new medications. *Arch Intern Med* 2006; 166: 1855-62.

[69]O'Leary K, Kulkarni N, Landler M, Jeon J, Hahn K, Englert K, Williams M. Hospitalized patients' understanding of their plan of care. *Mayo Clin Proc* 2010; 85(1): 47-52.

[70]Makaryus A, Friedman E. Patients' understanding of their treatment plans and diagnosis at discharge. *Mayo Clin Proc* 2005; 80(8): 991-4.

[71]Deuster L, Christopher S, Donovan J, Farrell M. A method to quantify residents' jargon use during counseling of standardized patients about cancer screening. *J Gen Intern Med* 2008; 23(12): 1947-52.

[72]Castro C, Wilson C, Wang F, Schillinger D. Babel babble: physicians' use of unclarified medical jargon with patients. *Am J Health* Behav 2007; 31 Suppl 1: S85-95.

[73]Sherman H, McGaghie W, Unti S, Thomas J. Teaching pediatric residents how to obtain informed consent. *Acad Med* 2005; 80(10 Suppl): S10-13.

[74]Angelos P, DaRosa D, Bentram D, Sherman H. Residents seeking informed consent: are they adequately knowledgeable? *Curr Surg* 2002; 59(1): 115-8.

[75]Medalie J, Zyzanski S, Langa D, Stange K. The family in family practice: Is it a reality? *J Fam Pract* 1988; 46(5): 390-6.

[76]Levine D. Communicating with chronic disease patients. Comment: A Newsletter from the Miles Council for Physician-Patient communication, 1989, 3(3), 1.

[77]Rosenberg E, Seller R, Leanza Y. Through interpreters' eyes: comparing roles of professional and family interpreters. *Patient Educ Couns* 2008; 70(1): 87-93.

[78]Diamond L, Schenker Y, Curry L, Bradley E, Fernandez A. Getting by: underuse of interpreters by resident physicians. *J Gen Intern Med* 2009; 24(2): 256-62.

[79]Rouf E, Chumley H, Dobbie A. Electronic health records in outpatient clinics: perspectives of third year medical students. *BMC Medical Education* 2008; 8: 13.

[80]Morrow J, Dobbie A, Jenkins C, Long R, Mihalic A, Wagner J. First-year medical students can demonstrate EHR-specific communication skills: a control-group study. *Fam Med* 2009; 41(1): 28-33.

[81]Lown B. Difficult conversations: anger in the clinician-patient/family relationship. *Southern Medical Journal* 2007; 100(1): 34-9.

[82]Walling A, Montello M, Moser S, Menikoff J, Brink M. Which patients are most challenging for second-year medical students? *Fam Med* 2004; 36(10): 710-4.

[83]Waddell A, Katz M, Lofchy J, Bradley J. A pilot survey of patient-initiated assaults on medical students during clinical clerkships. *Acad Psychiatry* 2005; 29(4): 350-3.

[84]Hojat M, Mangione S, Nasca T, Rattner S, Erdmann J, Gonnella J, Magee M. An empirical study of decline in empathy in medical school. *Med Educ* 2004; 38(9): 934-41.

[85]Benadapudi N, Berry L, Frey K, Parish J, Rayburn W. Patients' perspectives on ideal physician behaviors. *Mayo Clin Proc* 2006; 81(3): 338-44.

[86]Newton B, Barber L, Clardy J, Cleveland E, O'Sullivan. Is there hardening of the heart during medical school? *Acad Med* 2008; 83(3): 244-9.

[87]Ratanawongsa N, Wright S, Carrese J. Well-being in residency: effects on relationships with patients, interactions with colleagues, performance, and motivation. *Patient Educ* Couns 2008; 72(2): 194-200.

[88]Shanafelt T, Sloan J, Habermann T. The well-being of physicians. *Am J Med* 2003; 114: 513-9.

[89]Shanafelt T, West C, Zhao X, Novotny P, Kolars J, Habermann T, Sloan J. Relationship between increased personal well-being and enhanced empathy among internal medicine residents. *J Gen Intern Med* 2005; 559-64.

[90]Thomas M, Dyrbye L, Huntington J, Lawson K, Novotny P, Sloan J, Shanafelt T. How do distress and well-being relate to medical student empathy? A multicenter study. *J Gen Intern Med* 2007; 22: 177-83.

[91]Brownell A, Cote L. Senior residents' views on the meaning of professionalism and how they learn about it. *Acad Med* 2001; 76: 734-7.

Chapter 9

The New Rotation

"The clinical years, especially the third year, are in some ways a very harsh experience. It is frightening to feel you are ignorant in a setting where sick people are depending on you for care… You worry about making a mistake. You worry about hurting someone. On a different level, you worry about making a fool of yourself, about looking stupid on rounds."[1]

— From *A not entirely benign procedure: four years a medical student* by Perri Klass MD

Starting clinical rotations is very challenging. The skill set that you developed in order to be a successful basic science student is not the same one you'll need during clerkships. The basic science and clinical years of medical school are fundamentally different.

The challenges of moving from clerkship to clerkship are just as significant. Transitioning to a new team, a new environment, and a completely different field of medicine is a challenge for even the most intelligent and competent student. Issues include the basic, such as what resources to bring and how to learn proper charting. They range to the complex, including how to ascertain responsibilities and how to prioritize and accomplish numerous tasks. These challenges are significant, and many medical students don't feel prepared. Formal education in many of the areas required for clerkship success may be brief. In one study at a large urban medical school, curricular time spent on clinical skills during the first two years of medical school was documented. A total of 10 hours was spent learning how to write a progress note, 12 hours on how to do an oral case presentation, and five hours on generating a differential diagnosis and assessment.[2]

In this chapter, we present a number of practical suggestions on how to adapt and succeed in a new clerkship. You'll learn the basics of what resources to bring, and how to learn the chart and the electronic medical record. You'll learn the questions that you need to ask of your intern, resident, and attending at the start of every rotation to ascertain expectations and responsibilities. You'll also learn the practical, such as methods to organize vast amounts of patient data. In interviews conducted with 30 program directors, poor organizational skills were found to be a common struggle of interns. "We have been encountering more residents who have a difficult time multitasking…" stated one program director.[3] You'll learn other practical measures, including how to set up to a to-do list and how to prioritize the many patient care tasks you'll be expected to complete daily.

Key differences between the basic sciences and clinical years of medical school	
Basic sciences	**Clerkships**
Day starts at 8 AM or later	Day often well under way by 8 AM
Classes usually over by 5 PM	Day rarely ends at 5 PM
Flexible schedule	Structured schedule
Considerable control over time	Cede control over your time to others
Frequent breaks during the day	Few breaks during the day
Weekends always free	Weekend work responsibilities
Sleeping through the night	Working through the night (on call)
Few surprises during the day	Expect the unexpected
Expectations clear	Expectations often unclear
Intellectual challenge	People challenge (team members, patients)
Same routine from course to course (attending lecture, reading, studying, taking exam)	Varying routine from clerkship to clerkship, requiring the ability to adapt
Hearing about patients	Taking care of patients
Primary focus on learning and acquiring knowledge	Expected to apply this knowledge to patients
Lots of time to read and study	Lack of time to read and study
Professors	Supervisors (interns, residents, attendings)
Individual effort	Team effort
Less initiative required	Lots of initiative required
Can do it your way	Must do it the team's way
Objective grading (tests)	Subjective grading (evaluations)

Rule # 49   Arrive with the necessary electronic resources

The use of handheld computers, or personal digital assistants (PDAs), has exploded in recent years among medical students and other health-care professionals. Resources previously available only in print are now widely available in electronic formats. In a recent review of the psublished literature, up to 70% of medical trainees were found to use handhelds.[4] The most popular applications include medical calculators, electronic textbooks, drug databases, and patient-tracking software. Some commonly used applications are listed in the table on the following page.

Rule # 50   Arrive with the necessary books.

Have the books that you need in your hands before the rotation starts. Your classmates can tell you which books the clerkship requires or recommends. This information can also be found in the clerkship orientation material, which some rotations send to students before the start of the rotation or post online.

Your classmates, residents, or attending may tell you about other helpful books. Take a look at these books; if the information in the book fits well with the way you process information, then consider buying it. Many of these books are also available at the medical school or hospital library, or can be borrowed from a classmate.

Tip # 14

Publishers have increasingly made medical textbooks available electronically, and these resources are often available in medical school and hospital libraries. However, many students don't realize that they're available. For those who are aware, using these resources to answer patient care questions can still pose a challenge. Kathryn Skhal, Clinical Education Librarian at the University of Iowa School of Medicine Hardin Library, wrote that "medical student library education is often limited to the preclinical curriculum, but a new skill set is needed for the clinical environment. Searching must be focused, quick, and efficient to be feasible in a busy patient care setting."[5] If a library orientation isn't part of your clerkship, make it a point to visit the library to learn about the resources available.

Personal Digital Assistant Applications Commonly Used by Medical Trainees[1]

Application	Website
Calculators	
ACS risk	http://www.statcoder.com
Archimedes calculator	http://www.skyscape.com
Framingham calculator	http://www.statcoder.com
MedCalc	http://www.medcalc.be
MedMath	http://www.palmgear.com
MentSTAT	http://goldenratiodesign.com
Pneumonia Severity Index calculator	http://pda.ahrq.gov/clinic/psi/psi.htm
PregCalc	http://www.pilotzone.com/palm/previw/34754.html
STAT cardiac clearance	http://www.statcoder.com
STAT cholesterol	http://www.statcoder.com
TIMI risk calculator	http://criticalpathways.org.cnchost.com
Clinical Guidelines	
American Academy of Dermatology	http://aad.org/forms/mobile/clinicalguidelines/
American Academy of Neurology	http://www.aan.com/go/practice/technology/mobile
American Academy of Ophthalmology	http://www.apprisor.com
American Association for the Study of Liver Diseases	http://www.apprisor.com
American College of Cardiology	http://www.cardiosource.org
American College of Chest Physicians	http://www.apprisor.com
American College of Physicians	http://www.acponline.org
American Diabetes Association	http://professional.diabetes.org/CPR_search.aspx
Infectious Disease Society of America	http://www.idsociety.org/Content.aspx?id=16201
U.S. Preventive Services Task Force	http://epss.ahrq.gov/PDA/index.jsp
Electronic medical textbooks	
AccessMedicine	http://www.accessmedicine.com
eMedicine	http://www.emedicine.medscape.com
Five-minute Clinical Consults	http://www.skyscape.com
Cecil's	http://www.us.elsevierhealth.com/Medicine
Ferri's Clinical Advisor	http://www.us.elsevierhealth.com/Medicine
Handheldmed	http://www.handheldmed.com
Harrison's	http://www.skyscape.com
MD Consult	http://www.mdconsult.com
Merck Medicus	http://www.merckmedicus.com
STATRef	http://www.statref.com
Washington Manual	http://www.skyscape.com

Medication references	
A2zDrugs	http://www.skyscape.com
ABX guide	http://hopkins-abxguide.org
AHFS Drug Information	http://www.skyscape.com
Clinical Pharmacology OnHand	http://www.clinicalpharmacologyonhand.com
DrDrugs	http://www.skyscape.com
Epocrates	http://www.epocrates.com
Facts & Comparisons	http://www.factsandcomparisons.com
Immunizations	http://www.immunizationed.org
Internet Drug Reference	http://rxlist.com
Lexi-Comp ON-HAND	http://www.lexi.com
Medscape Mobile	http://www.medscape.com
Mobile Micromedex	http://www.micromedex.com
MobilePDR	http://www.pdr.net
Tarascon Pocket Pharmacopoeia	http://www.tarascon.com
Patient-Tracker	
Patient tracker	http://www.handheldmed.com
Patient keeper	http://patientkeeper.com
Pocket chart	http://gemedicalsystems.com

Partially adapted and expanded from Kho A, Henderson L, Dressler D, Kripalani S. Use of handheld computers in medical education. A systematic review. *J Gen Intern Med* 2006; 21(5): 531-7.

Rule # 51   Learn the chart.

The medical chart is the main avenue of communication between all healthcare professionals. It doesn't matter if you've ordered a stat consult from a subspecialty service; you probably won't be getting a phone call from the team. It is understood that they will communicate their findings to you via the chart. Charts may be written or electronic; their physical location and some specifics may vary from hospital to hospital. However, all charts are generally divided into the following areas:

• Orders
• Admission notes
• Progress notes
• Consultant notes
• Nursing notes
• Medication list
• Lab tests
• Radiology reports

On the first day of the rotation, spend the time to become completely knowledgeable about all components of the chart. Every morning, you will rely on the chart as well as the patient to update you on your patient's hospital course. It will help answer the question, "What happened to my patient while I was away from the hospital?" During the workday, you will turn to the chart to see what nurses, therapists, consultants, and other professionals have written or recommended.

Rule # 52   Learn the electronic chart.

> ### Did you know...
>
> In an effort to improve quality of care, numerous organizations, including the Institute of Medicine, have urged for widespread adoption and implementation of electronic medical records. Despite this, recent surveys of ambulatory care practices have shown that less than a quarter of such practices have implemented electronic medical records. In a 2006 survey of internal medicine clerkship directors at U.S. and Canadian academic medical centers, 58% reported use of an electronic medical record in the ambulatory setting.[6]

U.S. medical schools often have several affiliated hospitals and clinics through which students rotate. These practice settings often have their own electronic health record (EHR), each of which has its own idiosyncrasies. Students must learn the features of each of these different systems. At the start of a rotation, an orientation to the EHR is usually held for new students. Attend all such orientations. The medical record is critical to outstanding patient care, and you must be able to navigate it accurately and quickly.

    Dr. Jain, a faculty member at the Lehigh Valley Hospital, writes that "faculty and office staff should orient residents and students to each section of the patient chart in detail."[7] While important, this doesn't always happen, and therefore students must sometimes take the initiative. If necessary, enlist someone to go over the chart with you. If possible, spend extra time on the first day familiarizing yourself with the chart and each of its components.

Rule # 53   Know where to go and where to find things.

Learning the logistics of how things work is a common struggle for students. One student put it well: "The first week there were so many things that I was expected to know right off the bat that I just didn't feel comfortable with yet and a big thing was just getting oriented to the system, learning how documentation goes, how to read the electronic medical record, what different abbreviations mean, just how things run on the ward. So just some background things like that were difficult to get used to."[8]

    To reach a comfort level which allows you to do your best work, you must become familiar with the layout of the hospital and ward in which you will be working. If a tour of the hospital is offered as part of the orientation, then take advantage of it. If no such tour is offered, ask your resident or intern to give you one. If they are too busy, take yourself on a tour. Start with your ward. Locate:

- Supply rooms
- Dirty/clean utility rooms
- Staff bathroom

- Nursing conference room
- Patient rooms. Determine how patient rooms are numbered.

Then take a tour of the rest of the hospital. Locate:

- Lecture halls/rooms
- Call room
- Medical records
- Lab
- Radiology department, including the radiology file room where patient films/studies are kept
- Emergency room
- Library
- Vending machines
- Cafeteria
- Gift shop
- Resident/student lounge

Rule # 54   Meet with the resident and intern.

Obviously you'll be meeting your resident and intern on a new rotation, typically after orientation. However, just meeting them is insufficient. You should have a meeting to discuss the rules of the rotation, your responsibilities, and their expectations of you. In many cases, such a meeting won't occur unless you initiate it. When there's a lull in the action, ask the intern or resident if you can meet to discuss your upcoming month together. While you can meet with them together, we recommend separate meetings because their expectations will differ. Your goal is to meet and hopefully exceed the expectations of each and every team member.

    Some residents and interns understand the importance of this meeting and will take the time to fill you in on the specifics of the rotation. Others don't recognize the value of this meeting and have only brief discussions that lack structure and are short on useful specifics. Students may leave these meetings unclear about their work responsibilities. To ensure that you leave this meeting with the information you need, have a list of questions ready.

Questions to ask your resident and at your initial meeting

- Can you go over a typical day with me?
  - What time should I arrive in the morning?
  - What time do work rounds begin?
  - Where do we meet for work rounds?
  - What time are attending rounds? Where do they take place?
  - Do we have afternoon rounds? When and where do we meet?
  - How does this schedule differ on a weekend day?
- What is our call schedule?
- What are my responsibilities on call?
- What procedures do you expect me to perform?
- How would you like me to present patients during work rounds?
- Can you go over your preferences regarding the writing of the daily progress note?
- Is there a particular time of the day the progress note needs to be written by?
- Can you show me the paperwork I need to be familiar with (progress notes, lab request forms, x-ray request forms, consult requisitions, other)?
- Can you provide me with a list of important phone numbers (lab, x-ray, pharmacy, other)?
- Where can I safely keep my bag and other personal items?
- Where do you recommend that I work?

You may be overwhelmed by the amount of information you receive about ward logistics, the daily and weekly schedule, rules, and responsibilities. Take notes. Learn as much as you can about how things operate so that you can get off to a good start.

Tip # 14

Although you may want to know when your work day ends, take care in how you ask. You don't want to come across as someone who won't be working hard. You can, though, ask the resident or intern to describe a typical day's schedule. This will provide some idea of when the day will end.

Rule # 55   Meet with your attending physician.

Meeting with the attending physician some time during the first few days of a new rotation is a must. You need to learn about his expectations of you as a student. These expectations will differ from that of the intern and resident.

Ideally, this meeting should take place on the first day of the rotation. ~~s~~ with residents, not all attendings make it a point to have this meeting. If the attending doesn't initiate the meeting, simply approach him and ask, "Dr. Nguyen, do you have some time today to meet with me to discuss our upcoming month together?" Don't be afraid to initiate this meeting. I have yet to meet an attending who wouldn't be receptive to this approach.

If you're fortunate, your attending will spell everything out for you. More often, though, the meeting will be short on specifics. Have a plan in place to obtain the necessary information. Basically, you should ascertain what the attending considers to be the qualities of an ideal student. Listen for answers to the following questions:

- What are the attending physician's expectations for me as a student?
- What does the attending view as my clinical responsibilities?
- How will the attending evaluate my performance?
- How would the attending like me to present patients?
- Does the attending want me to turn in patient write-ups? If so, does he have any preferences regarding the write-up?

If some key information is lacking, ask. Too often, students don't ask questions because they don't want to seem ignorant. However, you want to know as much as possible up front, rather than being informed as problems arise.

Tip # 15

Make it clear that you want to learn as much as possible on this clerkship, that you wish to improve, and that you are open to suggestions.

Did you know...

Failure to meet with the attending may leave you feeling confused about the rotation and the attending's expectations of you as a student. This can impact your performance in a negative manner. In focus group sessions with over 80 students, researchers found that understanding roles, responsibilities, and others' expectations in clinical settings was the most common transition struggle for clerkship students.[8]

Rule # 56   First impressions matter.

As in any field of social or professional interaction, first impressions are critical. When meeting your team for the first time, treat this initial meeting as you would an interview. Your objective is to establish immediate rapport and trust.

Projecting a professional, confident appearance depends on a number of factors. Enter the room confidently and energetically. Non-verbal communication can be just as, if not more, powerful than spoken communication. Avoid a slumped posture or sagging shoulders, body language that suggests exhaustion or indifference. Maintain a professional appearance at all times.

Greetings are important, consisting of both the handshake and the verbal greeting. Wait momentarily for other team members to offer their hand. If they don't, then you may initiate the handshake. Shake hands using a firm grip. Your handshake shouldn't be weak or limp, but avoid a crushing grip. Since many students can't evaluate the quality of their own handshakes, solicit input from friends or colleagues. Direct eye contact and a strong handshake project confidence.

Did you know...

In the *Lancet* article, "Getting a grip on handshakes," Larkin reported the results of a study by Chaplin in which the handshake characteristics of men and women were evaluated.[9] Larkin wrote that "a strong correlation was found between a firm handshake – as evidenced by strength, vigor, duration, completeness of grip, and eye contact – and a good first impression…Given the power of first impressions, the researchers advise that women as well as men 'try to make that first handshake a firm one.'"

As you shake hands with team members, smile, speak clearly, and address each person by name. Don't address a team member by their first name unless you are clearly invited to do so. Repeat your own name.

> *Dr. Khan, I'm Josh Stein, a third year medical student assigned to your team. It's a pleasure to meet you.*

Rule # 57   Meet the entire team.

You don't just work with your intern, resident, and attending physician. You also work with nurses, ward clerks, medical assistants, pharmacists, social workers, radiology technicians, physical therapists, and others. You will be working with and relying on a variety of healthcare professionals during your clerkship. Dr. Greenberg, professor in the Department of Pediatrics at the George Washington University School of Medicine, wrote about the importance of developing collaborative relationships with all team members. "Working to develop relationships with team members such as unit secretaries, patient schedulers, nurses, and nurse practitioners is also important and sometimes difficult, in view of each student's short time in each clinical setting. Establishing such relationships may be extremely valuable to students in the short term, by helping them to care for their patients more efficiently. In the long term, these relationships may prove valuable in a different way, by teaching students the importance of collaboration."[10]

On your first day, meet as many of these individuals as you can. It can be as simple as:

Hello, my name is Amy Pamen. I'm the medical student working on Team A this month, and Dr. Reddy is my resident. It's nice to meet you, and I'm looking forward to working with you.

This simple effort on your part can help set the proper tone for your working relationship. In particular, you should meet:

- **Nurses**

  It's important to cultivate a good relationship with nurses because it can facilitate the care of patients. There are many physicians, including residents, who never understand this, always choosing to erect a barrier between themselves and the nursing staff. Some physicians take on an air of superiority with nurses, coming across as arrogant and condescending.

Did you know ...

In a survey examining the impact of physicians' disruptive behavior on nurses, 86% of nurses and 49% of physicians stated that they had witnessed disruptive behavior from a physician.[11] 22% of nurses stated that disruptive behavior occurred weekly. Over 50% of all respondents felt that there was a strong link between disruptive behavior and negative clinical outcomes, including patient safety, quality of care, and patient satisfaction.

Strive to be the student and future physician who treats nurses with respect. You may benefit in a number of ways. Because nurses spend more time with the patient than any other healthcare professional, they may share with you important information regarding your patient's condition. You may benefit from their teaching, even though, and especially because, their training and knowledge is different than yours. They may help you with blood draws, arterial blood gases, and placement of intravenous lines. These are procedures that students should be comfortable performing. Nurses can also be of great help early in the rotation when students aren't comfortable with their new environment. They can help you be more efficient.

How do you develop a solid working relationship with nurses? During the first few days of the rotation, introduce yourself to the nurses. Treat them with respect and encourage them to share their thoughts regarding your patients. When your team has decided on the diagnostic and treatment plan for the day, personally convey this to the nurse. It's through these types of interactions that a professional atmosphere is created, one which is essential to providing the best possible patient care.

- **Social workers**

  Social workers perform a variety of functions in the hospital setting. They may be responsible for:
  - Providing counseling for patients and family members to help them cope with the many issues that surround illness and hospitalization, including those that medical professionals are not adept at dealing with, including social, financial, and psychological issues
  - Identifying community resources
  - Treatment planning
  - Discharge planning/coordination of post-hospital services (e.g., home visits)

  The care provided by social workers is extremely valuable; medical students quickly realize this fact.

- **Radiology file clerks**

  These clerks can make your life easier by pulling x-rays and scans for you when needed for rounds and conferences.

- **Radiology technicians**

  If you establish good rapport with technicians, you may be more likely to have your x-rays and scans done sooner rather than later.

- **Lab personnel**

  The time will come when you need assistance. For example, you may need help reviewing a peripheral blood smear or performing a gram stain.

- **Pharmacists**

  Clinical pharmacists are a rich source of information, providing detailed information about the safe use of medications, including interactions and side effects. In a review examining the role of clinical pharmacists, Kaboli described the findings of two recent Institute of Medicine reports. These reports "recognized that pharmacists are an essential resource in safe medication use, that participation of pharmacists on rounds improves medication safety, and that pharmacist-physician-patient collaboration is important."[12] In some hospitals, clinical pharmacists round with the team. In other hospitals, a quick call to the pharmacist can provide the information needed to select the most appropriate medication, along with the correct dose and duration of therapy. Many students, not to mention residents and attendings, don't take advantage of this expertise.

- **Ward secretary/clerk**

  The ward secretary provides clerical support for the patients and staff on the ward. Responsibilities may include notifying residents when newly admitted patients have arrived on the floor, answering telephone calls to the ward, entering physician's orders into the computer system, calling transport to take patients for tests, and facilitating the discharge of patients.

By being aware of the responsibilities of these healthcare professionals, you will be able to call upon them when you require their assistance. When working with others don't forget to use the words "please" and "thank you." Being polite, respectful, and nice will go a long way in establishing a positive working relationship.

Rule # 58   To provide the best patient care, you must be organized.

Organization is a critical skill, not only in rotations and residency, but also throughout your entire career as a physician. With every new patient assigned, you are responsible for performing a thorough history and physical exam. You also need to gather the results of laboratory and imaging tests. After your evaluation, you will have collected a considerable amount of information, which may seem overwhelming. Take the example of a patient who comes in with diabetic ketoacidosis. A major part of the management of these patients is frequent laboratory testing, sometimes as often as every hour. The only way you can properly manage these patients is to stay highly organized.

There are many methods of staying organized, and you'll often hear others proclaim their method as the best. In the end, you have to decide on a system that works for you. Common methods include:

- Clipboard
- Blank or pre-made note cards/sheets
- Pocket-sized notebooks
- Digital devices [PDAs, Iphones]

There are advantages and disadvantages to each method. Clipboards, for example, are often lost because you have to put them down so many times a day. Note cards are popular with residents and interns because they're more portable. With both items, you should mark them with your name and beeper number in case they're lost. In recent years, a number of computing devices, such as Iphones, have become popular. Different applications are available to help you stay organized. Regardless of which method you choose, try to have your system in place on day one of the rotation.

There are myriad benefits to staying organized, one of which is the ability to relay important information to team members within seconds. Key information you should have at your fingertips:

- Patient name
- Medical record number
- Room number
- Date of birth or age
- Admission date
- Chief complaint

- History of present illness
- Medications, including frequency, route, and dosage as well as start and end dates
- Daily vital signs and I/O (input/output)
- Pertinent physical exam findings
- Results of lab/diagnostic studies
- Problem list (patient's active problems) along with management plan

The record you keep is not static. It will change on a daily basis as your patient's condition changes, new tests are ordered, and medications are started or stopped. No matter which system you choose, you must be able to add information to your record and keep it organized in such a way that it's readily accessible.

Your goal is to be the organized student with all patient data at her fingertips. Such students are regarded as efficient, competent, and thorough. Don't be the mess who fumbles around, flipping page after page looking for data, and in the process annoying the team. Without superb organization skills, you may lose track of important patient information. Your incompetence may affect the quality of care your patients receive.

Did you know ...

In a study evaluating problem students, clerkship coordinators, clinical faculty members, and residents were asked to identify the frequency with which certain problem types were encountered. Among 21 types of problem students, the disorganized student was the second most frequently encountered problem type in internal medicine and pediatrics. It was the third most frequently encountered problem type in surgery.[13]

Rule # 59   Create a to-do list.

Early in your day, you'll confer with the team to determine the day's plan for each of your patients. During this discussion, your intern and resident will ask you to take care of a number of tasks. Write down each and every task. The only exception is when you're assigned a task that requires immediate attention, in which case you drop everything and take care of it.

Making a to-do list is especially important when you're caring for many patients. Even with one patient it's a smart idea. Don't try to memorize tasks — even one forgotten patient care duty can prove disastrous. As you complete tasks, cross them off, and at the end of the day, review your list. You may not be lauded for getting everything done. However, if you fail to complete even a single task, you will appear unprofessional, your residents will be upset, and your patients may suffer.

Some students take a haphazard approach to keeping track of tasks. One action item may be written on a note card, another on a progress note, and yet another on a hand. Eventually, something will be forgotten or lost amidst a sea of papers. Keep your to-do list in one location.

> **Did you know ...**
>
> As you try to complete your work, you'll be frequently interrupted. These interruptions may impact care, even leading to medical error. In an observational time and motion study of 40 doctors, doctors were interrupted nearly seven times per hour.[14] Of note, "doctors failed to return to 18.5% of interrupted tasks."

Rule # 60   Prioritize tasks.

The team will evaluate patients in the morning, and then decide on the plan of action for the day. This involves a number of tasks, including ordering laboratory tests, performing studies, and requesting consultations. You must prioritize these tasks. Some are urgent and some are important, and the highest priority tasks are both. These need to be dealt with quickly. For example, if a CT scan isn't ordered early in the day, it may not be done until the next day, prolonging the hospitalization. You'll need to ascertain priority from discussion with your team, and then tackle the tasks of higher priority first.

> ### Tip # 16
>
> Do as much of your work as you can in the morning. If orders are written, tests are scheduled, and consults are placed in the morning, they are more likely to be done. If a task is particularly important, speak with the appropriate person to make sure it gets done.

It can be difficult for students to determine which tasks on the list are of higher priority. Interns and residents often don't make this clear, mistakenly assuming that their students are on the same page. If you aren't sure, you need to ask.

> ### Tip # 17
>
> Which tasks are most important? Which should be tackled first? Which can be delayed until later in the day? If your resident doesn't make this clear, you need to ask.

Did you know ...

In interviews conducted with 30 program directors, poor organizational skills were found to be a common struggle of interns. "We have been encountering more residents who have a difficult time multitasking…" remarked one program director.[3] According to Dr. David E. Meyer, director of the Brain, Cognition and Action Laboratory at the University of Michigan, "when people try to perform two or more related tasks either at the same time or alternating rapidly between them, errors go way up, and it takes far longer – often double the time or more – to get the job done than if they were done sequentially."[15]

Rule # 61   Get things done. On time.

On a daily basis, you'll be responsible for a number of tasks, each with different deadlines. Many of these tasks directly impact patient care, and are therefore a significant responsibility. It can be difficult to prioritize and accomplish so many different items. Given your limited time, you must stay focused. If you tell your intern that you'll have that CT with contrast ordered by 9 AM, with the proper forms and necessary documentation submitted, then make sure you meet that deadline. In some cases, unforeseen obstacles may interfere. If so, notify your intern right away.

As you tackle the items on your list, don't cross off a task until it is truly completed. Some items require the cooperation of others. If someone informs you that he'll help you finish a task, never assume that it's been done. Wait until you have confirmation.

I recall one student who was asked by the attending to check out films from the radiology department and have them ready for afternoon rounds. This student called the radiology department, spoke with the radiology file clerk, and arranged for the clerk to pull the films and have them delivered to the team's conference room just before rounds. He crossed the task off his list. When the team gathered for rounds, the films weren't there.

Rule # 62   Know everything about your patient.

Knowing a lot isn't enough. You need to know <u>everything</u> about your patient. Strive to be the team's expert on your own patients. This is easier said than done, due to a variety of factors.

As a student, important patient information may bypass you. You may be off the floor or away at conference when there is a change in your patient's hospital course. Interns are extremely busy, and while they'll take care of any immediate management issues, they may not remember to inform you. It's up to you to stay current.

- Keep in touch with your intern and resident throughout the day
- Read the chart frequently for new progress notes, consultants' notes, and new orders
- Stay aware of changes in vital signs, lab test results, and other studies

Rule # 63   Your attire is a reflection of your professionalism.

While students tend to dress conservatively on the first day of the rotation, some dress down. Some show up dressed in scrubs, and others forgo the tie. While a casual style may have worked on other rotations or for your classmates, dress conservatively for the first day of the rotation. Don't make any changes unless your attending informs you of what is and is not considered appropriate attire.

Even your lab coat may send the wrong message. I've seen too many medical students show up with dirty, unwashed white coats. Although that stain may only be iodine, to a patient it looks like blood. In the following box, we list some other professional appearance mistakes. Some may seem quite obvious, while others you may need to think about. Too many students continue to make these mistakes. I've seen female students arrive for an outpatient surgical procedure clinic in open-toed shoes. [Think about blood or falling instruments.] I still remember one student who arrived for an outpatient clinic in socks and Birkenstocks.

Professional appearance mistakes

- Too much make-up
- Heavy perfume/cologne/shaving lotion
- Flashy or excessive jewelry
- Dirty or unkempt hair
- Dirty fingernails
- Chipped nail polish
- Clothing that is too tight, stained, or wrinkled
- Provocative clothing (e.g., low neckline, see-through shirts, short skirts)
- Clothing that is too casual (e.g., jeans, sweatpants or shirts, tee shirts, loud ties, halters)
- Visible body piercing or tattoos
- Improper footwear, including dirty or scuffed shoes, tennis shoes, open-toed shoes, high heels
- Buttons or pins expressing political or social opinions or affiliations

---

Rule # 64   Ask questions.

As a newcomer, you aren't expected to know how things work in your new setting. Your goal is to complete all tasks correctly the first time. Avoid spending too much time on the task, and avoid having to repeat the task. From drawing blood to ordering a bone density scan to preparing the patient for their bone marrow biopsy, you need to get it right. Ask questions, listen carefully, and take notes. Don't be afraid or embarrassed to approach any team member for assistance.

Before performing a task, you must know ...

1) what you are supposed to do

2) how to do it

3) why you should do it

4) when to begin

5) when to finish

6) what the finished product should look like

7) how to do it the right way (the right way is their way)

8) the importance of the task, relative to your other responsibilities (priority)

After the task, you must receive specific feedback about your performance

Rule # 65   Move from observation to action mode as quickly as possible.

During the first few days, little is expected of students beyond familiarizing themselves with the rules, responsibilities, and expectations of the new clerkship. Team members sometimes assume that the best way for students to gain this familiarity is to simply observe.

While observing does have its merits, you can't truly reach a comfort level until you start doing what you are expected to be doing. In other words, you have to begin the work of patient care. For this reason, you should ask your intern, resident, or attending to assign you a patient on day 1 of the rotation. Once assigned a patient, you can proceed to perform the daily tasks involved in patient care, including writing progress notes, writing orders, obtaining lab test results, and so on.

References

[1]Klass P. *A not entirely benign procedure: four years as a medical student.* New York; Kaplan Publishers: 2010.

[2]Small R, Soriano R, Chietero M, Quintana J, Parkas V, Koestler J. Easing the transition: medical students' perceptions of critical skills required for the clerkships. *Educ Health* 2008; 21(3): 192.

[3]Lyss-Lerman P, Teherani A, Aagaard E, Loeser H, Cooke M, Harper G. What training is needed in the fourth year of medical school? Views of residency program directors. *Acad Med* 2009; 84(7): 823-9.

[4]Kho A, Henderson L, Dressler D, Kripalani S. Use of handheld computers in medical education. A systematic review. *J Gen Intern Med* 2006; 21(5): 531-7.

[5]Skhal K. A full revolution: offering 360 degree library services to clinical clerkship students. *Med Ref Serv Q* 2008; 27(3): 249-59.

[6]Mintz M, Narvarte H, O'Brien K, Papp K, Thomas M, Durning S. Use of electronic medical records by physicians and students in academic internal medicine settings. *Acad Med* 2009; 84(12): 1698-704.

[7]Jain S. Orienting family medicine residents and medical students to office practice. *Fam Med* 2005; 37(7): 461-3.

[8]O'Brien B, Cooke M, Irby D. Perceptions and attributions of third-year student struggles in clerskhips: do students and clerkship directors agree? *Acad Med* 2007; 82(10): 970-8.

[9]Larkin M. Getting a grip on handshakes. *Lancet* 2000; 356: 227.

[10]Greenberg L, Blatt B. Perspective: successfully negotiating the clerkship years of medical school: a guide for medical students, implications for residents and faculty. *Acad Med* 2010; 85(4): 706-9.

[11]Rosenstein A, O'Daniel M. Disruptive behavior and clinical outcomes: perceptions of nurses and physicians. *AJN* 2005; 105(1): 55-64.

[12]Kaboli P, Hoth A, McClimon B, Schnipper J. Clinical pharmacists and inpatient medical care. *Arch Int Med* 2006; 166(9): 955-64.

[13]Tonesk X, Buchanan R. An AAMC pilot study by 10 medical schools of clinical evaluation of students. *J Med Educ* 1987; 62(9): 707-18.

[14]Westbrook J, Coiera E, Dunsmuir W, Brown B, Kelk N, Paoloni R, Tran C. The impact of interruptions on clinical task completion. *Qual Saf Health Care* 2010; 19(4): 284-9.

[15]Wallis C. The multitasking generation. *Time.* March 19, 2006. http://www.time.com/time/magazine/article/0,9171,1174696,00.html. Accessed December 21, 2010.

Chapter 10

Admitting Patients

Rule # 66   Strive to function as the patient's intern, not just as a student.

Your goal isn't to function as a medical student. You should strive to function as the patient's intern. Become familiar with the intern's role in the evaluation and management of a newly admitted patient. The intern is responsible for:

- Obtaining the history
- Performing the physical examination
- Gathering the results of laboratory test data
- Gathering the results of other diagnostic studies (x-rays, electrocardiograms, other)
- Using the above information to determine the cause of the patient's symptom(s) or, if this is not possible, a list of possible causes (differential diagnosis)
- Deciding on which further diagnostic testing is needed to confirm the diagnosis and exclude other considerations
- Developing and instituting a treatment plan
- Writing the patient's admission orders
- Following through to make sure the orders are implemented
- Recording the history and physical examination in the patient's medical record (admission note or write-up)
- Preparing an oral case presentation which will be delivered to the attending physician on the following day (post-call day)
- Periodically checking in on the patient to assess the patient's condition and response to therapy
- Answering patient questions as well as the family's questions

Students who take it upon themselves to care for the patient as if they were the intern are presented with tremendous learning opportunities, as well as being held in high regard for substantial contributions to patient care.

Step-by-step approach to evaluating a newly admitted patient

Step 1: Have a patient information template available to collect all patient data. After you've been assigned a patient, enter the patient's name, room number, and medical record number on your template. You'll need this information to locate the patient and to access important patient information. Having the data on the template will help you organize the information for write-ups and oral case presentations.

Step 2: Check to see if there are previous medical records ("old charts") on your patient. Because it can take time for hospital personnel to pull medical records for review, it's a good idea to call the medical records department and request the records as soon as the patient is assigned to you. If you're rotating at a hospital which has adopted the electronic medical record, you may be able to access this information on your own. You will need this information to complete your work-up. If the records are available, see if they contain any information that's relevant to the patient's current reason for hospitalization. Record this information on your template. If the records aren't yet available, you can always look them over after you've performed the history and physical.

Step 3: Before seeing the patient, review the emergency room or clinic notes which prompted the admission. Patients will generally be admitted either through the emergency room or from their personal physician's office. Usually the chart will have a note reflecting this encounter.

Although the note may list a presumptive diagnosis, keep an open mind so that you don't focus too prematurely on the listed diagnosis. Doing so would keep you from carefully considering other causes of a patient's chief complaint, and the learning that comes from this evaluation. Note that presumptive diagnoses are often based on incomplete information. As the results of the full evaluation become available, you may reach a different conclusion.

Step 4: If you aren't familiar with the work-up of the patient's chief complaint, read about it quickly.

Step 5: See the patient and perform a complete history and physical examination.

Step 6: Gather all test results (laboratory, ECG, imaging, other). Record this information in your patient template.

Step 7: Review and organize the information you've collected. Consult books and other resources to help you formulate an assessment and plan. Ask yourself the following questions:

- What is the differential diagnosis?
- What is the most likely diagnosis (working diagnosis) and why?
- Why are other conditions in the differential less likely?
- What further evaluation is needed to support my working diagnosis?
- What treatment should I recommend?

The answers to these questions will help you create your own assessment and plan.

Step 8: Present the information and offer your assessment and plan to the resident. Present the case as you would to the attending physician. This is good practice for the next day's attending rounds. Ask the resident for feedback, especially regarding your assessment and plan.

Step 9: Write the admission orders. Have all orders reviewed and co-signed by your intern or resident.

Step 10: After the patient is "tucked in," read about the patient's issues using a variety of resources, including handbooks, textbooks, and the literature. This will allow you to prepare a high quality write-up and oral case presentation. You will also be better prepared for the attending physician's questions.

Reviewing an old chart efficiently

Old charts (see step # 2 above) are sometimes enormous. It can be challenging to review a chart of this size, especially with so much to do and so little time. Fortunately, you can usually obtain the necessary information with the following approach:

1) Look for the most recent hospitalization

2) Locate the discharge summary. Within the summary, you should be able to find:

- Reason for hospital admission
- Hospital course, including the results of important tests and response to treatment
- Medication list at the time of discharge
- Discharge diagnoses

3) If the discharge summary is not available or is lacking information, your job becomes harder. First, locate the admission note, which is usually the first note or two in the progress notes section. From there, read each progress note in chronological order to obtain the necessary information.

Rule # 67   Your evaluation should be more thorough than that of any other team member.

As a junior medical student, the expectation is that you will be extremely thorough, and perform a <u>complete</u> history and physical examination. Begin call with this mindset. Every part of the physical examination must be done, even if you don't think it's relevant to the issue that brought the patient into the hospital. Thorough patient evaluations performed by students have often revealed important information not obtained by other team members.

Tip # 18

Dr. Neveen El-Farra, director of the inpatient medicine clerkship at UCLA, stated it well.[1] "You will be expected to know your patients well. If you do this you will be the 'go to' person for your patients when anyone on your team has a question or wants something done. Sometimes, it is the medical student that obtains that one missing, essential piece of information that will affect patient management."

Since you will rarely be observed taking the history and performing the exam, you may wonder how others will know how thorough you've been. The thoroughness of your evaluation will be assessed by the attending during rounds the next day when you deliver your oral case presentations. Review of your patient write-up will provide further information.

Rule # 68   Evaluate the patient on your own.

When you are assigned a patient, you may be given the choice of seeing the patient alone or with the rest of the team. Although both options have merit, we encourage you to see the patient alone.

●   You must perform a thorough history and physical examination, while your intern and resident are more interested in a focused history and physical. If you see the patient together, you will usually have to come back to the patient's room to fill in the gaps.

●   If you do see the patient with the residents, they will often allow you to start the interview, but at some point will take over. While you only have a few patients to work up, they must evaluate many new patients. Because they're pressed for time, they may be forced to make you an observer. You can learn a great deal from watching experienced team members interact with a patient, but observation alone can only take you so far. To gain comfort evaluating a newly admitted patient, you must be an active participant.

●   At this early point in your career you are developing your own style and becoming comfortable with the process of performing the history and physical exam. Having your resident and intern next to you may be anxiety-provoking.

Try to evaluate the patient before the residents, but recognize that this may not be possible. If your patient is severely ill, your residents will need to evaluate the patient as soon as possible. They may ask you to either accompany them or evaluate the patient after they are through.

Tip # 19

Try to be the first team member who takes the patient's history and performs the physical exam. This allows you to make the most of the learning experience. Studies in inpatient settings have shown that students are often involved in patient evaluation after other team members have already acquired pertinent data, made diagnoses, and established treatment plans.

How often are students the initial investigator? In a study of students in a surgery clerkship, Southern Illinois University researchers found that students were the first to elicit the history of the chief complaint and perform the initial surgical physical exam in only 4.3% and 8.7% of inpatient encounters, respectively.[2] In only 2.2% of patient evaluations were students asked to generate the initial diagnostic hypothesis. By being involved as early as possible, you give yourself more opportunities to independently generate a diagnosis and management plan, critical thinking skills that are important to your development as a physician.

Tip # 20

The clinical status of a hospitalized patient can change quickly. If a patient appears seriously ill when you first see him, or if the patient worsens during your evaluation, call your resident or attending immediately. Do not wait until you present your patient to the resident. Do the same if you encounter a severely abnormal lab test, electrocardiogram, or imaging test result.

Rule # 69   **Learn how to gather information from the patient. Many physicians underperform in this critical area of patient care.**

Once the introductions are over, your goal is to determine the patient's chief complaint and delve into the history of present illness (HPI). In essence, the HPI is the patient's story of their problem. This history is essential to reaching an accurate diagnosis. In one study, 76% of diagnoses made by clinicians were suggested or established by the history.[3]

While obtaining a complete history is therefore critically important, doing so can be challenging, and some medical students perform poorly. In recognition of the importance of communication skills, medical schools now typically conduct comprehensive clinical skills assessment using standardized patients.

Faculty members who work with poorly performing students have noted several problems with history taking. "Many low-scoring students focused prematurely, failing to ask open-ended questions or adequately characterize the chief complaint. Respondents also observed students being too focused on the history of present illness, omitting or incompletely exploring the pertinent past medical, social, or family history, particularly as they related to the chief complaint." The patient's perspective on the illness was not explored by some students. The authors wrote that "these students treated standardized patients as symptoms or diagnoses rather than as people with feelings or concerns."[4]

Did you know...

In a study at the Feinberg School of Medicine at Northwestern University, nearly 700 medical students self-assessed their communication skills after viewing videotaped interactions of themselves with simulated patients.[5] Eliciting information was found to be the most frequently noted weakness, cited by 35% of participants.

Rule # 70   Medication histories are often more complicated than expected.

Obtaining and documenting the patient's medication regimen would seem to be straightforward. Even within this area, though, the potential exists for errors. Some patients rely on memory, while others bring in a typed list of their medications. Others may bring in their brown bag or plastic grocery bag full of medication bottles and hand them over to you. Don't just copy information about drug names and dosages from the list or bottles. Ask these questions each time:

- Which medications is the patient actually taking?
- Are they following the schedule as prescribed?
- If not, why not? Are they taking the medication less often due to side effects? Are they rationing their pills due to cost?
- Are they taking the medication more often than prescribed? Why? Do they feel it may be more effective that way?
- Are they taking any over-the-counter medications?
- Are they taking any nutritional supplements?
- Are they taking any herbal or natural medications, such as St. John's wort, gingko biloba, or colloidal silver?

It may be understandable that patients would leave out certain drugs. In the case of over-the-counter medications, nutritional supplements, herbal products, or "natural" medications, many patients just don't see these as medications. However, they have the potential to cause serious side effects, such as increased bleeding time or drug rashes. Some may lead to potentially dangerous drug interactions.

In the case of prescription medications, all physicians would agree that accuracy is paramount. However, researchers who looked at medication regimens among elderly patients found that family medicine faculty and residents didn't always document accurate information. In evaluating congruence, defined as agreement between the physician and patient regarding all prescription medications, dosages, and frequency, they found a rate of only 58% for residents.[6] As a medical student performing a thorough evaluation, strive for a congruence rate of 100%.

Tip # 21

Safe prescribing requires an accurate medication list. Unfortunately, inaccuracies are common, and may lead to duplication of medications, discontinuation of needed medications, and drug interactions. Since patients are often under the care of several physicians, always obtain the name and contact information of all providers. If the patient fills his or her prescriptions at a single pharmacy, contacting the pharmacy may help verify the accuracy of the medication list.

Rule # 71   Ask about relevant family and social history☐

Assumptions about a patient's social history [including alcohol intake or use of illicit drugs] based on superficial evidence aren't useful. However, asking intrusive questions is uncomfortable. For these, and a number of other reasons, students and physicians don't do well in this area. Research has shown that physicians often do not elicit key components of the history, including the family history, smoking history, and history of alcohol or illicit drug use. One reason cited for this failure is lack of confidence in obtaining this information. This may be the result of inadequate or insufficient training in the preclinical years, followed by poor reinforcement during clerkships and postgraduate training.

Elements of the history not often obtained by physicians	
Element of the history	**Deficiency**
Family history	Studies have shown that relevant family history information is often not obtained or, if obtained, not documented in the medical record: • In one study, over 50% of patients at higher risk for breast or colorectal cancer based on family history had no documentation of their risk in the chart. Among those whose higher risk was documented, age of cancer diagnosis for affected family members was only noted in 40%.[7] • In a study of randomly selected charts in a family practice residency, researchers discovered that family histories of certain conditions, including mental illness, emphysema, and alcoholism, were rarely recorded.[8] • In the Direct Observation of Primary Care study, 138 community physicians were observed in over 4,000 outpatient encounters. Family histories were only discussed in 51% of new patient visits.[9]
Alcohol or Illicit Drug Use	Physicians often fail to inquire about alcohol or illicit drug use: • In a survey of over 1,000 general internists, family physicians, psychiatrists, and obstetricians and gynecologists, researchers found that only 68% regularly inquired about illicit drug use among new outpatients.[10] Among the reasons cited for not obtaining information was lack of confidence in obtaining the history of drug use. • While up to 50% of ER visits involve illegal drugs or alcohol, Dr. Gail D'Onofrio, chief of emergency medicine at Yale-New Haven Hospital, states that typically "we don't ask it. It makes no sense whatsoever."[11] • In another study, only 18% of hospitalized patients were asked about illicit drug use based upon a review of patient charts. The authors concluded that "screening for drug abuse is not routinely performed and documented among hospitalized patients."[12]
Smoking	Many physicians fail to inquire about smoking. In one study, patients were asked if they smoked at only 67% of visits.[13]

Rule # 72   Ask to write the admission orders yourself.

Admission orders are written after a newly admitted patient is evaluated by the intern and resident. Admission orders are essentially instructions for nurses and other healthcare professionals in patient care. Orders are normally written by interns, but when students are involved in the care of the patient they are often allowed to write them.

If you aren't offered the opportunity to write orders, then you should ask. Keep in mind that interns may not be able to let you write orders, especially if there is a hospital policy against it. Also, if the patient's condition is such that orders need to be written promptly, then the intern won't have the luxury of waiting for you to complete your evaluation before writing orders. Even when you don't have the opportunity to write the admission orders yourself, you can always take an order sheet, write your own orders, and then compare yours with the intern's actual orders.

Did you know ...

In a survey of medical students, students wanted to enter 100% of orders for their patients. They strongly believed that placing orders made them feel as if they were the caregiver for their patients, and was an important way "to learn what tests and treatments are needed by patients."[14] Unfortunately, a variety of barriers exist. Scheduled conferences and teaching sessions may interfere. In other cases, students are unable to participate due to institutional policy, resident preferences, or inadequate training on the computer ordering system.

Rule # 73   **Prescribing errors are common and damaging. Take concrete steps to avoid these errors.**

Writing orders is a major responsibility, and each time you do so you need to ensure complete accuracy. One aspect of writing orders is prescribing medications. In this one aspect alone, the potential exists for multiple errors. In a study that looked at the incidence of adverse drug events and potential adverse drug events, researchers found that prescribing errors were common and contributed to over <u>half</u> of all significant adverse but preventable drug events.[15]

Prescribing errors are common. The issue for physicians and physicians-in-training is how to prevent them. Garbutt and colleagues studied the behavior of housestaff and medical students in regard to safe prescribing practices.[16] They describe in their article a number of safe prescribing behaviors that focus on different aspects of prescribing. These include confirming information about the medication itself (e.g., spelling), checking patient information (such as renal function), double-checking orders once completed, writing the orders correctly, and special considerations with verbal orders.

They asked respondents to report if they always followed specific safe prescribing practices. The results indicated that routine use of these behaviors was poor. Among students, they found that only:

- 85% reported always checking prescribing information before prescribing new drugs.
- 75% reported always checking for drug allergies before prescribing.
- 54% reported always double-checking dosage calculations.
- 52% reported always avoiding the use of dangerous abbreviations.
- 25% reported always checking for renal impairment before prescribing a medication that is renally excreted.
- 23% reported always checking for potential drug-drug interactions.

With every medication order you write, ask yourself:

1) Have I consulted a prescribing reference before writing a new medication order?
2) Is the patient allergic to this medication?
3) Is the medication contraindicated in this patient (e.g. beta-blockers in severe asthma)?
4) Is the medication teratogenic? If so, is the patient pregnant, trying to become pregnant, or breastfeeding?
5) Will this medication interact with any of the patient's other medications?
6) Does the dose need to be adjusted for renal dysfunction (including dialysis), liver dysfunction, weight, or age?
7) Have I spelled the medication correctly?
8) Have I avoided the use of abbreviations?
9) Is the dosage, route of administration (oral, intravenous, subcutaneous, intramuscular), and dosing schedule correct?
10) Did I date and time the medication order?
11) Have I signed and printed my name along with my beeper number?
12) Is my handwriting legible?
13) Does it need to be administered as soon as possible? If so, have I conveyed this to the nurse?

Always have your intern, resident, or attending review the order for accuracy prior to cosigning.

Adapted from Garbutt JM, Highstein G, Jeffe DB, Dunagan WC, Fraser VJ. Safe medication prescribing: training and experience of medical students and housestaff at a large teaching hospital. Acad Med 2005; 80(6): 594-599.

As a final note, I would like to emphasize that students must avoid the use of dangerous abbreviations.

Examples of dangerous abbreviations		
Dangerous abbreviation	Why?	Instead write out ...
Q.D.	The period after the "Q" may be misread as an "I." This may lead to four-times-daily dosing rather than the intended once daily dosing.	"every day"
MSO4	This abbreviation is often used for morphine sulfate but it may be misinterpreted as magnesium sulfate.	"morphine sulfate"
AZT	AZT has been used as an abbreviation for azidothymidine, an antiretroviral medication. This may lead to confusion with azathioprine, an immunosuppressant medication.	"azidothymidine"
U	"U" is often used as an abbreviation for units. However, when the "U" follows a number as in "Insulin 5U", it may be mistakenly read as a zero. This could lead to a tenfold increase in the drug dose.	"units"
HCT	HCT, a commonly used abbreviation for hydrocortisone, may be misinterpreted as hydrochlorothiazide.	"hydrocortisone"
μg	This is an abbreviation commonly used for micrograms. When handwritten, it may be mistaken for "mg."	"mcg"

References

[1]Orientation Outline: Third Year Inpatient Internal Medicine Clerkship at Ronald Reagan UCLA Medical Center. http://medres.med.ucla.edu/Policies/MS-3%20RR-UCLA%20Medical%20Center%20Orientation%20Outline-August%202009.pdf. Accessed January 30, 2011.

[2]Boehler M, Schwind C, Dunnington G, Rogers D, Folse R. Medical student contact with patients on a surgery clerkship: is there a chance to learn? *J Am Coll Surg* 2002; 195(4): 539-42.

[3]Peterson M, Holbrook J, Hales D, Smith N, Staker L. Contributions of the history, physical examination, and laboratory investigation in making medical diagnoses. *West J Med* 1992; 156: 163-5.

[4]Hauer K, Teherani A, Kerr K, O'Sullivan P, Irby D. Student performance problems in medical school clinical skills assessments. *Acad Med* 2007; 82(10 Suppl): S69-S72.

[5]Zick A, Granieri M, Makoul G. First-year medical students' assessment of their own communication skills: a video-based, open-ended approach. *Patient Educ Couns* 2007; 68 (2): 161-6.

[6]Bikowski R, Ripsin C, Lorraine V. Physician-patient congruence regarding medication regimens. *J Am Geriatr Soc* 2001; 49(10): 1353-7.

[7]Murff H, Greevy R, Syngal S. The comprehensiveness of family cancer history assessments in primary care. *Community Genet* 2007; 10(3): 174-80.

[8]Crouch M, Thiedke C. Documentation of family health history in the outpatient medical record. *J Fam Pract* 1986; 22: 169-74.

[9]Hayflick S, Eiff M, Carpenter L, et al. Primary care physicians' utilization and perceptions of genetics services. *Genet Med* 1998; 1: 13-21.

[10]Friedmann P, McCullough D, Saitz R. Screening and intervention for illicit drug abuse. *Arch Intern Med* 2001; 162: 248-51.

[11]Neergaard L. Helping doctors ask about drug, alcohol problems. http://www.physorg.com/news160675177.html. May 4, 2009. Accessed January 23, 2011.

[12]Stein M, Wilkinson J, Berglas N, O'Sullivan P. Prevalence and detection of illicit drug disorders among hospitalized patients: clinical note. *The American Journal of Drug and Alcohol Abuse* 1996; 22(13): 463-71.

[13]Thorndike A, Rigotti N, Stafford R, Singer D. National patterns in the treatment of smokers by physicians. *JAMA* 279(8): 604-8.

[14]Knight A, Kravet S, Harper M, Leff B. The effect of computerized provider order entry on medical student clerkship experiences. *J Am Med Inform Assoc* 2005; 12: 554-60.

[15]Bates D, Cullen D, Laird N, et al. Incidence of adverse drug events and potential adverse drug events. Implications for prevention. *JAMA* 1995; 274(1): 29-34.

[16]Garbutt J, Highstein G, Jeffe D, Dunagan W, Fraser V. Safe medication prescribing: training and experience of medical students of medical students and housestaff at a large teaching hospital. *Acad Med* 2005; 80(6): 594-9.

Chapter 11

On Call

The phrase "on call" refers to the period of time when a team is responsible for admitting new patients. Call structure varies from one institution to another, but in general it may occur either during the day or night. While students often approach their first call with trepidation, the experience of being among the first to work up a newly admitted patient is unique. Evaluating a patient, providing comfort, rising to the intellectual diagnostic and therapeutic challenges: all embody what it means to be a physician.

Rule # 74   Be prepared for call.

You can't be successful unless you have everything you need. Make sure these items are in your on call bag:

- Change of clothes
- Personal hygiene items
- Snacks (food/beverages)
- Medical equipment
- Books/resources

In order to perform at a high level, you have to take care of yourself. That's why we mention the obvious. Bring food. Know the cafeteria's hours of operation, but remember that your work on the wards may keep you from getting there before it closes.

Students are expected to perform a complete history and physical examination. In order to do so, you need to have the proper medical equipment. Don't assume that equipment will be easily available on the wards. Prior to your first call, speak with your intern and resident to determine what is, and what is not, available. If you don't have what you need to perform a specific aspect of the exam, then it won't get done. Inevitably, that's what the attending will focus on, and they just won't be impressed with your sad reply of "I didn't do the funduscopic exam because I didn't have access to an ophthalmoscope."

Rule # 75   Learn your responsibilities.

Many students approach call with apprehension, anxiety, or even dread, usually because they're unfamiliar with their role and expected responsibilities. The call experience varies from clerkship to clerkship, so prior experience may not help.

During orientation, most clerkship directors will review on call expectations. Prior to your first call, review this information. The information may be general; for example, students may be required to pick up and evaluate two new patients per call. For specifics, you'll need to meet with your intern and resident, who'll be on call with you.

Learn how you should spend your time on call. How many patients will you work up? Will you pick up the first patient, or will you shadow the intern until they assign a patient? Will you be helping the intern with subsequent admissions, or will you be released to read about your patient? What other responsibilities will you have?

Did you know...

In a study done by Virginia Commonwealth University researchers, internal medicine and pediatrics residents on call were observed for 106 nights from the hours of 7 PM to 7 AM.[1] Approximately 5 ½ hours per night were spent on activities such as eating, resting, chatting, and sleeping. Chart review and documentation accounted for 2 ½ hours per night. Discussion of the case with team members averaged 1 ½ hours per night. One and a half hours were also spent performing histories and physical examinations.

Another study shadowed surgical residents on call. Activities of daily living, which included eating, sleep, and hygiene, accounted for approximately 30% of the total time. This was followed closely by time spent in patient evaluation. However, only 30% of this time was spent performing the history and physical exam. The remaining time was devoted to charting and diagnostic review.[2] Of note, median sleep time was 201 minutes with frequent interruptions. The median uninterrupted sleep time was 39 minutes.

Rule # 76   Be visible and easily accessible when on call.

Students on call are presented with a variety of opportunities to learn, but only if they're visible or easily accessible. Many students express an interest in helping the team during call, asking the resident and intern to page them when needed. They then retreat to the call room or library to study while waiting for a page.

This approach doesn't work, because it doesn't take into account how call works for residents. Typically, call is very busy, with multiple competing demands placed on residents' time. Since every minute is precious, they may find it easier to take care of the matter themselves rather than page you, wait for your response, and then instruct you on what to do and how to do it. In the time that it takes to reach and instruct you, they may be able to accomplish not only that task but several others.

A far better approach is to be physically present. If your intern allows it, consider shadowing him. If shadowing is discouraged, plant yourself where the intern and resident can't help but notice you as they scurry around completing their work. The idea is to be around, but not in the way.

Rule # 77   Spend time with the patient, not in the library.

Once they're assigned a patient, students often read about the patient's symptom or condition before performing the history and physical. Reading about the patient's medical problems is beneficial, but save the bulk of your reading for later. When patients are admitted, there's a lot that needs to get done, often expeditiously. As a student, you should assume "ownership" of all newly assigned patients. You want to be an active participant, involving yourself in all aspects of the patient's initial care. That's hard to do if you spend considerable time in the call room or library reading. A better approach is to quickly review key aspects in the work up of the patient's symptoms and then proceed to evaluate the patient.

Rule # 78   Pick up a patient as soon as possible during call.

Pick up a patient as early as possible during call. The sooner you're assigned a patient, the sooner you can begin the evaluation. Evaluating a newly admitted patient takes considerable time, especially for students. You not only have to take a complete history and perform a thorough physical examination, you also have to read about the case, prepare the oral case presentation, and complete the patient's write-up. If you're expected to pick up more than one patient during call, then starting early becomes even more important.

Typically, the resident will be the one to assign patients. In assigning patients, residents sometimes have the tendency to wait for an "exciting case." This case may never come. You'll then be assigned a patient whose evaluation you could have started hours ago. Don't bypass a patient because the resident doesn't think it's a good enough case. In many cases, what residents consider boring may have great teaching value for students.

Rule # 79   Pick up the correct number of patients, according to the clerkship director.

Clerkships often have requirements that specify the number of patients that students should pick up while on call. This information is typically provided during clerkship orientation. However, residents aren't always

med of each and every clerkship requirement. It is your
to inform your resident of this requirement, and others,
t call. Your resident may feel that one new admit is suffi-
your attending the next day will wonder why you didn't pick up
enough patients.

Rule # 80   Meet with your intern or resident before attending rounds.

After you complete your history and physical examination, gather your thoughts. Working up a patient is like solving a puzzle – you have all these pieces of information and you have to see how they fit together. Once you do this, you'll be able to establish a diagnosis and then formulate an appropriate treatment plan. During this problem-solving process, questions will inevitably arise. For this reason, make it a point to sit down with the intern or resident to go over the case. If they don't initiate this meeting, you should, but don't forget how busy they are. While you may be ready to have your meeting, they may need to deal with other issues that take precedence.

During attending rounds, your attending will try to ascertain how well you understand your patient and his problems. If you have questions that remain unanswered from the on call day, there's a good chance that you'll be asked those very questions. Therefore, plan to meet with the intern or resident on the day that you admit the patient. During your meeting, present the case, including your assessment and plan, to see if it's in agreement with theirs. Your residents can often predict the questions the attending will ask.

Rule # 81   Don't ever leave for the day without first offering to help the team.

Medical students are often the first team members to finish, since they have fewer patients and less responsibility for patient care. When you complete your work, don't just leave. I've heard of medical students who make it a point to tell the team that their responsibility, per the clerkship director, is for a maximum of two patients while on call. Forget the "requirement." As a team player, you should be going above and beyond the minimum requirements. Offer to help other team members; the on call day is busy and stressful for the entire team. Any assistance that you can provide will be appreciated.

Tip # 22

Although you may have completed your work, don't leave without offering to help other team members.

Rule # 82   Don't arrive for rounds with that post-call look.

To avoid oversleeping after an overnight call in the hospital, set your alarm or your cell phone. If you didn't bring one, ask a colleague to page you or arrange a wake-up call.

After an overnight call, students don't always look their best. Call may be busy, but take the time to clean up. Avoid that post-call, disheveled look. Dress appropriately and be well groomed. Your appearance remains important in projecting the right degree of professionalism for your team and your patients.

References

[1]Moore S, Nettleman M, Beyer S, Chalasani K, Fairbanks R, Goyal M, Carter M. How residents spend their nights on call. *Acad Med* 2000; 75(10): 1021-4.

[2]Morton J, Baker C, Farrell T, Yohe M, Kimple R, Herman D, Udekwu P, Galanko J, Behrns K, Meyer A. What do surgery residents do on their call nights? *Am J Surg* 2004; 188(3): 225-9.

Chapter 12

Laboratory Tests

The state of lab testing in America can be summarized succinctly:

Physicians waste a lot of money on lab tests.

Many of us don't know enough about what we're doing.

This ignorance can lead to medical errors.

In its National Status Report, the Centers for Disease Control wrote that "medical education on laboratory testing is inadequate. Despite the integral role of laboratory testing in the practice of medicine, formal teaching of laboratory medicine is a relatively neglected component of the medical school curriculum."[1] In caring for patients, physicians must routinely order and interpret a wide variety of diagnostic tests. Unfortunately, many clinicians have received relatively little formal instruction in lab test ordering or interpretation.

The end result is that medical school graduates often "enter future practice with major gaps in this area of diagnosis and therapeutics."[2] Misinterpretation of test results may significantly impact patient care, increasing morbidity and mortality due to missed diagnoses or wrong diagnoses. From a monetary standpoint, according to the U.S. Congressional Budget Office, approximately $700 billion per year is spent on diagnostic tests that do not improve health outcomes.

Recognizing the importance of lab test interpretation, organizations such as the Clerkship Directors of Internal Medicine, Society of General Internal Medicine, and the Academy of Clinical Laboratory Physicians and Scientists have identified the selection and interpretation of appropriate diagnostic studies as key competencies for medical students.[3,4]

Abnormal lab test results are common, and you need to have a systematic approach in place to interpret these results. However, traditional textbooks of medicine are often lacking in this regard. Dr. George Lundberg, Editor in Chief Emeritus of Medscape and Former Editor of *JAMA*, wrote that "guidance on diagnostic testing in medical textbooks often consist of little more than listings of tests that may be abnormal in a given disease. Both the number and complexity of diagnostic tests have increased rapidly, requiring physicians to have not only considerable knowledge of the properties of individual tests but also a strategy for their sequential interpretation."[5] In this chapter, we introduce the principles of laboratory medicine. We then proceed to a review of lab test errors. Lastly, based on our own resources, we review a step-by-step approach to the interpretation of common lab tests.

Rule # 83   Abnormal lab test results are common. You must be prepared to interpret them.

The charts of patients admitted to the general medicine service at a city hospital in the Northeast were reviewed to determine the frequency of biochemical test abnormalities at the time of admission. Twenty-nine percent of the 5,328 tests obtained were abnormal.[6] In a retrospective chart review of over 500 patients admitted to an inpatient psychiatry unit, laboratory tests performed on admission were reviewed.[7] The prevalence of values outside the normal range is listed below.

Reviewing this list brings home the point that no matter what field of medicine you're in, you must be prepared to deal with abnormal lab test results. You have to know the differential diagnosis of an elevated LDH. You have to know if you need to investigate further, and how you would proceed to do so.

Prevalence of test results outside the normal range in psychiatric inpatients at the time of admission	
Test	**% of results outside the normal range**
Total cholesterol	36%
Lactate dehydrogenase (LDH)	25%
HDL-cholesterol	23%
Alkaline phosphatase	14%
Alanine aminotransferase (ALT)	13%
GGT	10%
TSH	7%
Calcium	5%
Potassium	4%
Sodium	3%
Free thyroxine	1%

Arce-Cordon R, Perez-Rodriguez M, Baca-Baldomero E, Oquendo M, Baca-Garcia E. Routine laboratory screening among newly admitted psychiatric patients: is it worthwhile? *Psychiatr Serv* 2007; 58(12): 1602-5.

Rule # 84   You will be involved in ordering lab tests. Before ordering any test, stop and ask if it's really necessary.

According to the U.S. Congressional Budget Office, approximately $ 700 billion per year is spent on diagnostic tests that <u>do not improve</u> health outcomes. This prompted the American College of Physicians to recently announce a major initiative – to eliminate improper use of diagnostic tests.

The preoperative setting is one well-studied arena in which excessive lab tests are common. In the latter half of the 20th century, a battery of laboratory tests was routinely ordered prior to surgery. It was not uncommon for test results to be abnormal. In one study of over 500 elderly surgical patients, the prevalence of abnormal creatinine, hemoglobin, glucose, potassium, and sodium values were 12%, 10%, 7%, 5%, and 2%, respectively.[8] However, research has shown that these results are seldom clinically significant. Hepner summarized it well[9]:

Untargeted testing should be avoided. An unexpected result will probably not be clinically significant for the surgery and will only lead to more needless testing, unnecessary anxiety for the patient, and delays in proceeding to the operating room. The more tests that are ordered, the higher the likelihood of having an abnormal result by chance: for a test with 95% specificity, results for 1 out of 13 ordered tests will likely be abnormal without there being a true underlying physiologic abnormality.

A more targeted approach is possible if the ordering clinician carefully considers the need for the test.

Criteria for determining whether a preoperative test is indicated[9,10]

1. Does the test correctly identify abnormalities?
2. Will the test change your diagnosis?
3. Will the test change your management?
4. Will the test change your patient's outcome?

Numerous studies have shown that clinicians often order tests that are not clinically indicated. In one study, researchers examined the ordering patterns and clinical indications for the prothrombin time (PT) and activated partial thromboplastin time (aPTT). Over 80% of all admitted patients had these tests ordered. "At least 70% of these tests were not clinically indicated," costing over $60,000 in one year at the hospital studied.[11] As a medical student, you will routinely order lab tests as part of a team. Before ordering any test, ask yourself how the results will impact the patient's diagnosis, management, or outcome.

Rule # 85   Lab test errors are common.

Recently, Dr. Michael Laposata, pathologist-in-chief and director of laboratory medicine at Vanderbilt University Hospital, wrote that "medical error from incorrect laboratory test selection and result interpretation is rapidly becoming a more serious problem as the test menu becomes larger and more complex."[12] Reviews of malpractice claims have shown that incorrect interpretation of laboratory test results is a major cause of missed or delayed diagnoses. In one study, Gandhi reviewed 307 closed malpractice claims in the ambulatory setting.[13] Fifty-nine percent involved diagnostic errors. Failure to order appropriate diagnostic or laboratory tests accounted for 55% of the breakdowns in care. Thirty-seven percent of the errors were related to incorrect interpretation of diagnostic or laboratory tests. Some key studies are summarized below, highlighting these issues.

Studies of lab test errors	
Study	**Findings**
Survey of internists, medical specialists, and emergency physicians	Respondents were asked to describe cases involving diagnostic error. Analysis of the 583 cases revealed that errors occurred most frequently in the testing phase, defined as failure to order, report, and follow-up laboratory results (44%).[14]
Study evaluating the assessment and management of severe hyponatremia in a large teaching hospital	Incorrect diagnoses were found in 42% of patients and significant management errors in 33%. Among patients with management errors, a significant percentage died (41%).[15]
Study of patients referred to an autoimmune disease center	Misdiagnosis of autoimmune disease by primary care physicians was common. "Of those referred with SLE, 29% were seropositive for antinuclear antibodies but did not have autoimmune disease." In many cases, ANA positive patients who were incorrectly diagnosed with autoimmune disease were treated with high-dose corticosteroid therapy.[16]

Rule # 86   If you are asked to draw blood, realize that errors in specimen collection are common, and have the potential to impact patient care and management.

Do you know how to draw blood? Most students enter clerkships with the assumption that the hardest part of the blood draw is finding the vein. It's not. The entire blood draw must be done correctly, or else a pre-analytical lab test error may occur. These can be serious, especially since they're hard to recognize. Even something as seemingly irrelevant as the order that the tubes are filled is important. If you draw blood without paying attention to the order in which you fill the different tubes, the patient may be harmed.

Since lab test results impact 60-70% of all critical patient care decisions, it is imperative that test results reflect the patient's actual physiology. However, results may be affected by improper specimen collection. If this isn't recognized, clinicians may misdiagnose or mismanage patients. These errors may even be life-threatening.

As a student, you will be asked to draw blood. You must realize that errors can and do occur during blood collection and processing. Blood may be drawn from the wrong patient. The specimen tube may be mislabeled. The wrong tube may be sent to the lab. Blood may be drawn at an improper time of the day. A test that is thought to be a fasting value may be performed after an inadequate period of fasting. Blood cultures may be drawn without careful attention to sterile site preparation. Venipuncture technique may be suboptimal, leading to hemolysis with significant alteration of lab test results.

This list goes on and on, but all are examples of the types of pre-analytical errors that commonly occur in hospitals on a daily basis. In fact, it's estimated that pre-analytical errors may cost a 400-bed hospital over $200,000 per year.[17] Putting cost aside, the real concern is how clinicians act upon the test results. Will the physician recognize the error? Or will it be viewed as a true abnormality? If the latter, the actions or inactions of the clinician may place the patient at serious risk of harm. An awareness of common pre-analytical errors will allow you to take steps to avoid these errors.

Did you know...

Lab tests performed on blood drawn from an extremity being infused with intravenous fluids can be drastically altered. The diluted blood specimen may yield test results that are not at all representative of the patient's actual physiology. If the clinician acts on wrong information with a change in treatment, the ensuing actions may seriously harm the patient.

Did you know...

Specimen collection tubes containing additives must be filled to the proper level. Underfilling of tubes is a common pre-analytical error that can significantly alter test results. For example, if sodium citrate or blue stopper tubes are underfilled, the result may be a falsely prolonged PT or aPTT levels, due to an inappropriate proportion between blood and anticoagulant. Laboratories screen specimens to make sure they are acceptable before performing testing. However, despite these safeguards, underfilled tubes may still be accepted. If the clinician doesn't recognize the error, and instead acts on the test results, the patient is in danger. In one study, 464 of 15,335 prothrombin time samples received by a laboratory were rejected.[18] The most common reason for specimen rejection was underfilling (60%).

Did you know...

When multiple specimen tubes are needed, take care not to violate the rules governing the order of draw. Some blood collection tubes contain an additive, and carry-over of the additive from one tube to another can significantly alter test results.[19] This happens when the needle used to fill one tube transfers some of the blood-additive combination into the next tube. For example, if anticoagulant in one tube is transferred to a blue top tube for measurement of coagulation studies, it can falsely lengthen coagulation times. This may prompt an evaluation for a coagulation disorder in a patient with normal coagulation. For patients receiving anticoagulation therapy such as heparin, the clinician may interpret the falsely elevated result to mean that the patient is overmedicated with heparin. The result may be a decrease in heparin dosage and an increased risk of clotting. Carry-over may also make an under-medicated patient receiving heparin therapy falsely appear therapeutically anti-coagulated.

You should always follow your institution's protocol for order of draw. For more information, visit the Clinical and Laboratory Standards Institute website (http://www.clsi.org/). The organization has developed a standard order in which tubes must be filled.

Did you know...

Hemolysis during blood specimen collection can occur, and is a common reason for specimen rejection in the lab. The destruction of red blood cells with release of their contents into the serum or plasma can lead to falsely elevated potassium, AST, ALT, phosphorus, magnesium, and LDH levels. Following centrifugation, hemolysis is readily apparent because it leads to a red tinge.

Did you know...

After you draw blood, take the specimens to the lab as soon as possible. After blood collection, cells remain metabolically active. A delay in specimens reaching the lab is a major cause of abnormal results. The best example is with arterial blood gases, where even a slight delay can lead to significant changes in test results.

Rule # 87   Develop an approach to determine the cause of the abnormal test result.

Abnormal lab test results may either be related to the patient's chief complaint or may be unrelated to the patient's current illness. We recommend the following with abnormal test results:

Step 1: Look up and learn the differential diagnosis of every one of your patient's abnormal test results.

Step 2: Determine if the abnormal test result supports any of the conditions in the differential diagnosis of your patient's complaints.

Step 3: If the abnormal test result isn't supportive of any of the conditions in the differential diagnosis, consider the possibility that it is unrelated to the patient's current illness.

Step 4: If it is unrelated, develop an approach to determining the etiology.

Tip # 23

Proper interpretation of lab test results requires that you consider sensitivity, specificity, and likelihood of disease.

Step 4 is the most challenging for students, because traditional textbooks of medicine seldom describe approaches or strategies to determine the cause of an abnormal test result. Dr. George Lundberg, Editor in Chief Emeritus of Medscape, describes the situation well. "Guidance on diagnostic testing in medical textbooks often consists of little more than listings of tests that may be abnormal in a given disease." He goes on to state that it is crucial that clinicians have a strategy for interpretation.

This difficulty is recognized by most clinicians. In response to these challenges in lab test interpretation, and in recognition of their importance in patient management and medical errors, we developed a targeted guide to lab test interpretation. This resource, the *Clinician's Guide to Laboratory Medicine: Pocket*, offers a step-by-step approach to lab test interpretation. In the following pages we have reproduced the book's approach to the patient with hyponatremia.

Hyponatremia

Causes of hyponatremia	
Type	**Causes**
Spurious	Drip arm hyponatremia, dead space hyponatremia
Isotonic	Hyperlipidemia, hyperproteinemia, bladder irrigation
Hypertonic	Hyperglycemia, mannitol, maltose
Hypotonic	Hypovolemic • Extrarenal (GI fluid loss [nasogastric suction, vomiting, diarrhea], skin loss of fluid [excessive sweating, burns], third-space fluid loss [bowel obstruction, pancreatitis, peritonitis, trauma]) • Renal (salt-losing nephropathies, diuretic therapy, osmotic diuresis [glucosuria], mineralocorticoid deficiency, ketonuria, bicarbonaturia, cerebral salt-wasting syndrome) Euvolemic – (syndrome of inappropriate antidiuretic hormone [SIADH], adrenal insufficiency, hypothyroidism, primary polydipsia, ↓ intake of solutes [beer drinkers' potomania, tea and toast diet], reset osmostat) Hypervolemic - (CHF, cirrhosis, nephrotic syndrome, acute renal failure, chronic renal failure)

Approach to ↓ Na$^+$:

Step 1: Consider spurious hyponatremia

Hyponatremia is common, occurring in 15 to 22% of hospitalized patients. Before beginning the evaluation of hyponatremia, consider the possibility of spurious hyponatremia.

• Drip arm hyponatremia → when serum Na$^+$ is measured from sample taken upstream from IV infusion of hypotonic fluid.

• Dead space hyponatremia → when blood is taken from central venous line without discarding of the dead space.

If spurious hyponatremia is possible, repeat the serum Na$^+$ level taking care to avoid the above.
If the repeat test result is normal, stop here.
If spurious hyponatremia is not present, proceed to step 2.

Step 2: Measure the plasma osmolality

The evaluation of the hyponatremic patient begins with measurement of the serum osmolality. The serum osmolality can be used to categorize the patient into one of three groups:

- Hypertonic hyponatremia (> 290 mOsm/kg)
- Isotonic hyponatremia (275 – 290 mOsm/kg)
- Hypotonic hyponatremia (<275 mOsm/kg)

If the patient has hypertonic hyponatremia, proceed to step 3.
If the patient has isotonic hyponatremia, proceed to step 4.
If the patient has hypotonic hyponatremia, proceed to step 5.

Step 3: Determine the cause of the hypertonic hyponatremia

Hypertonic hyponatremia is seen with increased glucose or administration of hypertonic mannitol. For every 100 mg/dL increase in the serum glucose over 100 mg/dL, the serum sodium falls by 2.4 mEq/L. If the serum Na+ concentration is decreased to a value lower than expected, evaluate for an additional cause of hyponatremia.

End of section

Step 4: Determine the cause of the isotonic hyponatremia

Causes of isotonic hyponatremia (pseudohyponatremia) include severe hyperproteinemia and hyperlipidemia. These are rare causes of hyponatremia today because of changes in lab methodology used to measure serum sodium levels.

End of section

Step 5: Assess the patient's volume status

Most hyponatremic patients will have hypotonic hyponatremia. To determine the cause of hypotonic hyponatremia, begin by assessing the patient's volume status. Based upon the volume status, the patient can be categorized into one of three groups, as shown in the following table.

Physical exam findings used to assess volume status	
Finding in physical examination	Volume Status
Orthostatic changes in blood pressure and heart rate Dry mucous membranes Flat jugular veins Absence of axillary sweat	Hypovolemic
Peripheral edema Elevated jugular venous pressure Ascites Other signs of CHF, cirrhosis, or nephrotic syndrome	Hypervolemic
No exam findings consistent with hypervolemia or hypovolemia	Euvolemic

These three types of hypotonic hyponatremia are discussed below.

Hypovolemic hypotonic hyponatremia

Causes can be divided into renal and extrarenal (see causes above). If the cause is unclear, obtain urine Na^+ level:

- Urine Na^+ < 20 mEq/L → extrarenal cause
- Urine Na^+ > 20 mEq/L → renal etiology

Hypervolemic hypotonic hyponatremia

Causes include CHF, cirrhosis, nephrotic syndrome, ARF, and CRF. If the cause is unclear, obtain urine Na^+ level:

- If urine Na < 20mEq/L → consider CHF, cirrhosis, and nephrotic syndrome
- If urine Na > 20mEq/L → consider ARF, CRF

Euvolemic hypotonic hyponatremia

In these patients, the urine osmolality can be used to help determine the etiology. Urine osmolality < 100 mOsm/kg should lead to consideration of primary polydipsia or beer drinkers' potomania. The other causes are associated with urine osmolality > 100 mOsm/kg.

Criteria for SIADH, the most common cause of this type of hyponatremia, are listed in the following table.

Essential criteria for SIADH	
Plasma osmolality < 275 mOsm/kg	Normal acid-base balance
Euvolemic volume status	Normal adrenal function
Urine osmolality > 100 Osm/kg	Normal renal function
Urine Na$^=$ level > 40 mEq/L	Normal thyroid function

To diagnose SIADH, hypothyroidism and adrenal insufficiency should be excluded (obtain thyroid function tests and cosyntropin stimulation test).

It can be difficult to differentiate subtle volume depletion from SIADH. SIADH is more likely if the plasma uric acid < 4 mg/dL, BUN < 10 mg/dL, FENA > 1%, and fractional urea excretion > 55%. Failure to correct hyponatremia after administration of 0.9% saline is also supportive of SIADH diagnosis.

Once the diagnosis of SIADH is established, search for the cause.

Causes of SIADH	
Type	**Cause**
Lung disease	Abscess, chronic obstructive pulmonary disease, pneumonia (bacterial, viral), tuberculosis, aspergillosis, asthma, bronchiectasis, empyema, cystic fibrosis, pneumothorax, respiratory failure with positive pressure ventilation
CNS disease	Brain tumor, cerebrovascular accident, infection (encephalitis, meningitis, abscess, Rocky Mountain spotted fever, AIDS), subarachnoid hemorrhage, subdural hematoma, acute psychosis, head trauma, cavernous sinus thrombosis, multiple sclerosis, acute intermittent porphyria, Guillan-Barre syndrome, delirium tremens, hydrocephalus, Shy-Drager syndrome
Medications	Chlorpropamide, cyclophosphamide, opiates, carbamazepine, tricyclic antidepressants, vincristine, vinblastine, selective serotonin reuptake inhibitors, oxytocin, ifosamide, desmopressin, lysine vasopressin, clofibrate, prostaglandin synthesis inhibitors, nicotine, antipsychotics, acetaminophen, NSAIDs, bromocriptine, MDMA
Malignancy	Lymphoma, leukemia, lung (small cell, mesothelioma), oropharyngeal carcinoma, GI (duodenal cancer, pancreatic, stomach), genitourinary (bladder, ureter, prostate, endometrium), thymoma, sarcoma
Other	Stress, pain, endurance exercise, nausea, general anesthesia, idiopathic

HYPONATREMIA

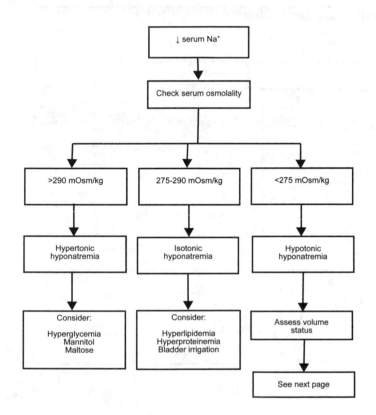

HYPONATREMIA (continued)

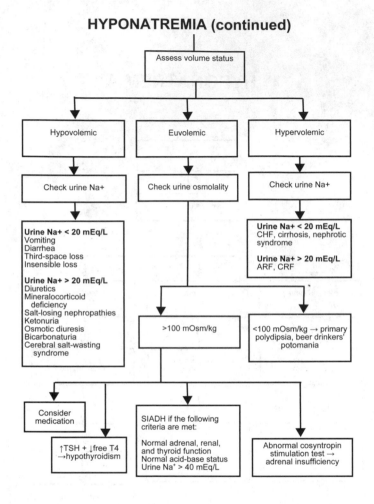

Assess volume status

Hypovolemic → Check urine Na+

Urine Na+ < 20 mEq/L
Vomiting
Diarrhea
Third-space loss
Insensible loss

Urine Na+ > 20 mEq/L
Diuretics
Mineralocorticoid
    deficiency
Salt-losing nephropathies
Ketonuria
Osmotic diuresis
Bicarbonaturia
Cerebral salt-wasting
    syndrome

Euvolemic → Check urine osmolality

>100 mOsm/kg

<100 mOsm/kg → primary polydipsia, beer drinkers' potomania

Hypervolemic → Check urine Na+

Urine Na+ < 20 mEq/L
CHF, cirrhosis, nephrotic syndrome

Urine Na+ > 20 mEq/L
ARF, CRF

Consider medication

↑TSH + ↓free T4 →hypothyroidism

SIADH if the following criteria are met:

Normal adrenal, renal, and thyroid function
Normal acid-base status
Urine Na+ > 40 mEq/L

Abnormal cosyntropin stimulation test → adrenal insufficiency

References

[1]Division of Laboratory Systems, Centers for Disease Control and Prevention. Patient-centered care and laboratory medicine: national status report: 2008-2009 update. https://www.futurelabmedicine.org/ reports%5CLaboratory_Medicine_National_Status_%20Report_08-09_Update-- Patient-Centered_Care.pdf. Published May 2009. Accessed May 18, 2010.

[2]Park Y, Marques M. Teaching medical students basic principles of laboratory medicine. *Clin Lab Med* 2007; 27: 411-24.

[3]Clerkship Directors in Internal Medicine (CDIM) and Society of General Internal Medicine (SGIM). Core Medicine Clerkship Guide: A Resource for Teachers and Learners, Version 3.0. http://www.im.org/Resources/Education/Students/ Learning/Documents/OnlineCDIMCurriculum.pdf. Published 2006. Accessed May 18, 2010.

[4]Smith B, et al. Educating medical students in laboratory medicine: a proposed curriculum. *Am J Clin Pathol* 2010; 133(4): 533-42.

[5]Wong E, Lincoln T, Lundberg G. Ready! Fire!...Aim! An inquiry into laboratory test ordering. *JAMA* 1983; 250 (18): 2510-13.

[6]Ferguson R, Kohler F, ChavezJ, Puthumana J, Zaidi S, Shakil H. Discovering asymptomatic biochemical abnormalities on a Baltimore internal medicine service. *Md Med J* 1996; 45(7): 543-6.

[7]Arce-Cordon R, Perez-Rodriguez M, Baca-Baldomero E, Oquendo M, Baca-Garcia E. Routine laboratory screening among newly admitted psychiatric patients: is it worthwhile? *Psychiatr Serv* 2007; 58(12): 1602-5.

[8]Dzankic S, Pastor D, Gonzalez C, Leung J. The prevalence and predictive value of abnormal preoperative laboratory tests in elderly surgical patients. *Anesth Analg* 2001; 93(2): 249-50.

[9]Hepner D. The role of testing in the preoperative evaluation. *Cleve Clin J Med* 2009; 76 (Suppl 4): S22-7.

[10]Silverstein M, Boland B. Conceptual framework for evaluating laboratory tests: case-finding in ambulatory patients. *Clin Chem* 1994; 40: 1621-7.

[11]Erban S, Kinman J, Schwartz J. Routine use of the prothrombin and partial thromboplastin times. *JAMA* 1989; 262: 2428-32.

[12]Laposata M. CDC Website. http://wwwn.cdc.gov/cliac/pdf/Addenda/cliac0906/ AddendumL.pdf. Accessed January 30, 2011.

[13]Gandhi T, Kachalia A, Thomas E, Puopolo A, Yoon C, Brennan T, et al. Missed and delayed diagnoses in the ambulatory setting: a study of closed malpractice claims. *Ann Intern Med* 2006; 145: 488-96.

[14]Schiff G, Hasan O, Kim S, Abrams R, Cosby K, Lambert B, Elstein AS, Hasler S, Kabongo M, Krosnjar N, Odwazny R, Wisniewski M, McNutt R. Diagnostic error in medicine. *Arch Intern Med* 2009; 169 (20): 1881-7.

[15]Huda M, Boyd A, Skagen K, Wile D, van Heyningen C, Watson I, Wong S, Gill G. Investigation and management of severe hyponatraemia in a hospital setting. *Postgrad Med J* 2006; 82: 216-9.

[16]Narain S, Richards H, Satoh M, Sarmiento M, Davidson R, Shuster J, Sobel E, Hahn P, Reeves W. Diagnostic accuracy for lupus and other systemic autoimmune diseases in the community setting. *Arch Intern Med* 2004; 164(22): 2435-41.

[17]Paxton A. Stamping out specimen collection errors. *CAP Today* 1999; 13(5): 1, 14-16, 18.

[18]Goswami B, Tayal D, Chawla R, Mallika V. Pre-analytical factors that influence the interpretation of prothrombin time in the clinical laboratory: one year experience in a super specialty hospital in India. *Clin Chim Acta* 2009; 410(1-2): 93-4.

[19]Calam R, Cooper M. Recommended "order of draw" for collection blood specimens into additive-containing tubes. *Clin Chem* 1982; 28: 1399.

Chapter 13

Ancillary Tests

For a medical student directly involved in patient care, the correct interpretation of electrocardiograms (ECG) and chest radiographs (CXR) is a vital skill. These are commonly ordered tests, and they provide a wealth of important information in the evaluation and management of patients with a wide variety of disease.

Medical educators agree, and have made ECG and CXR interpretation a priority during clerkships. In a survey of internal medicine clerkship directors, 89% and 81% of respondents agreed that ECG and CXR interpretation, respectively, were important clinical skills for medical students.[1, 2]

Rule # 88   Errors in ECG and CXR interpretation are common. Take advantage of all opportunities to read these studies.

In a study of resident proficiency, 120 internal medicine and emergency medicine residents were asked to take a test containing 12 electrocardiograms.[3] For each ECG, residents were instructed to write a diagnosis and record their level of certainty. Residents had considerable difficulty making critical diagnoses such as myocardial infarction, ventricular tachycardia, and complete heart block. Surprisingly, 58% of residents wrongly diagnosed complete heart block. Only 22% of residents were certain in their diagnosis of ventricular tachycardia.

Residents find CXR interpretation difficult as well. In one study, researchers had third year medical students, IM interns, IM residents, and fellows from the divisions of cardiology and pulmonary/critical care view ten chest x-rays.[4] The chosen x-rays included common conditions as well as 3 examples of radiographic emergencies – pneumothorax, misplaced central venous catheter, and pneumoperitoneum. Participants were asked to record the diagnosis along with their certainty in that diagnosis. Median overall score for the entire group is shown in the following table.

Overall Score by Level of Training	
Learner (number)	Overall score (0-20)
Medical student (25)	8.0
Internal medicine intern (44)	10.0
Internal medicine resident (45)	12.8
Fellow (16)	15.0
Radiology resident (15)	17.5

From Eisen L, Berger J, Hegde A, Schneider R. Competency in chest radiography. A comparison of medical students, residents, and fellows. *J Gen Intern Med* 2006; 21(5): 460-5.

While the overall score did increase with increased level of training, the results of this study were extremely concerning. In the three emergency situations, pneumothorax was misdiagnosed by 91% of participants overall. Misplaced central venous catheter was misdiagnosed by 74%, while pneumoperitoneum was misdiagnosed by 54%.

As a student, you will receive instruction in the interpretation of ECGs and CXRs during your third year of medical school. ECG instruction is provided in 92% of internal medicine clerkships, either through lectures, teaching rounds, or both.[1] Most internal medicine clerkships (76%) also offer instruction in CXR interpretation.[2]

Did you know...

The Department of Radiology at the Indiana University School of Medicine writes that "no matter what specialty they go into, medical students need to acquire a basic understanding of radiology and its use in contemporary medical practice. First, they need to know what tests to order....Students also need to acquire basic skills in image interpretation so that they are adequately prepared for postgraduate training."[5]

Electrocardiogram

Rule # 89   You will be asked to perform ECGs. Learn the proper lead placement to avoid errors.

As a student, you may be asked to perform ECGs. This may not appear technically difficult, but proper lead placement is critical. Misplacement of leads can lead to misinterpretation of ECGs. This may result in incorrect diagnoses and subsequent mismanagement.

The results of one study indicated that "nurses and doctors do not know the correct positions for ECG electrodes." To ascertain the reliability of ECG precordial lead placement, researchers recruited a group of physicians, nurses, and cardiac technicians.[6] Study participants were asked to mark on diagrams of the chest where they would place leads V1-V6. Tremendous variation in lead placement was found. Although most cardiac technicians (90%) correctly identified the position of V1, only 49% and 31% of nurses and physicians, respectively, were able to do so. Of particular concern was the changes in ECG that incorrect lead placement introduced, placing patients "at risk of potentially harmful therapeutic procedures."

The possible consequences of lead misplacement were examined in a study of both healthy volunteers and patients with ECG signs of inferior myocardial infarction. Deliberate, defined lead misplacement was able to introduce ECG findings of inferior ischemia in the healthy volunteers.

Researchers were also able to show that abnormal ECGs in patients with ischemic heart disease could be turned to normal with lead misplacement. "Such artifacts can probably reach clinical importance in evaluating patients. For example, recognition of ischemic heart disease is important in a preoperative assessment because these patients need peri- and post-operative treatment with beta-blockers."[7]

Tip # 24

Lead misplacement is common. In one study of over 11,000 ECGs, lead misplacement was found in 2% by automated electrocardiogram analysis software.[8] Suspect lead misplacement if you note one of the following: positive P wave in lead aVR, negative P waves in lead I and/or II, QRS axis between 180 and -90 degrees, abnormal R wave progression in the precordial leads, and very low amplitude in an isolated peripheral lead (<0.1 mV).[9]

Recently, an excellent review was published of the technical mistakes that occur during the acquisition of the electrocardiogram.[10]

Garcia-Niebla J, Llontop-Garcia P, Valle-Racero J, Serra-Autonell G, Batchvarov V, de Luna A. Technical mistakes during the acquisition of the electrocardiogram. *Ann Noninvasive Electrocardiol* 2009; 14(4): 389-403.

Tip # 25

The ECG tracing is often accompanied by a computer generated diagnostic interpretation. The analysis by the computer is often but not always correct, and should not replace your own systematic review. In one study, there was significant disagreement (10% of ECGs) between cardiologist and computer interpretation.[11] The most common computer interpretation errors involved diagnosis of arrhythmias, conduction disturbances, and electronic pacemakers.

Rule # 90   Analyze every ECG systematically.

To catch critical information, it is essential that you analyze every study systematically. If you haven't been introduced to a system, check with your intern or resident. Below is one systematic approach to the ECG. No matter which system you adopt, use your approach consistently.

Systematic Approach to ECG Interpretation

Rate
Rhythm
Intervals (PR, QRS, QT)
Blocks
Axis
Hypertrophy
Conduction disturbances
Myocardial injury/infarction
ST-segment changes
T-wave changes
Q waves
Changes from previous ECG

Don't be surprised if the attending asks you to interpret an ECG during rounds, especially with your own patients. Prepare for this in advance:

- Interpret the study on your own in a systematic manner.

- Review the ECG with your resident or intern. Ask them to comment on your interpretation.

- Know the criteria for any ECG abnormalities that are present (e.g., left bundle branch block), as well as the clinical significance of the findings.

- Establish a differential diagnosis. Dr. J. Willis Hurst writes that "a differential diagnosis should be created when the electrocardiogram is abnormal. The statement that there is bundle-branch block, or some other electrophysiologic-anatomic abnormality, is not a clinical diagnosis. The clinical differential diagnosis should include the diseases that might be responsible for the abnormal ECG."[12]

Chest radiograph

Rule # 91   Before interpretation, assess the technical quality of the film.

If the technical quality of the film isn't examined, clinicians can easily draw the wrong conclusions. Key questions to ask:

- Is there adequate penetration?
- Is the film taken in full inspiration?
- Is there adequate rotation?

With underpenetrated and overpenetrated chest films, pulmonary markings may appear to be more or less prominent than they really are. This can easily lead you to believe that there is disease, when there is not, or miss disease when it is present. A chest film with poor inspiration effort can cause compression of the lung markings, incorrectly suggesting pneumonia or another process.

Rule # 92   Analyze every CXR systematically.

As with the ECG, a systematic approach is best. Below are two systematic approaches to the CXR. No matter which system you adopt, use your approach consistently.

Systematic Approach to Chest X-ray Interpretation	
One approach[13]	ABC approach[14]
Patient name	Patient name
Date of study	Date of study
Comment on:	Comment on:
- whether it is a PA or AP film	- whether it is a PA or AP film
- rotation of the patient	- rotation of the patient
- adequacy of inspiration	- adequacy of inspiration
- penetration of the film	- penetration of the film
- exposure of the film	- exposure of the film
Soft tissues	A – airway and adenopathy
Trachea	B – bones and breast shadows
Bony thorax/ribs	C – cardiac silhouette
Intercostal spaces	D – diaphragm
Diaphragm	E – everything else
Structures below diaphragm	F – fields (lung)
Pleural surfaces	G – gastric air bubble
Mediastinum	H – hilum
Hila	Comparison with previous chest film
Lung fields	
Catheters, tubes, wires, lines	
Comparison with previous chest film	

The attending will often ask you to interpret a chest film during rounds, especially with your own patients. Prepare for this in advance:

- Interpret the study on your own in a systematic manner.
- Review the chest film with your resident or intern. Ask them to comment on your interpretation.
- Review imaging studies with the radiologist.
- Establish a differential diagnosis for the radiographic abnormalities that are present.
- Interpret the findings in the context of the patient's clinical presentation.

Tip # 26

You may also be asked to interpret the study of a patient that you aren't following. While some students freeze, remember that you aren't expected to be proficient with ECG or chest film interpretation. The attending has involved you because you only improve with experience and practice. When asked to interpret a study, allow yourself 15 to 20 seconds to simply look at the study. Then proceed to describe the findings using a systematic approach.

Rule # 93   X-rays are a tool. They're a valuable tool, but you have to recognize their limitations.

Imaging studies provide valuable information that supplements your clinical findings. However, they are a tool, and must be utilized properly. This includes recognizing their limitations.

A colleague on the pediatrics faculty related the case of a young child who presented with a tender abdomen. The child had already been in the emergency room for hours when she evaluated the patient. The abdomen was tender when the child presented, but imaging studies weren't conclusive. While the surgeon wasn't sure, he was ready to take the child to the OR if she hadn't improved. On exam, however, the child was showing signs of respiratory distress. She moved straight to the pulmonary exam, and auscultation and percussion all indicated a pulmonary effusion. "This was the frustrating part-the staff just wasn't buying it. 'But the chest x-ray's completely clear!" She had the staff proceed with treatment anyway, and when the chest x-ray was repeated several hours later, the pneumonia was glaringly obvious. It's known in pediatrics that pneumonia can present as an acute abdomen. The other rule: x-ray findings can lag behind clinical findings.[15]

References

[1]O'Brien K, Cannarozzi M, Torre D, Mechaber A, Durning S. Training and assessment of ECG interpretation skills: results from the 2005 CDIM survey. *Teach Learn Med* 2009; 21(2): 111-5.

[2]O'Brien K, Cannarozzi M, Torre D, Mechaber A, Durning S. Training and assessment of CXR/basic radiology interpretation skills: results form the 2005 CDIM Survey. *Teach Learn Med* 2008; 20(2): 157-62.

[3]Berger J, Eisen L, Nozad V, D'Angelo J, Calderon Y, Brown D, Schweitzer P. Competency in electrocardiogram interpretation among internal medicine and emergency medicine residents. *Am J Med* 2005; 118(8): 873-80.

[4]Eisen L, Berger J, Hegde A, Schneider R. Competency in chest radiography. A comparison of medical students, residents, and fellows. *J Gen Intern Med* 2006; 21(5): 460-5.

[5]Gunderman R, Siddiqui A, Heitkamp D, Kipfer H. The vital role of radiology in the medical school curriculum. *AJR* 2003; 180: 1239-42.

[6]Rajaganeshan R, Ludlam C, Francis D, Parasramka S, Sutton R. Accuracy in ECG lead placement among technicians, nurses, general physicians and cardiologists. *Int J Clin Pract* 2008; 62(1): 65-70.

[7]Rudiger A, Schob L, Follath F. Influence of electrode misplacement on the electrocardiographic signs of inferior myocardial ischemia. *Am J Emerg Med* 2003; 21(7): 574-7.

[8]Heden B, Ohlsson M, Edenbrandt L, et al. Artificial neural networks for recognition of electrocardiographic lead reversal. *Am J Cardiol* 1995; 75: 929-33.

[9]Rudiger A, Hellerman J, Mukherjee R, Follath F, Turina J. Electrocardiographic artifacts due to electrode misplacement and their frequency in different clinical settings. *Am J Emerg Med* 2007; 25(2): 174-8.

[10]Garcia-Niebla J, Llontop-Garcia P, Valle-Racero J, Serra-Autonell G, Batchvarov V, de Luna A. Technical mistakes during the acquisition of the electrocardiogram. *Ann Noninvasive Electrocardiol* 2009; 14(4): 389-403.

[11]Guglin M, Thatai D. Common errors in computer electrocardiogram interpretation. *Int J Cardiol* 2006; 106(2): 232-7.

[12]Hurst J. Electrocardiographic crotchets or common errors made in the interpretation of the electrocardiogram. *Clin Cardiol* 1998; 21(3): 211-6.

[13]Siela D. Chest radiograph evaluation and interpretation. *AACN Adv Crit Care* 2008; 19(4): 444-73.

[14]Crausman R. The ABCs of chest x-ray film interpretation. *Chest* 1998; 113: 256-7.

[15]Nield L, Mahajan P, Kamat D. Pneumonia: update on causes – and treatment options. *Consultant for Pediatricians*. http://www.consultantlive.com/pediatrics/content/article/10162/12019. Accessed January 31, 2011.

Chapter 14

Attending Rounds

Attending rounds are a formal meeting of the team, led by the attending physician, that centers on patient care. A secondary goal of rounds is medical education. Your main interactions with attendings will occur during rounds. In earlier times, rounds meant physically rounding on the patient and incorporated more bedside teaching. Now, the bulk of rounds may occur while sitting down in the team room. In this chapter, we discuss aspects of rounds that center on patient care and patient comfort. This chapter also includes rules that enhance your clinical education as well as ensure rotation success in your interactions with attendings.

Rule # 94   Prepare.

Preparation for rounds begins the evening before. Since attending rounds usually take place on a daily basis, this means working every evening. If you're post-call, you'll present newly admitted patients, and may be asked to provide updates on established patients. If you haven't admitted, then the entire rounds may focus on issues pertaining to established patients on the service. Usually the attending will ask the student or intern for an update on the hospital course. In general, patients who are severely ill or have complex medical issues are almost always discussed, and usually before any other issues are tackled. If you're involved in the care of such a patient, the attending will be hearing from you.

   Other activities may also occur, such as talks given by team members, including students. The key point here is to anticipate what's likely to take place during the next day's rounds, and focus your preparation accordingly.

Did you know...

In an observational study of pediatric rounds at a university-affiliated hospital, much more time was spent discussing new patients than established patients (14.9 minutes versus 2.5 minutes per patient). In most sessions, rounds began with a discussion of all new admissions. The greatest amount of time was spent on the first patient discussed.[1]

Rule # 95   **While critical to your education, bedside teaching should first and foremost ensure the comfort of the patient.**

Bedside teaching is any teaching that occurs in the presence of a patient. Over the years, studies have shown that the percentage of time spent in attending rounds at the bedside is on the decline. In fact, some attendings don't conduct any bedside rounds whatsoever, preferring to round solely in the conference room. Most, however, will split teaching time between the conference room, the hallway, and the bedside.

Did you know...

As the years have passed, less and less time is spent teaching at the bedside. In the 1960s, 75% of attending rounds occurred at the bedside.[2] This percentage has fallen considerably, with one observational study from the 1990s showing that only 11% of attending physician time was spent at the bedside.[3]

Students worry about the impact of bedside rounds on their patients, especially with regard to patient comfort. A patient's comfort level will depend on a number of factors, including what's done at the bedside and how it's done. Several studies have shown that patients generally enjoy bedside visits from the team. However, this is only if team members conduct themselves appropriately, with respect and sensitivity. These rules should govern your conduct at the bedside:

- Inform your patient, in advance, that you'll be returning with the team for bedside rounds. Let the patient know what will happen during rounds.
- After the team enters the patient's room, close the door to ensure privacy.
- Introduce all team members, including the attending physician.
- Make the same introductions with any family members present. Ask the patient if he would like family to stay.
- Before interacting with the patient, wash your hands.
- If the patient is sharing the room, pull the bedside curtain to ensure privacy.
- If the television or radio is on, ask for permission to turn it off.
- If you are paged during bedside rounds, don't answer using the patient's telephone or other phone in the room.
- Don't carry on side conversations with other team members.
- Don't laugh at anything the patient says, unless it is, without a doubt, a joke.
- Don't bring coffee, soft drinks, or other beverages into the patient's room.
- Don't chew gum while in the patient's room.
- Don't lean against the wall.

- Don't sit on the patient's bed or place any of your items on the patient's furniture unless you have permission to do so.
- Before leaving the room, ask the patient if he has any questions.

At the bedside, attendings will usually ask the patient questions to clarify and confirm what they've heard from the team. They do so to ensure that they have an understanding of the patient's story, which is essential to patient care. Don't be surprised when the patient's story of his illness differs from your own. Attendings see this all the time, and it doesn't necessarily reflect poorly on your abilities. It's happened to everyone at some point, and often on more than one occasion. While this is frustrating, repeated questioning can bring forth new information that has bearing on the diagnosis and management.

During the physical exam, the attending will determine if the physical findings documented by the team are, in fact, present. They may also uncover new findings. If there are aspects of the physical exam that gave you difficulty, inform the attending beforehand so that he can demonstrate the proper exam technique. As always, keep the patient appropriately draped during the exam.

Tip # 27

In one study of medical students and residents, 89% of respondents reported that two or fewer physical diagnosis skills were taught or reviewed per day of rounds.[4] Forty-five percent reported less than 1 skill taught per day. Attending physicians understand the importance of teaching physical exam skills, but sometimes find it difficult to do so because of multiple demands placed on their time during rounds. Sometimes, a gentle request is all that's needed. "Dr. Bernstein, one area that I'm having trouble with is assessing JVP. Do you think you might be able to help me with this sometime over the next few days?"

Rule # 96   **Bedside presentations must be made with a constant awareness of the patient next to you.**

Usually you'll present the patient before you reach the bedside. Some attendings, though, prefer that you present at the bedside. Bedside presentations require a number of changes:

- Present with sensitivity.
- Don't ignore the patient during your presentation. Periodically make eye contact with the patient, especially when repeating the story of their illness.
- Don't refer to the patient by first name.
- Present in such a way that the patient understands what you are saying.

- Avoid using the words "denies" or "admits" as in
  abdominal pain" or "patient admits to drinking 5 b
- Avoid detailed discussions of differential diagnos
  confuse or even frighten the patient. Save these
  discussions for the team room.
- Avoid use of the word "cancer" unless the attending has given
  permission in advance.

Always find out in advance the attending's ground rules for bedside presentations. In particular, you need to know what can and cannot be discussed at the bedside.

Rule # 97   Strive to function at the highest student level.

Within the past few years, a new method of evaluating students has
gained popularity in clerkships across the country. This system is called
the RIME method and stands for

Reporter	**I**nterpreter	**M**anager	**E**ducator

Dr. Pangaro, who developed the RIME method, describes four stages in
a student's development.[5]

In the first or lowest stage, students are reporters. Students are said
to have mastered this stage if they:

- Consistently and reliably take an excellent history and physical
  exam
- Present patients or report patient data consistently, reliably,
  concisely, and in an organized manner, clearly communicating
  the key issues (oral and written communication)

Note that you've already been introduced to your function as a reporter
during your basic science years. Your physical diagnosis course focused
on developing your ability to perform a history and physical exam. Now, in
your clerkships, your goal is to master this role and then proceed to the
next stage, that of an interpreter.

It is vital that you master the reporter stage, because educators
believe that by the end of a clerkship, at the very least, students should
reach this level. Students who have mastered their role as a reporter, but
haven't yet mastered the next stage, are generally given a pass for the
rotation, assuming that there are no problems with their professionalism.

For most students, making the transition from reporter to interpreter
is quite difficult. In order to be an interpreter, you must be able to:

- Identify problems (requires the ability to recognize normal and
  abnormal). Problems can include symptoms, physical exam
  findings, abnormal lab tests, and so on
- Prioritize among these identified problems
- Create a differential diagnosis for each problem

- Rank the entities in the differential diagnosis in terms of likelihood

As an example, consider the student who learns that his patient's platelet count is low. He must recognize that thrombocytopenia is a problem. Then he must develop a differential diagnosis for the thrombocytopenia. The term "differential diagnosis" refers to a list of conditions that could account for the problem.

In this example, a student functioning only as a reporter would state:

I just checked to see if today's lab test results came back for Mr. Kim. His platelet count is 110. Yesterday it was 250.

Contrast this with the student functioning as an interpreter:

I just checked to see if today's lab test results came back for Mr. Kim. His platelet count is 110. Yesterday it was 250. **There are many causes of thrombocytopenia but the most likely causes, in Mr. Kim's case, are heparin-induced thrombocytopenia, bone marrow depression due to the effects of alcohol, and splenomegaly. Since I didn't palpate a spleen tip on exam, I believe that bone marrow depression due to alcohol and heparin-induced thrombocytopenia are more likely. I believe that heparin is the cause - he didn't have thrombocytopenia when he was first admitted and it developed five days after starting heparin therapy.**

Students who consistently perform as an "interpreter" are generally given a high pass evaluation. By the end of a clerkship, most students will either be in the reporter or interpreter stage. Some students, however, are able to move past these two stages to reach the "manager" level. These students usually receive the highest evaluation of honors.

Students who are at the "manager" level are able to recommend a particular diagnostic test or course of treatment tailored to their patient's clinical situation. This is an example of a student functioning as a manager:

I just checked to see if today's lab test results came back for Mr. Kim. His platelet count is 110. Yesterday it was 250. There are many causes of thrombocytopenia but the most likely causes, in Mr. Kim's case, are heparin-induced thrombocytopenia, bone marrow depression due to the effects of alcohol, and splenomegaly. Since I didn't palpate a spleen tip on exam, I believe that bone marrow depression due to alcohol and heparin-induced thrombocytopenia are more likely. I believe that heparin is the cause since he didn't have thrombocytopenia when he was first admitted and it developed five days after starting heparin therapy. **I propose that we discontinue the heparin and switch to another form of therapy for DVT prophylaxis. If the platelet count returns to normal after stopping the heparin, then we'll have confirmed the diagnosis.**

Most of the statement describes reporting and interpretin
tion. In the bolded portion, the student takes it a step furt
strating that he's also managing the patient.

Functioning as a manager isn't easy for students. Soi
culty has to do with inexperience. As a student, you simpl, ...
a condition as often as the rest of the team. Your lack of experience, however, shouldn't prevent you from making efforts to manage your patient's
problems. Always try to come up with a plan, and share it with the team.
They won't expect that your plan will always be correct, but they will be
pleased with your efforts to manage the patient. Since many students
stop at the reporter or interpreter stage, your attempts to manage the
patient will set you apart.

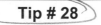

Tip # 28

Even when unsure, outstanding students will offer a plan. Team members are impressed with students who have given a problem considerable thought and are brave enough to recommend a course of action.

It's rare for a student to reach the educator stage during a clerkship. At
the "educator" level, students demonstrate that they are the team's expert
in the area by:

- Being able not only to identify knowledge gaps but also to
  address them
- Reading deeply and sharing new information with others
- Probing the literature to find the evidence that backs up a
  particular course of therapy, diagnostic test, or other action

Share what you learn with the team, and remember that all team members, including the attending, are learners.

While gaining in popularity, the RIME method may not be officially
used in your clerkship. However, many attendings, even if they've never
heard of the RIME method, use the same principles in the evaluation of
their students.

Rule # 98   Pimp questions are a fact of life. Regard them as an opportunity to demonstrate your knowledge and capabilities.

Wear defined pimping "as the clinical practice where persons in power
ask questions of their junior colleagues."[6] In one study, 4th year medical
students were interviewed to determine their views on pimping. All,
except for one, divided pimping into two groups - malignant [or bad] versus benign [or good]. Any question that was asked to embarrass or
humiliate students was viewed as malignant pimping. Although the entire
group of students had witnessed such behavior, they all felt that it was
the exception rather than the rule. It seemed that, in most cases, pimping
had been of the good variety.

As a third year medical student, you will be pimped. Students generally view it as a means for attendings to evaluate their knowledge base. They feel that pimping is a way for attendings to ensure that they're reading about their patients' problems and are knowledgeable about these problems. While this has an evaluative function, there are other reasons why attendings ask questions. Doing so allows the attending to determine your learning needs to enable teaching to your level. Attendings also ask questions to stimulate students, keep them engaged, and monitor their progress.

Embrace these teaching sessions. While you may be anxious, recognize that these sessions are a great opportunity to demonstrate your knowledge and capabilities.

Did you know...

According to Brancati, the origins of the term *pimping* can be traced back to 17th century London.[7] The practice made its way to North America in the 20th century, and was documented by Abraham Flexner in his observations of rounds led by Osler at Johns Hopkins.

Did you know...

Detsky described the typical pimping process. "...the faculty member selects 1 or more of the participants to respond. If the first student cannot correctly answer, another student is chosen, and so on until someone answers the question correctly. If no one answers the question correctly, the attending does."[8]

Rule # 99   **Prepare for both clarifying and probing questions.**

You have a much higher chance of answering questions correctly if you prepare properly. Start the evening before rounds by anticipating the next day's questions. If you'll be presenting a newly admitted patient, then expect questions about that patient's illness. Questions generally fall into one of two categories:

Clarifying questions

A clarifying question is one that an attending asks to ensure his understanding of the patient's clinical presentation. Examples include "How did he describe his pain?" and "How has the serum creatinine changed since his last visit to his primary care physician?" Your odds of answering these questions increase significantly if you perform a thorough history and physical examination, organize the data, and have it readily accessible.

Probing questions

A probing question is one that an attending may ask to gauge your knowledge and understanding of the patient's medical problems. Examples include "What are the physical exam findings of aortic stenosis?" and

"What does S3 indicate to you?" To field these questions you must be well read about your patient's medical problems.

Rule # 100   Answer questions with confidence. Avoid the "I think that," "I may be wrong but," "I'm not sure but" .... and the killer question mark.

Your goal is to answer the attending's questions with confidence. It's not possible to have the answers to every potential question, and you may not always be confident about your answers. However, many students answer correctly, but ruin the effect of their correct answer with their phrasing. A classic example is the student who phrases his response in the form of a question:

Attending: What are the two major causes of acute pancreatitis in the United States?
Student: Aren't alcohol and gallstones the two major causes?

Some students will preface their response with the words "I think" when, in fact, they know.

Attending: What are the two major causes of acute pancreatitis in the United States?
Student: I think alcohol and gallstones are the two major causes.

Don't diminish the strength of your responses with the words "I think." Also, avoid responses that begin with:

"I may be wrong but ..."
"I'm not sure but ..."

Both are examples of how students discount their response before they ever provide it. In her book *Thinking on Your Feet,* Marian Woodall said that when asked questions, "Many people give mediocre responses with superb delivery; they generally fare better than those with good responses and mediocre delivery skills."[9]

Rule # 101   It's not enough to answer questions with confidence. Obviously, you have to be right.

Of course, it's not enough to answer questions confidently – you must also answer them correctly. How can you maximize your chances of doing so? First, utilize multiple sources of information to learn about your patient's medical conditions. Too often, students rely heavily or entirely on handbooks. While these are helpful, you should also utilize the larger, more authoritative texts, as well as checking online sources for the recent medical literature on the subject. Handbooks are often geared to students and residents. However, your attending will have a deeper working knowledge of the patient's problems based on his reading of larger texts, the literature and years of practical experience.

Tip # 29

Among students, small handbooks are popular because they are concise and relatively inexpensive. However, many handbooks lack the depth and breadth of information required to take care of patients on a day-to-day basis. For this reason, it's important that you use one of the larger textbooks of that field, recognizing that it too, at times, may fail to provide you with the necessary information. If you need the most current information, then you need to perform a Medline search.

An attending's initial questions may not be all that difficult. Many will begin with questions that they would expect an average student to answer. These questions generally require simple recall of factual information. In fact, some data indicates that 70% of questions asked by teachers involve simple recall.[10] Handbooks are particularly useful in helping you answer these questions. As you field these initial questions successfully, the attending may then ask more difficult questions. Often, these are open-ended questions such as "What do you think about...?", "What would you do at this point?", and "What if this patient were 70 instead of 35?" For example, Dr. Samuels, a faculty member at the Penn State University College of Medicine, engages students by "asking them questions...what are you thinking...how do these two go together...if this were different what would you do?"[11]

Although these may be questions that he would expect an intern or resident to answer, they may be posed to you first. These questions require that students offer an explanation, and cannot be answered by simply recalling a fact. You can increase your chances of answering these questions correctly if you turn to the larger texts and the recent literature. Especially useful are recent review articles.

Did you know...

In an observational study of pediatric rounds at a university-affiliated hospital, when medical students spoke, it was most often to present patient data and answer questions. Most questions asked by the attending physician dealt with the factual details of the case under discussion. However, nearly 20% of questions "required analysis of data or the demonstration of deeper thinking processes."[1]

Many attending questions deal with different aspects of the patient's diagnosis. For example, if your patient has acute pancreatitis, you should be prepared to answer questions about the incidence, epidemiology, pathogenesis, risk factors, differential diagnosis, clinical features (symptoms and signs), laboratory studies, imaging and other diagnostic tests, prognosis, complications, and therapy of this condition.

While you may be tempted to focus your reading only on the illness that prompted the hospitalization, you should read about the patient's other medical problems as well. This will enhance patient care if and when they become active. For example, a patient may come in with asthma exacerbation. The past medical history reveals a history of diabetes mellitus. In such a case, the student typically becomes very well informed about asthma exacerbation, but spends little or no time reading about diabetes. When the patient is placed on corticosteroids as therapy of the asthma exacerbation, the blood sugar may increase. Some students can't handle this effect, because they didn't review the management of diabetes.

Did you know...

The UCLA Department of Medicine encourages students to "read about every diagnosis your patient has and understand why they have received each of the therapies provided to them in the past and present."[12] The reasons for this recommendation are:

1) Learning and understanding everything about your patient is expected of you by your team.

2) Understanding every detail will allow you to deliver stronger patient presentations and write better notes.

3) It is easier to remember material when you can tie it to a patient you have followed.

As you read, try to anticipate questions the attending may ask. Make a list of possible questions and prepare answers to those questions. Practice by feeding questions to yourself or having someone else do so. Unlike standardized exams or basic science exams, you won't be given a choice of five different answers. Too often, students remember reading about something but aren't able to retrieve the information and express it properly.

Tip # 30

If another student can't answer a question, refrain from jumping in, no matter how tempting it may be. Wait until you are asked the question or it is thrown out to the entire group. Never make a colleague look bad.

Rule # 102   Deliver your responses concisely.

Your goal in answering questions during rounds is to deliver your responses as concisely as possible. If you're asked a question and have no idea of the correct answer, you should simply say, "I don't know, but I will find out." Sometimes students ramble on in a variety of directions, in the hope that they'll stumble upon the right answer. They end up providing a long-winded response that's usually incorrect. If you don't know the answer to a question, say so. Part of being a good physician is recognizing limitations in your knowledge and having the confidence to say, "I don't know."

While many questions are open-ended, others can be answered with either a "yes" or "no." When asked such a question, respond appropriately. If further information is needed, the attending can ask you for it. It's particularly important to answer questions concisely when you're in the operating room. Surgical attendings, at some point in the case, will ask questions about the patient and his problems. If questions are met with long-winded responses, he may cease to ask further questions. As one attending physician told me, "I wish students would avoid diarrhea of the mouth."

Did you know...

Dr. Farhood Farjah, chief surgical resident at the University of Washington School of Medicine, offers advice to students on answering questions. "If you do not know the answer to a question, it is better to say, 'I don't know, but I will look it up.' Some people suggest stating everything you know about the general topic. In my experience, most people don't have the attention span or patience for this approach. Also, never make up an answer. You will be setting yourself up for heavier interrogation."[13]

Rule # 103   Unanswered questions that arise during rounds should always be addressed. By you.

During rounds, a question may arise for which no one has the answer. This happens often, and these questions often remain unanswered. In one study, 1,101 questions were asked by family physicians during over 700 hours of observation in clinical settings.[14] Only 2 questions led to a formal literature search. In a study of residents, Green found that 280 questions were generated during 404 patient encounters. Over 70% of questions were not pursued, most often due to a lack of time and forgetting the question.[15]

In some cases, the attending may turn to a team member and ask him to research the issue. If no one is asked, you need to do so yourself. You don't need to wait until you're asked - take the initiative to explore the issue on your own. Share your findings with the team, along with a copy of a relevant article.

Tip # 31

Questions that arise in rounds are often not easily ⌐
handbooks or even textbooks. A literature review is ofte
useful sources to begin with include ACP Journal Clu
Database of Systematic Reviews, and UpToDate. All are examples of
easy to search resources that are regularly updated with information from
the recent literature.

Rule # 104   Ask questions at the correct time.

While it's not necessary to always seek permission before asking a question, sometimes it can be difficult to know if the time is right. You have to take into account all sorts of factors, ranging from your attending's frame of mind to any time pressures. For example, don't ask questions when a patient's condition has taken a sudden turn for the worse, or during a delicate moment in the operating room.

If you're not sure, you can seek permission. "Dr. Gonzalez, I wanted to ask you about testing for pulmonary embolism. Would now be a good time, or should I wait until later in the week?"

Did you know...

The Department of Surgery at the University of North Carolina School of Medicine offers this advice: "The more you show yourself to be interested, the more people will involve you. By asking questions and asking for opportunities to participate, you show that you are interested in learning. People respond positively to this and whether intentionally or not, they will end up involving you more."[16]

Rule # 105   Read about all of the team's patients.

Although you won't be directly involved in the care of all patients assigned to your team, these other patients will be discussed during attending rounds. You stand to learn much more from these discussions if you read about these patients' problems beforehand. This helps your performance during rounds, as well as in preparation for the clerkship exam. During a two-month clerkship you won't personally encounter all of the medical issues that may be included on the exam.

When other team members are presenting patients, pay close attention. This is not the time to let your mind wander - you never know when the attending may involve you in the discussion. Attendings commonly ask students questions about patients they're not following.

106   Three words: Be On Time.

It is extremely important to arrive on time for attending rounds. Arriving late on just one occasion has been known to negatively impact a student's evaluation. Arriving late indicates that you are inconsiderate, careless, or disrespectful.

Unfortunately, this is one of those obvious mistakes that students manage to make time and time again. Many students find themselves becoming complacent as the rotation progresses. Many attendings don't adhere to their own rules, arriving well past their designated start time. If this happens frequently, team members begin to mirror the attending's bad habit. In an effort to take advantage of the time available, residents will scurry in and out of the team room instead of waiting for rounds to begin. While it may be tempting to leave the team room to take care of a task on your to-do list, don't do it. Some attendings operate with the idea that rounds begin when they arrive, in which case your absence will be noticed. Be punctual not only at the beginning, but also throughout, the rotation.

Rule # 107   If you're late to rounds, or if you have to leave early, for any reason, explain yourself.

While attendings expect the entire team to arrive on time for rounds, considerably more leeway is afforded to interns and residents. They have many more demands on their time, some of which may arise just before rounds. While students are also responsible for patient care, it's felt that these responsibilities are seldom pressing enough to interfere with attending rounds. Exceptions to this rule include:

- There may be a time when a patient problem prevents you from being on time (i.e., Mr. Smith develops chest pain five minutes before starting rounds). In these cases, patient care takes precedence.

- The resident may realize that she forgot to check out patient films from the radiology file room for the attending's review. If she realizes this five minutes before rounds begin, she may send you in her place.

- It is common for a conference or lecture to extend past its scheduled time. This leads to problems when rounds immediately follow the end of the conference. Students can either leave the conference early or inform their attending of the conference schedule, allowing the attending an opportunity to adjust the start time of rounds. Once informed of the schedule, some attendings will simply ask students to join rounds after the conference ends.

In these situations, your attending will understand your reasons for being late. Do not, however, assume that a team member has talked to the attending. Inform the attending yourself at the end of rounds. If you may be delayed because of a conference, it's always better to inform the attending before it happens.

Tip # 32

On the first day of the clerkship, inform your attending of your conference schedule, especially mandatory lectures. Often, attendings aren't familiar with the schedule, let alone which conferences are mandatory.

As a general rule, you also shouldn't leave rounds early. Sometimes, however, it can't be avoided. Certain conferences or lectures are mandatory, even taking precedence over attending rounds. If so, inform your attending ahead of time. Discuss your conference schedule with the attending on the first day of the rotation. If it seems likely that rounds will extend into mandatory lecture time, tell the attending, preferably before rounds, that you have to leave at a specific time. Also apologize for any inconvenience this may cause.

References

[1]Walton J, Steinert Y. Patterns of interaction during rounds: implications for work-based learning. *Med Educ* 2010; 44: 550-8.

[2]Reichsman F, Browning F, Hinshaw J. Observations of undergraduate clinical teaching in action. *Acad Med* 1964; 39: 145-63.

[3]Miller M, Johnson B, Greene H, Baier M, Nowlin S. An observational study of attending rounds. *Med Educ* 1993; 27(6): 503-8.

[4]Gonzalo J, Masters P, Simons R, Chuang C. Attending rounds and bedside case presentations: medical student and medicine resident experiences and attitudes. *Teach Learn Med* 2009; 21(2): 105-10.

[5]Pangaro L. A new vocabulary and other innovations for improving descriptive in-training evaluations. *Acad Med* 1999; 74: 1203-7.

[6]Wear D, Kokinova M, Keck-McNulty C, Aultman J. Pimping: perspectives of 4th year medical students. *Teach Learn Med* 2005; 17(2): 184-91.

[7]Brancati F. The art of pimping. *JAMA* 1989; 262(1): 89-90.

[8]Detsky A. The art of pimping. *JAMA* 2009; 301(13): 1379-81.

[9]Woodall M. *Thinking on your feet, how to communicate under pressure*. Lake Oswego; Oregon Professional Business Communications: 1996.

[10]Williamson K, Ya-Ping K, Steele J, Gunderman R. The art of asking: teaching through questioning. *Acad Radiology* 2002; 9(12): 1419-22.

[11]Taylor E, Tisdell E, Gusic M. Teaching beliefs of medical educators: perspectives on clinical teaching in pediatrics. *Med Teach* 2007; 29: 371-6.

[12]Orientation Outline: Third Year Inpatient Internal Medicine Clerkship at Ronald Reagan UCLA Medical Center. http://medres.med.ucla.edu/Policies/MS-3%20RR-UCLA%20Medical%20Center%20Orientation%20Outline-August%202009.pdf. Accessed January 30, 2011.

[13]Farjah F. Primer For Third Year Surgical Clerkship. http://depts.washington.edu/surgstus/CLERKSHIP/TIPS.html. Updated November 15, 2007. Accessed January 18, 2011.

[14]Ely J. Analysis of questions asked by family doctors regarding patient care. *BMJ* 1999; 319(7206): 358-61.

[15]Green M. Residents' medical information needs in clinic: are they being met? *Am J Med* 2000; 109(3): 218-23.

[16]University of North Carolina Medical Student's Guide to Surgery. http://www.med.unc.edu/surclerk/overview/guide. Accessed January 30, 2011.

Chapter 15

Oral Case Presentations

Developing proficiency in oral communication skills can prove challenging for medical students in many ways. To begin with, you may have limited training in the formal oral case presentation. In one study at a large urban medical school, curricular time spent on clinical skills during the first two years of medical school documented a total of only 12 hours on the oral case presentation.[1]

However, these skills are integral to success as a physician. Every aspiring physician knows the importance of memorization, especially in the basic science years. As you advance in your career, however, communication skills come to the forefront. Physicians with poor communication skills are more likely to be sued.[2] They are more likely to be disciplined by the medical board. They may not receive as many professional referrals from colleagues or word-of-mouth referrals from patients.

Poor communication skills have the potential to directly impact patient care. In a study of malpractice claims, researchers found that incomplete or inaccurate transfer of clinical information frequently occurred between residents and attending physicians. Transfer of information resulted in a patient care error in 32% of cases.[3]

These skills are considered so important that the Association of American Medical Colleges (AAMC) considers the development and acquisition of communication skills a core learning objective for medical students.[4]

In this chapter, you will learn how to effectively transfer important clinical information between team members. During an oral case presentation [OCP] of a newly admitted patient, your goal is to convey the story of the patient's illness, along with the findings of your evaluation, an assessment of the patient's clinical status, and the treatment plan. The term "present" means to tell someone about a case, usually in a formal manner. Most case presentations take place the day following the patient's admission, during attending rounds. In order to make informed decisions about the appropriate diagnostic work-up and therapeutic plan, the attending physician must be given an OCP that is accurate, complete, and concise.

You'll learn the mechanics of the OCP, as well the different facets of oral presentations that affect their quality. In short, you'll learn how to deliver high quality oral case presentations, the type that facilitate patient care, improve team efficiency, become a valuable learning experience, and best reflect your excellence in patient care.

Rule # 108   Follow the correct format when presenting.

There is a proper order to the presentation of patient information. This was highlighted in a survey of internal medicine clerkship directors. An OCP that was "organized systematically according to usual standards" was rated as "very important" by 85% of clerkship directors.[5] OCPs that don't adhere to the expected order are difficult to follow and considered disorganized. A fourth year medical student at UCSF described it:[6]

> Early on, I learned rule one: heed syntax. As one professor put it, "Never order dessert before the salad." In other words, in any presentation, adhere to the chronology that your listeners expect. Hospital training wires physicians to think in the structure and rhythm of the H & P. One swap made, and a student confuses the team. For example, if I give the patient's sodium level before the vital signs, the residents will be wondering, "What was the temperature? Is he hypotensive? I wonder why she gave the labs before the vitals..." And by then I've lost my audience.

The order and content, to some extent, varies by clerkship. During the pediatrics clerkship, you'll be expected to present the patient's birth, neonatal, and feeding history. These elements aren't required during internal medicine.

Even within a clerkship, you may encounter differences when working with different attendings. An order that worked with one attending may not fit the needs of another. Learn your own attending's style and follow a format that suits his preferences. This is the traditional format of the oral case presentation:

Component	Important points for oral case presentation
Patient identification	Start your presentation with the name of the patient, location of the patient, and any other identification required to access medical records (medical record number)
Chief complaint	Keep it one sentence long Include duration of the complaint
History of present illness (HPI)	Make sure it is chronological Discuss chief complaint in more detail (onset, intensity, severity, precipitating factors, relieving factors, progression of illness, other) Include associated symptoms Include pertinent positives and negatives (let your differential diagnosis guide what you include) Include elements of past medical/surgical history, medications, social history, and family history that are relevant to the present illness Include degree of impairment caused by the patient's illness Include any therapy instituted by patient and/or physician along with response to treatment

Past medical/ surgical history	Relevant or pertinent past medical or surgical history should be included in the HPI Include only important PMH/PSH Leave out minor diagnoses Do not repeat previously stated information
Medications	Group together any medications given for the same condition Include PRN, over-the-counter or herbal medications
Allergies	For drug allergies, include the type of reaction
Social history	Pertinent social history should be included in the HPI and need not be repeated here
Family history	If the information obtained is not relevant to the patient's current illness, you may state "the family history was noncontributory."
Review of systems	If the information obtained is not relevant to the patient's current illness, you may state "the review of systems was noncontributory." Do not repeat previously stated information
Physical examination	Begin with brief description of patient's general appearance followed by vital signs Follow expected order* Include both pertinent positives and negatives If an aspect of the physical examination is normal, it may be acceptable to say that it is "normal" or "unremarkable" (ask attending for preferences)
Lab/imaging/ other studies	Ask attending if he wants all results or only abnormal lab test results Start with basic lab tests first Bring electrocardiogram, x-rays, CT scan with you for the attending to review
Summary	Generally a three to four sentence summary of the patient's clinical presentation, including the most important complaints, physical exam findings, studies, and lab values
Assessment/ plan	This is your opportunity to demonstrate your reasoning skills and fund of knowledge Use information obtained (history, physical exam, labs, other) to argue for a particular diagnosis Discuss other possibilities (differential diagnosis) and why these are less likely Offer diagnostic and therapeutic plan

*A commonly used order: general appearance → vital signs → HEENT (head, eyes, ears, nose, throat) → neck → thorax → heart → lungs → abdomen → rectal → pelvic/genital → extremity → neurological/musculo-skeletal

As you progress through each aspect of the presentation, don't jump around. Physical examination findings should not be included in the history of present illness.

Tip # 33

Don't stop your oral case presentation when you reach the assessment and plan, as some students do, because you're worried that your assessment and plan may be incorrect. Present your conclusions with confidence. Even if you're wrong, the fact that you committed to a diagnosis and provided support for it is impressive.

Did you know ...

55 verbal case presentations of house officers and medical students were observed during an inpatient ward month.[7] Students reported the chief complaint in only 61% of their presentations.

Rule # 109   Utilize headings during transitions.

As you progress through your presentation, keep your listeners oriented by using standard headings. When you reach the patient's past medical history, you may start by saying, "The past medical history was remarkable for ..." Before delving into the physical exam, say, "On physical examination ..."

Rule # 110   Learn and utilize the qualities of an outstanding oral case presentation.

If you talk to enough attendings, they'll describe some common features of outstanding oral case presentations.

Characteristics of an outstanding oral case presentation

- Well organized
- Clear and concise
- Complete
- Follows the expected order or format
- Includes relevant aspects of the history, physical exam, laboratory testing, and other data, including pertinent negatives
- Free of irrelevant information
- Thorough but not overly laden with detail
- Allows the listener to develop a coherent and accurate picture of the patient's problems
- Accurate
- Shows knowledge of major and minor issues
- Minimal use of notes
- Good eye contact
- Excellent assessment and plan

Certain features are universally regarded as signs of a poor presentation.

Characteristics of a poor oral case presentation

- Includes irrelevant facts
- Rambling
- Disorganized
- Ill-prepared
- Major omissions
- Unclear
- Skipping around (e.g. lab data is included in the HPI)
- Inattention to detail

Your goal is to consistently deliver outstanding oral case presentations. The following rules provide a framework to help you reach this goal.

Rule # 111   The oral case presentation is often used as a surrogate for direct observation of a history and physical.

Your attending may not have been anywhere near the patient's room while you were completing your evaluation. He may instead draw conclusions about your abilities to evaluate and treat patients based on your oral presentation. An evaluation of your fund of knowledge may be based on the same presentation. The oral case presentation, therefore, becomes a surrogate for direct observation of a history and physical. Some attendings also utilize it to learn how competent, reliable, and thorough you are. As such, it substantially impacts your clerkship evaluation.

Tip # 34

No matter how well you understand your patient's illness, if you can't clearly and confidently convey your thoughts during the oral case presentation, you won't be seen as competent or effective.

Did you know ...

In their article titled "Identification of Communication Apprehension in Medical Students Starting a Surgery Rotation," Lang and colleagues wrote that "much of a student or resident's evaluation is based on oral presentations: case presentations ..."[8]

Did you know ...

In their article titled "Assessing student performance on a pediatric clerkship," Greenberg and Getson found "a highly significant relationship between students receiving a final grade of honors and an 'A' on their case grade."[9]

Did you know ...

In a recent article, researchers from the University of Colorado wrote that "we believe that the majority of the student interactions with attending physicians in EM [emergency medicine] occur during oral presentations...other interactions, such as direct patient contact...are often not observed by superiors. Thus, the majority of the resident and attending's impression of a student, and ultimately the student's evaluation, is directly linked to how well the student presents."[10]

Similar conclusions were reached through research at Cornell on oral case presentations during the internal medicine clerkship. The authors wrote that "a predictable result is that student's skills in case presentation would predominate in the teacher's assessment of his/her overall performance and that performance in case presentation would predominate in overall clinical performance assessment. Since performance assessment by residents and faculty constitutes a major portion of the grade in clerkships, stronger performance in case presentation would predictably be associated with higher final grades."[11]

Rule # 112 Know how much time you have before you begin.

The duration of the OCP varies depending upon the preferences of the attending, but typically ranges between 5 and 15 minutes. At the start of the rotation, ask the attending how much time you have to deliver your presentation. While your attending has a preconceived notion as to how much time your presentation should take, he's unlikely to volunteer it. Ask early in the rotation, preferably before you ever present.

Rule # 113 Don't present for longer than the allotted time.

Once you know how much time you have, your goal is to prepare and practice your presentation, making sure that it doesn't exceed the allotted time. It is very easy to do so. If you were to include every piece of infor-mation that you obtained during your patient encounter, the presentation would easily exceed your time limit.

Unfortunately, many students don't adhere to the time limit imposed by the attending. This is a sure-fire way to annoy team members. Long presentations take time away from other activities that need to be done during rounds. With so many tasks to accomplish in a relatively short period of time, it is imperative that the team stays on schedule.

Tip # 35

While rehearsing the oral case presentation, you need to time yourself.

Rule # 114   Avoid a presentation that includes too little or too much detail.

Most students tend to include too much detail in their presentations. Successful students must communicate an organized and succinct history, physical exam, assessment, and plan without losing the attending's attention. This can be a challenge, considering how much material there is to convey on any given patient. Students often fear that they'll leave out key details if they don't present all of the data learned. They also worry that they're too new to medicine to be the judge of what should and shouldn't be included.

It can be difficult to determine whether a detail is relevant or not. While experience will help, here are some tips:

- Include the detail if it helps build your case. With every OCP, your goal is to convey patient information that provides support for the diagnosis.

- Include the detail if it helps your listener take care of the patient.

- If you aren't sure whether the detail is relevant, omit it. Be prepared to provide the information if your listener asks for it.

- If your attending keeps asking for the same type of information during your presentation, then include it in the next one.

Rule # 115   Avoid a verbatim reading of the patient's write-up.

The OCP should not be a verbatim reading of the patient's write-up. Instead, it should be a carefully edited version of the write-up. Oral and written case presentations have different purposes. The latter is much more comprehensive. Oral presentations, however, are meant to rapidly convey key information.

It's also difficult, if not impossible, to keep the attention of your audience when reading verbatim. Your goal during a presentation is to keep the audience engaged and interested. Lesser reliance on notes allows you to maintain eye contact with your listeners. It also conveys to the attending that you have a firm grasp on your patient's medical problems. It is acceptable to glance at your notes occasionally, such as when reporting medication dosages and laboratory data.

Rule # 116   Practice, practice, practice.

Practicing over and over ensures you know your patient information. It's also one of the best ways to combat anxiety. Practice entails giving your presentation out loud. Practicing it silently in your mind robs you of the opportunity to hear yourself say the words. By hearing yourself say the words, you become more confident in your delivery.

To deliver a polished OCP, you should practice on your own and with others. Practice before family, friends, or fellow students. One student wrote about how she benefited from feedback given by her classmate:[6]

> We were practicing in the nurses' room, with a few minutes to go
> before the big performance. My classmate Julie and I ran
> through our lines and critiqued each other. "You have the history
> and differential diagnosis down," she said, "but you look half
> asleep. Sit up straight, for goodness' sake."

It's particularly important to practice with your resident or intern before presenting to the attending. If your resident doesn't ask you to present the case to her beforehand, ask if you may. She may offer suggestions on how to polish the presentation, or may identify problems. Since residents have considerable experience delivering OCPs, their advice should be taken seriously.

Tip # 36

Videotaping is an underutilized but very effective way of improving the quality of your oral case presentations.

Rule # 117   Pay close attention to your volume.

In normal conversation, we generally speak in a softer voice. During an oral presentation, however, you need to adjust the volume of your voice, depending on the setting and circumstances. If you're presenting in a larger room with team members spread throughout, your goal is to be heard clearly by the person sitting farthest away.

At other times, you may be asked to present in the hallway between patient rooms. In this more intimate setting, your focus will again be on making sure that all team members can hear you. However, you don't want to speak so loudly that you compromise patient privacy.

In our experience, the most common problem for students is that of speaking too softly. For some, this is the natural way they speak. For others, this stems from fear or anxiety. Since we often have difficulty evaluating the volume of our own voice, solicit feedback from others and make changes if necessary.

Rule # 118   Speak at the correct pace.

In delivering your presentation, your goal is to speak slowly enough to be easily understood by the audience. If you speak too slowly, however, you'll lose their attention. If you speak too rapidly, you enunciate each word clearly and distinctly, which impa sion.

Speaking too quickly seems to be the more common dents. With so much information to convey in a fixed am dents will sometimes increase the pace of their speech so they can finish on time. Rushing through a presentation is also a common sign of anxiety. Again, advance preparation can help.

The most interesting presentations are given by students who vary their rate of delivery. By speeding up and slowing down when necessary, they are able to emphasize certain points. You can learn about your rate of delivery by recording your presentation, reviewing it, and making adjustments where you see fit.

Rule # 119   Avoid the monotone.

To really learn about effective presentations, you should listen closely to a dynamic speaker. One of their hallmarks is that they vary the pitch and tone of their voice during a speech.

Utilizing a monotone voice can make even the most interesting content come across as boring. Recording and listening to your presentation is a useful way to evaluate your own pitch and tone. Also, as with other aspects of your OCP, seek feedback.

Tip # 37

The tone of your voice conveys feelings and attitudes. Be aware of how you sound by recording your presentation and listening to it. Students who are known for monotonous presentations often don't realize it until they hear themselves speak.

Rule # 120   Learn the correct pronunciation of all the words you use.

While practicing your presentation, make sure you know how to pronounce all words. Students commonly make pronunciation errors, and these mistakes can affect your credibility. A student who is knowledgeable about his patient may not be perceived as such when words are mispronounced.

Students and physicians frequently encounter unfamiliar words. Consult a medical dictionary or team member who can educate you on the proper pronunciation. In other cases, you may be unaware that you are pronouncing a word incorrectly. This is yet another reason to present your case to the resident first.

These errors are particularly common during the medication section. I can't tell you how many times my students have mispronounced medication names such as tamsulosin, carvedilol, irbesartan, and rosiglitazone.

Tip # 38

Students want to be seen as intelligent and competent. To be perceived as such, you must speak well. Students who deliver polished oral case presentations understand the importance of voice quality (volume, rate, pitch, and tone) and correct pronunciation.

Rule # 121   Avoid, umm, annoying speech habits.

OCPs should be polished and free from extraneous words or phrases. Do not use the classic "uhh," "um," "like," or "you know." The use of these phrases, also known as fillers, is distracting. Their use also detracts from the polished, competent image you wish to portray. These annoying habits are typically used unconsciously or manifest due to anxiety.

Most students are unaware of their own use of fillers. When practicing in front of others, you should specifically seek feedback on the use of fillers. Replace any fillers with a short, silent pause.

Did you know ...

In one study, faculty members from the Department of Internal Medicine independently viewed the same 17 videotaped student case presentations. Most raters placed high value on three communication skills: economy, fluency, and precision of language. In the article, these skills were defined as:

> Economy - "the information's relevance and avoiding unnecessary content"
>
> Fluency – "the student's ability to articulate without verbal tangles, with a minimum of qualifiers and hesitations"
>
> Precision in language – "unambiguity in phrasing, appropriate use of terms, and avoidance of lay jargon"

This study demonstrated that the faculty's assessment of oral case presentation quality was regularly influenced by the way in which the information was conveyed by the student.[12]

Rule # 122   As with any type of presentation, nonverbal communication is an important part of your message.

With any presentation, communication occurs in two main ways. Verbal communication is what students focus on the most - "what should I say?" However, your audience receives a strong message from your nonverbal

communication as well - "how should I say it?" To mak
able impression, you should:

- Maintain eye contact with team members. Rotate y
  to keep all listeners engaged. Students who are at
  contact are seen as more credible, competent, and confident.

- Display good posture, whether you are standing or seated. Students who slouch give the impression that they're not interested, even if they feel otherwise. With good posture, you're also likely to speak more clearly.

- Never invade a colleague's space. If you're presenting in a large room, this won't be a problem. In a hallway, though, a team is often huddled close together. Adjust your body position so that you're at a comfortable distance for interaction.

- Avoid distracting behaviors such as playing with your hair, jewelry, or tie. Most students don't know that they do this. During your dress rehearsal, ask your resident or friend if they notice any distracting habits.

Rule # 123   Project confidence.

The most polished presenters are able to project confidence throughout their presentation. To exude confidence, you must feel confident, and to feel confident, you must prepare well. Barbara Linney in her article, "Presentations that hold you spellbound", said "presentation content is important but even more so body language and voice quality because the best of messages will fall on deaf ears if you don't look and sound confident."[13]

Rule # 124   Utilize appropriate techniques to minimize anxiety.

Anxiety is natural, and in fact can be helpful. A certain degree of adrenaline can spur you into delivering a better performance. However, uncontrolled anxiety will damage your performance. Some suggestions to reduce anxiety:

- Anxiety is not necessarily a negative. You need that burst of adrenaline to perform well.

- Practice. Practice again. The best way to avoid anxiety is to feel confident about your presentation. You gain this confidence from practice.

- While practicing, visualize the room, the audience, and yourself during the presentation. Picture yourself impressing the team. Studies have actually demonstrated that positive thinking in "speech-anxious subjects" can reduce subjective anxiety and cardiovascular responses.[14]

Your anxiety is not as apparent to your audience as it is to you. From speaking to many students, I know this to be the case.

- Get off to a good start by knowing your introduction (typically the history of present illness) very well. If you're able to convey the first part of your presentation with poise, you'll gain confidence during the rest of the presentation.

- You know more about your patient than any other team member. Remember this.

Did you know ...

In a survey of preclinical students at a single medical school, proficiency in OCPs was considered to be one of the three most essential skills requiring mastery before beginning clerkships. Students also reported being most anxious about their oral case presentation skills.[1] Some of this anxiety stems from the fact that time spent learning how to present is limited during the preclinical years. In the study, only 12 hours of time was spent on the OCP during the first two years. Of note, OCPs were among the least anxiety-provoking areas when students nine months into their clerkship year were surveyed.

Rule # 125   Interruptions are common. Plan for them.

In the perfect student world, an attending would never interrupt. The reality is that many attendings do interrupt with questions or comments. These can throw off your train of thought, and while some students are able to handle this with poise, others become flustered and disoriented. Some students are unable to recover.

As you prepare and practice your presentation, recognize that most of the time you will be interrupted. Students tend to assume that an attending will only interrupt if there is something lacking in the presentation. However, an attending may interrupt to ask questions simply because it's his style. He may interrupt to ask for a clarification or because he missed something you said. Questions or comments may also indicate that your attending is interested in what you have to say.

How do you handle these interruptions? First, understand that an interruption does not mean you're presenting poorly. In fact, it usually indicates that your attending is paying close attention. If the attending asks a clarifying question, answer it and move on. If the attending asks a question to gauge your knowledge base, then answer it to the best of your ability. In many cases, your reading will allow you to answer the question. If you don't know the answer, say so and move on. You aren't expected to have the answers to every question.

Rule # 126 Monitor audience response.

As you deliver your presentation, pay close attention to how it's received. This requires that you make eye contact with your listeners. Watch for body language cues that indicate approval, confusion, frustration, or other emotions. It's up to you to read these nonverbal cues and then respond appropriately. If you sense that your listeners are growing impatient with the length of your presentation, shorten the remainder by cutting out the less important details.

Rule # 127 Assess your performance.

As you're practicing, and then again following your presentation, you should assess how well you did. The form on the next page outlines some of the important points to review.

Some attendings will initiate a discussion with you shortly after your OCP, reviewing mistakes and areas for improvement. In most cases, though, you'll have to ask for feedback from your attending and resident, and you should try to do so soon after you present.

	Below Average	Average	Above Average	Excellent
The patient was clearly identified (name, age, gender, race, pertinent past medical history)				
Clearly stated chief complaint				
Chronologically organized HPI				
Pertinent positive information was included				
Pertinent negative information was included				
Physical exam included general appearance				
Physical exam included vital signs				
Physical exam was presented in logical order				
All pertinent physical exam findings were presented accurately				
No extraneous information was presented				
Pertinent/significant labs/studies were included				
A problem list was conveyed				
Problem list was presented in descending order of importance				
Plan was presented - not just an assessment				
Presents with minimal use of notes				
Voice volume, quality appropriate				
Accurately pronounces words				
Presents in a way that holds attention				
Good time management				
Adequately responds to questions and requests for clarification or additional information				
Is knowledgeable about illness or topic, including up-to-date literature				

Rule # 128   Don't lie.

The literature does show that students engage in unethical behavior while taking care of patients. In a survey of students at Johns Hopkins University School of Medicine, 13 to 24% admitted to cheating during the clinical years of medical school.[15] Examples included "recording tasks not performed" and "lying about having ordered tests." In another study performed at the University of New Mexico School of Medicine, students were asked whether they had heard of or witnessed unethical behaviors on the part of their student colleagues. In response, 21% had personal knowledge of students "reporting a pelvic examination as 'normal' during rounds when it had been inadvertently omitted from the physical examination." Another 35% had personal knowledge of students "reporting a lab test or x-ray as 'normal' when in actual fact there had been no attempt to obtain the information."[16]

When presenting a patient to your attending, do not lie. There are many times when you may be tempted to stretch the truth or outright lie in an attempt to make your history and physical exam more complete than it actually was. If your attending asks you about the patient's dorsalis pedis pulses and you didn't check them, don't say they were normal. Tell the attending that you didn't examine the pulses and learn from your mistake. It's not possible to deliver the best possible care to patients unless team members are scrupulously honest.

Did you know ...

In a survey of incoming interns at two major academic medical centers, participants were asked about their participation in unprofessional behaviors. Ten percent reported presenting patient information (test results, examination results) as normal when, in fact, they were uncertain of the true results.[17]

The following article, originally published on www.studentdoctor.net, describes the importance of oral communication skills, and includes additional tips on delivering oral case presentations.[18]

The Successful Match: Oral Communication Skills

Every aspiring physician knows the importance of memorization, especially in the basic science years. As you advance in your career, however, communication skills come to the forefront. Physicians with poor communication skills are more likely to be sued.[2] They are more likely to be disciplined by the medical board. They may not receive as many professional referrals from colleagues or word-of-mouth referrals from patients.

Successful communication requires establishing a connection and imparting a message. Successful patient care does not end with gathering data from your patient. It revolves around imparting that information to the entire team that is involved in patient care: your team members, the consulting physicians, the nurses, the patient and family members, and even the cafeteria, among others. ("The patient's allergies include a history of anaphylaxis to shrimp.")

Third year students, in the midst of early clinical rotations, quickly recognize the importance of communication. Memorization may be a crucial skill for those taking exams and receiving grades based on an objective test score. However, when receiving a subjective grade based on your ability to take care of patients, one's ability to communicate with patients, to establish rapport with colleagues, and to impart medical information, become important indicators of communication skills.

How exactly do medical schools determine a student's ability to provide excellent patient care? A student's grade in core clinical rotations is determined by several factors, including subjective ratings and objective test scores. One study examined the evaluation techniques of 97 US medical schools.[19] Faculty and resident ratings accounted for 50-70% of a student's grade in core clinical rotations.

How do faculty and residents arrive at their subjective rating of a student's abilities? Clerkship evaluation forms ask faculty to rate students on specific skills, such as a student's ability to take a history and perform a physical examination. However, attending physicians rarely or infrequently observe students in these areas. In fact, in a survey of 322 University of Virginia medical students at the end of their third year, 51% reported never having a faculty member observe them while taking a history; 81% had never been observed performing a complete physical exam.[20] Therefore, many faculty draw conclusions about a student's ability in these areas from the quality of the oral case presentation.

In a study of surgical faculty, Pulito found that it was rare for faculty members to directly observe a student taking a history or doing a physical examination.[21] In fact, only one of nine faculty members surveyed had done so. Despite this, five of the nine faculty participants rated students in this area. They inferred the rating of this characteristic from other factors, particularly the oral case presentation. Pulito wrote that "in the clinic setting, for example, if a student presents a patient to an attending and is verbally facile, succinctly describing a focused history and physical examination, the inference may be drawn that the student expeditiously obtained the relevant history and performed an appropriate examination."

In one study focusing on communication apprehension among medical students starting a surgery rotation, Lang wrote that "much of a student or resident's evaluation is based on oral presentations."[8] In another study assessing student performance on a pediatrics clerkship, Greenberg found "a highly significant relationship between students receiving a final grade of honors and an 'A' on their case grade."[9]

In oral case presentations, students aim to effectively transfer important clinical information between team members. When done well, these presentations facilitate patient care, improve team efficiency, and become a valuable learning experience. Since they also serve an evaluative function, students hope to deliver high-quality presentations to prove their competence. While some students are inherently gifted in the area of making presentations, all would benefit from practice and the following suggestions:

- Expectations for the oral case presentation vary from clerkship to clerkship, attending to attending, and resident to resident. For this reason, always meet with your attending and resident on the first day or two of the clerkship to ascertain their expectations.

- Your goal is to leave this discussion knowing the attending or resident's personal preferences (preferably before your first presentation). Ask specific questions about time limits, the order in which to present information, and so on. "Do you want me to report the entire physical exam or just pertinent positives?" "Which labs would you like to hear, or would you prefer to hear all of them?"

- What worked well with one attending or resident may not work well with another. You may have internalized a certain set of "presentation rules." With the start of a new clerkship or arrival of a new attending, recognize that these rules may not meet their needs.

- Be aware of the context in which you are presenting. Your presentation to a resident with whom you evaluated the patient should be different than the presentation given to an attending who is hearing about the patient for the first time.

- Make your presentation flow like a story. Your goal, many times, is to make an argument for a particular condition. Put the details of the case together in such a way as to lead the listener to a diagnosis.

- As a novice clinician, your inexperience makes it difficult to decide what to include and what to leave out. The easy way out, and the route that many students take, is to simply read the written H & P word for word. However, the oral case presentation should be a carefully edited version of the written record. The key is to communicate only what's relevant. For a new clerk, that can be very difficult. Don't be afraid to ask for help in this area.

- Use residents as a resource. Residents are often familiar with attending preferences and can help polish your presentation before you have to deliver it to the attending.

- Seek feedback after each and every one of your presentations. The best feedback is that which is explicit and timely. Many attendings won't automatically provide feedback; you may have to specifically ask for it. "Dr. So, do you have any suggestions on how I can improve my presentation?"

- Uncertainty is normal with oral case presentations. Because of the evaluative function of these presentations, it can be tempting to bluff or lie in an effort to look good. As hard as it can be to say "I don't know," honesty and accuracy in the transfer of clinical information is vital to patient care. In a survey of Johns Hopkins medical students, 13% to 24% admitted to cheating during the clinical years of medical school.[15] Examples included "recording tasks not performed" and "lying about having ordered tests."

- Projecting confidence is important. Your choice of words, the manner in which you speak, and your body language are all factors that will be used to judge the quality of your presentation.

- It is rare to present a patient without any interruptions. In one study of emergency medicine faculty and students, the mean number of interruptions was 2.49 per oral case presentation.[22] Although students often view interruptions as a sign that their presentation is lacking, this is often not the case. Attendings find it difficult to balance the need to teach with the need to care for a service full of sick patients. In addition to interruptions due to time constraints, you may be asked to repeat information or clarify a certain point. Unfortunately, many students let interruptions derail their presentation, and find they can't recover.

- Many students stop short of offering an assessment and plan, especially novice clinicians who don't feel qualified to do so. Always offer your own assessment and plan. Attending physicians are impressed with students who take the initiative to do so.

- Read extensively about your patients' problems using a variety of resources, including handbooks, specialty textbooks, and the recent literature. As you read, make it a habit to ask "why?" Why did we order this test? Why did we choose this particular antibiotic? Such questions further your understanding of the disease – not to mention prepare you for the attending questions that are sure to come during or following your presentation.

Because of the complexity of the oral case presentation and the varied needs and expectations of residents and attendings, delivering high-quality presentations can be difficult. Is it worth the effort? Absolutely. First, presentation quality is a major factor used in the evaluation of students. Second, the development and acquisition of communication skills is important for your future career as a physician. That's precisely why, in recent years, organizations such as the Association of American Medical Colleges (AAMC), Clerkship Directors of Internal Medicine (CDIM), and the Accreditation Council for Graduate Medical Education (ACGME) have emphasized its importance. In fact, the AAMC considers the development and acquisition of communication skills a core learning objective for medical students.

References

[1]Small R, Soriano R, Chietero M, Quintana J, Parkas V, Koestler J. Easing the transition: medical students' perceptions of critical skills required for the clerkships. *Educ Health* 2008; 21(3): 192.

[2]Virshup B, Oppenberg A, Coleman M. Strategic risk management: reducing malpractice claims through more effective patient-doctor communication. *Am J Med Qual* 1999; 14(4): 153-9.

[3]Singh H, Thomas E, Petersen L, Studdert D. Medical errors involving trainees. A study of close malpractice claims from 5 insurers. *Arch Intern Med* 2007; 167(19): 2030-6.[7]

[4]AAMC Medical School Objectives Project. American Association of Medical Colleges Web Site. https://www.aamc.org/initatives/53198/msop/. Accessed January 22, 2011.

[5]Green E, Durning S, DeCherrie L, Fagan M, Sharpe B, Hershman W. Expectations for oral case presentations for clinical clerks: opinions of internal medicine clerkship directors. *J Gen Intern Med* 2009; 24(3): 370-3.

[6]Sobel R. MSL – Medicine as a second language. *N Engl J Med* 2005; 352: 1945.

[7]Marinella M. Residents and medical students noting the chief complaint during verbal presentations. *Acad Med* 2000; 75(3): 89.

[8]Lang N, Rowland-Morin P, Coe N. Identification of communication apprehension in medical students starting a surgery rotation. *Am J Surg* 1998; 176 (1): 41-5.

[9]Greenberg L, Getson P. Assessing student performance on a pediatric clerkship. *Arch Pediatr Adolesc Med* 1996; 150 (11): 1209-12.

[10]Davenport C, Honigman B, Druck J. The 3-minute emergency medicine medical student presentation: a variation on a theme. *Acad Emerg Med* 2008; 15(7): 683-7.

[11]Kang Y, Bardes C, Gerber L, Storey-Johnson C. Pilot of direct observation of clinical skills (DOCS) in a medicine clerkship: feasibility and relationship to clinical performance measures. *Med Educ Online* 2009; 5: 14: 9.

[12]Elliott D, Hickam D. How do faculty evaluate students' case presentations? *Teach Learn Med* 1997; 9(4): 261-3.

[13]Linney B. Presentations that hold you spellbound. *Physician Exec* 2000; 3: 72-5.

[14]Hu S, Bostow T, Lipman D, Bell S, Klein S. Positive thinking reduces heart rate and fear responses to speech-phobic imagery. *Percept Mot Skills* 1992; 75 (3 Pt 2): 1067-73.

[15]Dans P. Self-reported cheating by students at one medical school. *Acad Med* 1996; 71 (1 Suppl): 70-2.

[16]Anderson R, Obenshain S. Cheating by students: findings, reflections, and remedies. *Acad Med* 1994; 69(5): 323-32.

[17]Arora V, Wayne D, Anderson R, Didwania A, Humphrey H. Participation in and perceptions of unprofessional behaviors among incoming internal medicine interns. *JAMA* 2008; 300(10): 1132-4.

[18]Desai S, Katta R. The Successful Match: Oral Communication Skills. October 23, 2007. http://www.studentdoctor.net/2007/10/the-successful-match/. Accessed January 30, 2011.

[19]Kassebaum D, Eaglen R. Shortcomings in the evaluation of students' clinical skills and behaviors in medical school. *Acad Med* 1999; 74(7): 942-9.

[20]Howley L, Wilson L. Direct observation of students during clerkship rotations: a multiyear descriptive study. *Acad Med* 2004; 79 (3): 276-80.

[21]Pulito A, Donnelly M, Plymale M, Mentzer R Jr. What do faculty observe of medical students' clinical performance. *Teach Learn Med* 2006; 18(2): 99-104.

[22]Yang G, Chin R. Assessment of teacher interruptions on learners during oral case presentations. *Acad Emerg Med* 2007; 14 (6): 521-5.

Chapter 16

Write-Ups

"They don't teach you how to do documentation in the first two years. So when you hit a clinic or a hospital you're completely at sea unless someone pities you and shows you how to write notes."

> - From "Perceptions and Attributions of Third-Year Student Struggles in Clerkships," published in *Academic Medicine*[1]

Communication skills are of vital importance in patient care. The Association of American Medical Colleges issued a report stating that schools must ensure that, prior to graduation, students "have the ability to communicate effectively, both orally and in writing, with patients, patients' families, colleagues, and others with whom physicians must exchange information in carrying out their responsibilities."[2]

In response to the AAMC mandate, schools have made examination of the student's written record a major area of emphasis during core clerkships. Recognizing the importance of written communication, the USMLE Step 2 Clinical Skills Examination evaluates the ability of students to *document* the findings of encounters with standardized patients.

The development of written communication skills is emphasized heavily in core clerkships. The written case presentation, or write-up, is a detailed account of the patient's clinical presentation. One of the major purposes of the write-up is to help you develop the written communication skills needed to take care of patients. Being able to communicate patient information in an organized and succinct way, either orally or written, is important throughout a medical career.

Most students are introduced to the process of writing a case presentation during the physical diagnosis course. During clerkships, the impact of these write-ups quickly becomes apparent. These are important documents which impact patient care and patient outcomes. During rotations, you'll be asked to prepare write-ups on the patients you admit. Your write-ups may be placed in the medical record, along with those of the resident and attending. You may also be required to submit one or more write-ups to your attending or clerkship director as part of your clerkship grade.

Rule # 129 **Your patient write-up may be placed in the medical chart, and is likely to be referenced by other health care professionals. Don't underestimate its importance in patient care.**

Documentation of your clinical encounter with a newly admitted patient is an important task. In your write-up, you will record clinical data, chronicle important findings and results, and end with an assessment and plan. Your write-up, along with your daily patient progress notes, will be the vehicle through which essential patient information is conveyed from one healthcare provider to another. Therefore, it is vital that you prepare a well-organized, complete, and accurate write-up.

Did you know ...

Written documentation of patient information obtained from a physician encounter is also used for billing, in epidemiological research, and as evidence during malpractice litigation.

Did you know ...

Faculty at the Mount Sinai School of Medicine and Penn State College of Medicine recently wrote about how some institutions do not permit students to write or enter information in the patient medical record.[3] "Institutional disincentives to student documentation include insurance regulations that restrict student documentation from substantiating billing claims, concerns about the legal status of student notes, and implementation of electronic medical records that do not allow or restrict student access." The authors warned that this trend "may have wide-ranging consequences for student education, from delaying the learning of proper documentation skills to limiting training opportunities."

Rule # 130 **The write-up often serves as a surrogate for an observed history and physical.**

The website www.usmle.org describes an interesting aspect of medical education on the wards: "During recent field trials, 20 percent of the fourth-year students who completed a survey said they had been observed interacting with a patient by a faculty member two or fewer times. One in 25 said they had never been observed by a faculty member."[4]

If you aren't observed while taking care of patients, how can attendings evaluate your ability to perform a thorough history and physical? The oral case presentation and written case presentation become proxies for direct observation.

Students are often asked to turn in write-ups for formal evaluation. In most cases, the attending will review them. At some schools, the clerkship director may also review write-ups. The reviewers will evaluate your ability to perform a comprehensive patient evaluation and appropriately record the result of this evaluation. In addition to your ability to collect information, reviewers will assess your ability to identify and evaluate problems, generate an accurate differential diagnosis, demonstrate clinical reasoning, and formulate a management plan.

Did you know ...

Kogan and Shea wrote that "Assessment of the write-up is believed to be important because it evaluates a student's ability to collect information; identify, prioritize, and evaluate problems; demonstrate clinical reasoning; develop management plans; and communicate through a written record. These are important clinical skills that students are expected to be proficient in prior to graduation."[5]

Tip # 39

The quality of your write-ups will significantly contribute to the attending physician's impression of your clinical performance.

Rule # 131   Utilize the proper format and order for a write-up.

There is a proper order to the presentation of patient information. Write-ups that don't adhere to the expected order are considered disorganized and are difficult to follow. The order in which information is presented is the same as that of the oral case presentation.

Write-ups begin with subjective data, followed by objective data (physical examination, lab test results), assessment, and plan. Components of the subjective portion of the write-up include the identifying data, chief complaint, history of present illness, past medical history, medications, allergies, social history, family history, and review of systems.

The content of the write-up will differ, to some extent, from specialty to specialty. For example, while the prenatal, birth, and neonatal histories are important in the pediatric patient, this information generally has no bearing on the adult patient.

Rule # 132   Record an accurate and thorough history of present illness.

The history of present illness, or HPI, is a description of why the patient is here now. It is considered the most important element of the history. As such, it should flow like a story, giving the reader a clear idea of the events that transpired before the patient sought medical attention from you. A well-constructed HPI:

- Begins with an introductory statement that includes the patient's age, race, gender, and relevant past medical history
- Is chronological. The story should begin when the patient was last in his usual state of health (baseline), and trace the development of symptoms from onset to the current time
- Identifies time of symptom onset
- Identifies duration of symptom
- Addresses why the patient has sought medical attention now
- Explores the patient's chief complaint thoroughly, including onset, precipitating/palliative factors, quality, region/radiation, severity, and timing/temporal aspects
- Includes pertinent positives and negatives
- Includes any therapy initiated by the patient, as well as therapy prescribed by other caregivers. Also includes response to therapy
- Includes relevant features of the past medical history, social history, medications, family history, and review of systems
- Includes patient's concerns, fears, and thoughts about what may be accounting for his symptoms
- Includes the degree to which the illness is affecting the patient's quality of life

Rule # 133   Record a complete problem list.

Clerkships often prefer that the write-up include a problem list, which is a compilation of the patient's active medical problems. To identify problems that should be included on the list, a useful technique is to start at the beginning of the write-up and circle all symptoms, known illnesses, abnormal physical exam findings, and abnormal test results (laboratory, ECG, imaging, etc.). Everything that is circled should be listed as a problem, with the exception of inactive problems. An inactive problem is one that has no bearing on the present illness or the patient's future health. An example would be tonsillectomy performed as a child in an adult patient.

Rule # 134   All write-ups should include an appropriate assessment and plan.

No other area of the write-up causes students as much distress as the assessment and plan. New clerks tend to write a brief assessment and plan section.

A – *Unstable angina*

P – *Rule out myocardial infarction with enzymes and treat with aspirin, beta-blocker, and heparin*

What's wrong with this assessment and plan? The student doesn't describe what led him to believe that unstable angina was the most likely diagnosis. He doesn't include any information from the patient's history, physical exam, or testing that supports his assessment. There is also no discussion about other conditions (differential diagnosis) that could cause similar symptoms. The plan is also very brief, with no rationale given.

It's very important to remember that the attending physician will assess your understanding of the patient's disease, including your knowledge of appropriate management and therapy, based on the quality of your assessment and plan. In this section, it is not only important that you commit to a diagnosis (even if you are less than 100% certain) but also that you provide support for it. You must also offer a differential diagnosis and explain why other conditions in the differential are less likely. End this section with the diagnostic and therapeutic plan.

Tip # 40

In the assessment and plan, explain your thoughts. Explain how you came to a particular diagnosis, why other conditions in the differential diagnosis are less likely, and the rationale for the diagnostic and therapeutic plan you are recommending.

To assist you in the development of this important section, below is a step-by-step approach.

Step-by-step approach to developing the assessment and plan

Step 1 – From the patient's problem list, determine the patient's most important problem. List it as problem # 1 under the assessment and plan section.

Before listing the problem, ask yourself if you've made it as specific as possible. If the patient is admitted for chest pain and the etiology of the chest pain isn't clear, then you would list it as:

> *1. Chest pain*

If, on the other hand, your initial evaluation of the patient's chest pain reveals that he is having a myocardial infarction, then you would list it as:

> *1. Acute myocardial infarction*

Step 2 – Provide a differential diagnosis

The differential diagnosis is a list of conditions that could account for a patient's illness. Start your assessment with a statement that provides your reader with the differential diagnosis that you've considered.

1. Chest pain

> *While the differential diagnosis for chest pain is extensive, in this hospitalized patient, we will first consider the potentially life-threatening and common etiologies. Life-threatening causes of chest pain include unstable angina, myocardial infarction, pulmonary embolism, aortic dissection, pneumonia, pneumothorax, esophageal rupture, and pericardial tamponade.*

Note that thus far the assessment and plan only includes a differential diagnosis. It's always a good idea to comment on the life-threatening causes of a patient's symptom, since that's what concerns physicians the most in a newly admitted patient.

Did you know ...

Faculty at the University of Minnesota Medical School were asked which aspects of student performance discriminated better between average and superior medicine clerks.[6] Formulation of a reasoned differential diagnosis and plan was found to be more discriminating than any other aspect of student performance.

Step 3 – State the most likely diagnosis (working diagnosis)

A definitive diagnosis may be established in some patients immediately after your work-up. More often, though, you'll have what's known as a working diagnosis. In other words, you and your team will make a likely diagnosis based on the patient's clinical presentation and the results of testing. As the patient's hospital course is observed, the results of further testing become available, and the response to therapy is assessed, a definitive diagnosis may be established. Before you reach that point, though, you'll have to complete your write-up. Therefore, you have to commit to a working diagnosis.

With that in mind, you'll have to determine which of the entities in the differential diagnosis is the most likely (or working) diagnosis. You'll accomplish this by reading about each of the considerations in the differential diagnosis. As you read, determine which of these conditions best accounts for your patient's presentation. That becomes your working diagnosis (see example below).

1. *Chest pain*

> *While the differential diagnosis for chest pain is extensive, in this hospitalized patient, we will first consider the potentially life-threatening and common etiologies. Life-threatening causes of chest pain include unstable angina, myocardial infarction, pulmonary embolism, aortic dissection, pneumonia, pneumothorax, esophageal rupture, and pericardial tamponade. **Of these possibilities, unstable angina or myocardial infarction is the most likely diagnosis.***

Tip # 41

You may be hesitant to commit to a particular diagnosis because you fear you're way off track. It's always better, however, to commit. Those who commit demonstrate that they've thought about the case.

Step 4 – Provide support for your working diagnosis

After you've stated what you believe to be the most likely diagnosis, you should proceed to inform your reader how you came to that conclusion.

> *In support of this is his history of coronary artery disease. Up until one week prior to admission, the patient described only exertional chest pain. He then began experiencing more frequent episodes of chest pain, lasting longer in duration and even occurring at rest. These episodes of pain are otherwise similar in nature to his previous episodes of stable angina. Although his physical exam did not reveal any findings consistent with ischemia or infarction, the patient was examined when he was free of pain. ECG findings revealed ST-segment depression in the inferior leads, which were not present on an old tracing. When chest pain becomes more frequent, lasts longer, or occurs at rest, it raises concern for unstable angina and myocardial infarction. Lending further support to our working diagnosis is the ECG changes.*

Note that in providing the reader with support for the diagnosis, data from the patient's history, physical exam, and testing are weaved in to make a strong argument.

Step 5 – Inform the reader why other considerations in the differential diagnosis are either not the cause or are a less likely cause of the patient's illness

After stating the working diagnosis and providing support, discuss other considerations in the differential diagnosis and why they are less likely to account for the patient's illness.

> *Aortic dissection is quite unlikely given the description of the pain (pressure sensation in the center of his chest rather than a sharp, tearing pain), lack of radiation (pain of aortic dissection often radiates to the back), lack of physical exam findings (pulses symmetric and normal in all extremities), and normal mediastinal size noted on chest x-ray. Pneumothorax was also considered but, again, the description of the pain was not typical (pressure sensation rather than a sharp, pleuritic pain), shortness of breath was absent (shortness of breath is common in patients with pneumothorax), classic physical exam findings*

were not present (decreased breath sounds, hyperresonance to percussion), and the chest x-ray was normal. Pulmonary embolism always needs to be considered in the differential diagnosis of chest pain, especially given the fact that most diagnoses of this condition are made at autopsy. Therefore, we must always think of it as a possibility. This patient has no risk factors for pulmonary embolism, lacks symptoms and signs of deep venous thrombosis in the lower extremities, and does not have any other findings supportive of this diagnosis. Pericardial tamponade ... Pneumonia ... Esophageal rupture ...

In discussing other considerations in the differential diagnosis, provide reasons why you think they are less likely. Incorporate data from the history, physical exam, and testing to support your argument.

Step 6 – Provide your diagnostic and therapeutic plan

Many attendings prefer that students write the plan as a list or outline. Include both the diagnostic and therapeutic plan.

The diagnostic and therapeutic plan for this patient with chest pain due to an acute coronary syndrome includes:

1) Bed rest with continuous ECG monitoring

2) Oxygen

3) Serial cardiac enzymes (CK, CK-MB, troponin) to rule out myocardial infarction

4) Aspirin

- *Aspirin therapy has been shown to reduce the risk of death or MI in patients with unstable coronary artery disease not just in the acute setting but also long-term.*

- *Chewable 325 mg aspirin given in the ER*

- *Will continue aspirin therapy at a dose of 81 mg po daily*

5) Clopidogrel

- *In combination with aspirin, clopidogrel has been shown to reduce the rate of cardiovascular death and reinfarction to a greater effect than aspirin used alone*

- *Loading dose of 300 mg po given*

- *Will continue clopidogrel therapy at a dose of 75 mg po daily*

6) Metoprolol

- *Beta-blocker therapy has been shown to reduce mortality in patients with myocardial infarction*

- *Metoprolol 5 mg IV given and then repeated twice for a total of 15 mg. This was followed by 25 mg of metoprolol given orally with this dosing to continue every six hours.*

7) Heparin

- *Studies have shown that the addition of heparin to aspirin will lead to a further reduction in the risk of death and myocardial infarction in patients with unstable coronary artery disease.*

- *Will use low-molecular-weight heparin in this patient*

8) Ramipril

- *In the HOPE trial, ramipril was shown to reduce mortality and myocardial infarction in all patients with coronary artery disease.*

- *Will begin ramipril at a dose of 2.5 mg PO daily*

9) Atorvastatin

- *Several studies have shown that the early use of statins in patients with LDL-cholesterol levels above 100 mg/dL has beneficial effects in reducing ischemic events.*

- *Begin atorvastatin 20 mg po daily*

Tip # 42

Clerkship evaluation forms often ask evaluators to comment on a student's use of the literature. Because many students don't realize this, they fail to show their team that they are reviewing the literature. One place to demonstrate your use of the literature is in the write-up, particularly in the assessment and plan. Note that in step 6 above, I mention the HOPE trial under "ramipril" to demonstrate how you can incorporate recent literature findings into an assessment and plan.

Step 7 – Determine which one of the patient's problems is 2nd in importance and list it as problem # 2.

After listing problem # 2, ask yourself if it's a known (established) or unknown diagnosis. For example, if the patient has had gout for 10 years, then that's an established diagnosis. For established diagnoses, you don't need to discuss a differential. However, you should provide the reader with reasons as to why this diagnosis can be accepted in this patient, the current status of the problem, and the treatment plan.

2. Gout

    Patient was diagnosed with gout ten years ago when he developed acute right knee pain and analysis of the synovial fluid revealed the presence of needle-shaped, negatively birefringent monosodium urate crystals. Since then he has had several more attacks, but none over the past five years. Because the gout is currently stable, we will continue his current therapy of allopuri-nol.

If, on the other hand, problem # 2 is thrombocytopenia of unclear etiology, then it isn't an established diagnosis but rather an "unknown." With an "unknown," the assessment and plan should include a differential diagnosis, the most likely diagnosis, the diagnostic plan, and the therapeutic plan.

Step 8 – Complete the assessment and plan section, making sure that you deal with each problem on the problem list in the manner described in step 7.

Rule # 135   The assessment and plan must be in your own words. Using other sources, and quoting them without acknowledgement, is plagiarism.

The assessment and plan section of the write-up is difficult for all students. Some are tempted to take shortcuts. One involves copying the intern's or resident's assessment and plan verbatim. While attendings may want the student to review the assessment and plan with their residents, no attending expects to read one that is identical to the house officer's. While the basic diagnostic and therapeutic plan is unlikely to differ, the student's version should be more detailed. It should be written in such a way that the attending is able to understand the student's thought process. And, of course, it should always be written in the student's own words.

Do not copy information directly from a text or journal article. While students are expected to turn to a variety of resources, the information learned should be stated in your own words. Synthesizing and applying information is a critical skill for a physician. Applying information to your own patient demonstrates this skill, and demonstrates that you have a firm understanding of the patient's illness. If you must copy information from a text, you must include references. In general, it's a good idea to include references regardless.

The prevalence of plagiarism has not been well studied in American medical schools. However, over the past five years in conversations with faculty at different medical schools, a handful have raised concerns about this issue, citing examples in which student plagiarism occurred and how it came to light. Recently, a colleague related a story about one of his third year medical students. As he read through the student's write-ups, he suspected that the words and ideas expressed in the discussion didn't belong to the student. He punched in portions of the discussion into an internet search engine, and found a website that contained sections of the discussion word for word. The website was never referenced by the student. This was immediately brought to the attention of the clerkship director and others in the administration, and the student faced disciplinary action.

Tip # 43

Medical schools have policies in place to deal with the student who passes off another's work as his own. The punishment is often severe. The website for the Internal Medicine Clerkship at the University of Wisconsin School of Medicine states that "if plagiarism is identified, disciplinary sanctions will be taken...at a minimum this will include a lower grade for the course. Sanctions can include expulsion from the university."[7] Attendings expect that you will turn to a variety of resources to analyze and understand your patient's problems. You should always cite these sources in the write-up.

Rule # 136 **Cutting and pasting text is often used in the EMR as a shortcut while documenting the clinical exam. Some physicians consider this plagiarism, and some clerkships prohibit it.**

Electronic medical records (EMR) often allow for easy copying and pasting of text. It's not uncommon for a physician to read another's note, only to discover that his own words have been copied. In a recent article, Drs. Hartzband and Groopman, faculty members at the Harvard Medical School, wrote "Many times, physicians have clearly cut and pasted large blocks of text, or even complete notes, from other physicians; we have seen portions of our own notes inserted verbatim into another doctor's note. This is, in essence, a form of clinical plagiarism with potentially deleterious consequences for the patient."[8]

Physicians have even copied the clinical exams of other physicians. University of Washington researchers used specialized software to detect copied clinical exams in a set of over 167,000 VA records.[9] Exam copying was noted in 25% of patient charts. In interviews with faculty and residents, Embi found that study participants had concerns about the reliability of electronic charting, mainly because of the frequent use of copy and paste.[10] "Many felt that the use of such features sometimes resulted in the propagation of misinformation or even in frank errors."

Drs. Hartzband and Groopman also recognize the potential impact of copying and pasting of text on trainees. "This capacity to manipulate the electronic record makes it far too easy for trainees to avoid taking their own histories and coming to their own conclusions...Writing in a personal and independent way forces us to think and formulate our ideas." To combat this growing problem, clerkships have implemented firm rules. For example, the Department of Medicine at the University of Florida writes that "cutting and pasting anything other than online medication lists and lab data is plagiarism."[11]

Rule # 137   Avoid improper abbreviations.

Physicians frequently use abbreviations in their write-ups. In a review of abbreviations in pediatric notes, Sheppard noted 3,668 abbreviations in 168 sets of medical notes.[12] Only about half of these abbreviations were understood by other healthcare professionals. In a chart review in a neonatal unit, Manzar found the following in a progress note written by a junior physician:[13]

> *Prem 32 WOG, F & G, Problems: RDS, IVH II, S/P SVT, Stable on RA, TPR normal, PU, BO, Chest, CVS & Abdomen: NAD*

Were you able to decipher this line? In order, the abbreviations used are: premature, weeks of gestation, feeder and grower, respiratory distress syndrome, intraventricular grade 2 hemorrhage, status post supraventricular tachycardia, room air, temperature plus respiration, passed urine, bowel open, cardiovascular system, and no abnormality detected.

While convenient, the use of medical abbreviations may lead to misinterpretation and serious patient error. Confusion can easily occur, since abbreviations can stand for more than one word. For example, CP may be used as an abbreviation for chest pain, chicken pox, cleft palate, and cerebral palsy. Kuhn wrote how a query of an on-line dictionary of medical abbreviations yielded 79 medical phrases for the abbreviation CP.[14] Another problem is that abbreviations may be unfamiliar to those outside of the specialty. In a study of physicians who were not otolaryngologists, researchers found that six of 13 commonly used abbreviations in the field of otolaryngology were unclear to 90% of the physicians.[15]

Concern about medical abbreviation use and its potential to harm patients led the Joint Commission on Accreditation of Healthcare Organizations to introduce an official list of <u>Do Not Use</u> abbreviations, acronyms, and symbols in 2004.[16]

List of Abbreviations <u>Not</u> to Use

U, u
IU
Q.D., QD, q.d., qd
Q.O.D., QOD, q.o.d, qod
Trailing zero (X.0 mg)
Lack of leading zero (.X mg)
MS
MSO_4
$MgSO_4$

In 2005, The Institute for Safe Medical Practice published a list of error-prone abbreviations, available at http://www.ismp.org/tools/errorproneabbreviations.pdf.[17]

Institutions have made it a priority to avoid these abbreviations. Many institutions have even developed their own list of approved abbreviations. Make sure that the abbreviations you use are approved, preferably by your own institution.

Rule # 138   Accuracy is paramount.

Student write-ups are generally the most detailed document in the chart, and therefore are likely to be referenced by other healthcare professionals. Your write-up may be referenced during the patient's present admission or during subsequent admissions. Therefore, accuracy is paramount.

While everyone would agree that all aspects of the medical record should be accurate, studies involving a variety of healthcare professionals indicate that this is not the current reality. In a chart review of resident physician progress notes in a neonatal intensive care unit, researchers found discrepancies in 61.7% of notes with respect to weight, vascular lines, or medications.[18] Discrepancies in the documentation of medications were found in 27.7% of notes, including omission of information as well as documentation of inaccurate information. The authors concluded that "daily progress notes written by resident physicians in the neonatal intensive care unit often contain inaccurate, or omit pertinent, information."

The accuracy of student documentation has also been studied. In a study done at the University of Texas Medical Branch at Galveston, senior medical students were videotaped examining standardized patients.[19] The patient encounter was then compared to the information documented by students in the patient note. Researchers found that only 4% of the notes accurately reflected what occurred during the encounter. The problems identified included underdocumentation, overdocumentation, and inaccurate documentation. The authors offered some potential explanations for why students underdocumented physical exam maneuvers, including forgetting that they had done the maneuver, forgetting to record it, or deciding that the maneuver didn't need to be recorded because of lack of relevance.

Did you know ...

Physicians may document information in patient records that they have not personally observed. In a survey of internists and internal medicine subspecialists, 59% reported personally engaging in a questionable documentation behavior.[20] These behaviors included "writing the admitting history and physical exam on patients without personally obtaining all information that was written in the chart, copying observations (signs and symptoms) made by other health care givers as one's own findings in notes" and writing notes on patients without personally seeing or examining them. A substantial percentage also reported witnessing such behavior in their colleagues. This practice has also been noted among students, some of whom embellish their notes after realizing that they'd forgotten to elicit information or perform maneuvers that should have been done.

Did you know ...

Once you have written and placed the write-up in the patient's medical record, it cannot be changed. It has the potential to be used as evidence in legal proceedings, such as a malpractice case.

Did you know ...

To determine the accuracy of medication histories, researchers evaluated 115 hospital medical records.[21] The written record was compared to a structured history taken by a member of the study's research staff. An error was defined as "either the failure to record the use of a medication the patient claimed to use or the recording of a medication that the patient denied using." At least one such error was found in 83% of all patients.

Rule # 139   Every write-up must be complete.

Your write-up should be very detailed, reflecting a thorough patient evaluation on your part. If you look closely at your clerkship evaluation form, you'll find that the highest marks for written communication are given to students who consistently produce *complete* patient write-ups or notes.

     The literature has shown that even practicing physicians have a high rate of inadequate or incomplete documentation. In a survey of 655 internists and family practitioners, while 99.8% reported documenting prescription drugs in the medical record, fewer physicians reported documenting over-the-counter drugs (68%), nutritional supplements (63%), and herbal treatments (47%).[22]

These findings are consistent with what Dr. S. Scott Tauber has observed.[23] "It has been my experience that oftentimes physicians do not take the appropriate amount of time during the initial office visit to thoroughly document their patient's history...One of the fundamental purposes of the initial patient history is to form the foundation for all the subsequent clinical procedures (examinations, radiographs, etc.) and treatment(s). Without this solid foundation, your treatment and procedures may easily become clinically unsupported."

Underdocumentation of patient information has also been reported in medical students. Jefferson Medical College researchers had students examine standardized patients.[24] Following the encounter, students documented their findings. Patients were asked to also complete checklists identifying the history and physical exam elements performed by students. When students' notes and patients' checklists were compared, an underdocumentation rate of 29% was found, a rate that is similar to experienced physicians.

Does incomplete documentation impact the quality of care given to patients? Dalhousie University researchers performed a direct chart audit of patients admitted with myocardial infarction or heart failure. They assessed documentation of cardiac risk factors and cardiac history, which would have obvious impact on the management of these patients.[25] Surprisingly, key information wasn't documented in a significant percentage of cases. Among patients admitted with myocardial infarction, lack of documentation for diabetes, hypertension, and hyperlipidemia was 22%, 18%, and 38%, respectively. Among patients hospitalized with heart failure, lack of documentation for previous myocardial infarction and heart failure was 42 and 35%, respectively. The authors wrote that "lack of adequate documentation of information that has direct bearing on the diagnosis and treatment of common clinical conditions is a concern...Risk factor assessment...is also a prerequisite for optimal patient management."

Did you know ...

In a study in which three student write-ups were evaluated by seventeen faculty members, incompleteness was the most common error students made.[26] Many clerkship evaluation forms ask evaluators to grade students on their ability to perform a comprehensive history and physical exam. As discussed, attending physicians are typically not present while you perform a patient evaluation. Therefore, the write-up becomes a stand-in for direct observation. The chief means by which you can demonstrate the thoroughness of your patient work-up is by turning in a comprehensive, complete, and detailed write-up.

Did you know ...

After videotaping clinical interviews performed by medical residents, the contents of each videotape were compared with the medical record to determine the adequacy of medical history documentation. Researchers found that "residents recorded a little over half of all medical history information observed on the videotapes."[27]

Rule # 140   The ability to write legibly is an underappreciated, yet vital, skill.

Doctors and their poor handwriting skills are the subject of many jokes. Are they really any different from the general population? Studies have shown mixed results. An early study examining the handwriting of doctors and community volunteers showed that doctors wrote more malformed individual letters when asked to write a standard sentence.[28] In another study, no difference was found in the legibility of handwriting between doctors and administrators.[29] Recently, University of Kansas researchers had right-handed men and women working in diverse areas (law, auto repair, builder, engineer, doctor, scientist) write the following sentence in 17 seconds or less:[30] *The quick brown fox jumps over the lazy dog.* No difference in legibility was noted between occupations.

Regardless of whether doctors actually write less legibly than other occupations, the fact remains that 7,000 deaths a year in the United States are attributed to medication errors, some of which are the result of poor penmanship.

> *A Texas cardiologist wrote a prescription for 20 mg of Isordil to be taken every six hours. However, the pharmacist filled the prescription with Plendil, a medication which has a maximum daily dosage of 10 mg. The patient died after suffering a heart attack related to medication overdosage. A court of law found both the cardiologist and pharmacist culpable in the death of this patient, with the former being blamed for the illegible handwriting that led to the pharmacist filling the order with the wrong medication.[31]*

A number of efforts are under way to eliminate the adverse effects of poor legibility, including e-prescribing and electronic medical records. However, many aspects of patient care still rely on the handwritten note or order.

Poorly legible handwriting prevents other healthcare professionals from understanding or accessing key information. Their inability to read your work wastes time. If information is misconstrued or simply missed because handwriting is indecipherable, then the patient may be harmed. Even as a student, you will feel the pressures of time. This can lead to hastily written notes, write-ups, and orders. To avoid compromising patient safety, recognize that poor penmanship can have serious consequences, and review your work to ensure complete legibility.

Did you know ...

In the article "Don't be a target for a malpractice suit," Dr. Zurad writes that "the idea that illegible notes reduce risk because they obscure evidence is a common misconception. Not only do they provide no protection, plaintiffs' attorneys and juries view them as evidence of sloppy care."[32]

Rule # 141 Even a write-up must have perfect grammar and flawless spelling.

Poor grammar and incorrect spelling are often found in student write-ups, and will substantially detract from an otherwise solid write-up. This rule is imperative for your future career as well. Should you ever be named in a lawsuit, you will want your documentation to be free of these errors. Even if the care provided was sound, poor documentation with spelling errors, poor grammar, and sloppy penmanship creates an impression of carelessness.

Did you know ...

In a study in which student write-ups were evaluated by faculty members, poor readability/misuse of language was the second most frequent problem type.[26]

Tip # 44

Appearance makes a difference. If you hold your write-up out in front of you, does it look good? Is it pleasing to the eye? Before the attending physician begins reading the write-up, his first impression will be based on how professional it looks. Coffee stains, crossed-out lines, endless paragraphs, and poor spacing appear unprofessional.

Rule # 142 Respect all deadlines.

You will be given a deadline for submission of your write-up. Always meet this deadline. Clerkships usually make the deadlines, as well as the consequences of missing these deadlines, very clear in their orientation materials.

Consequences stemming from failure to submit write-ups in a timely manner	
Medical school department	**Write-up deadlines**
Department of Pediatrics at the Uniformed Services University of the Health Sciences	"2 complete written history and physicals required on pediatric inpatients. The write-ups will comprise 7.5% of the total clerkship grade. Both write-ups are due by close of business each Monday that you are on the ward. Write-ups turned in late will be considered a sign of poor professionalism and may result in grade reduction."
Department of Surgery at the Wright State University Boonshoft School of Medicine	"Each student must complete a minimum of 3 H&P's during the general surgery clerkship and submit their write-up via e-mail to the clerkship director for evaluation and grading. H&P's will be graded on format, content, and appropriateness of the differential diagnosis. These workups may be general surgery or subspecialty cases (excluding orthopedics) and should represent 3 different problems."
Department of Obstetrics/Gynecology at Michigan State University College of Human Medicine	"At least one write-up per week must be turned in every Monday starting the 3rd week of your clerkship. The final write-up is due on the last Friday of your clerkship. Failure to submit the write-ups in the required time frame will result in the student receiving a No Pass grade on the clinical performance portion of the clerkship."

A late write-up <u>will</u> affect your evaluation. You may also miss out on useful feedback that would improve your next write-up.

While you would think that late submission is rare, our conversations with clerkship directors indicate otherwise. Students miss submission deadlines for a variety of reasons. One of the most common is perfectionism, since a write-up could always be better.

Tip # 45
Turn in write-ups on time. There's always going to be something you want to change, word differently, or explain better. At some point, you have to let it go.

Did you know ...

Timeliness of documentation is also an issue for physicians. At the time of discharge, physicians are expected to complete a discharge summary, which is a clinical report that summarizes the reason for admission, diagnostic findings, therapy administered, hospitalization course, and recommendations on discharge. This document is important in maintaining continuity of care as the patient transitions from the hospital to the outpatient setting. In a review of literature on communication between hospital-based and primary care physicians at hospital discharge, researchers found that discharge summaries were often unavailable at the time of the first visit following discharge (only 12-34% were available). The authors wrote that this affected "the quality of care in approximately 25% of follow-up visits."[33]

Another study showed a trend towards decreased risk of readmission when summaries were available before the patient's outpatient follow-up visit.[34] According to Dr. Thomas Bodenheimer, a UCSF physician, "Discharge is a critical time for the patient. When we don't know about discharge, no one has charge of their care, and these patients get dropped in a major crack."[35]

Rule # 143   Seek feedback on the quality of your write-ups.

Write-ups are very useful for learning. They're even more valuable when faculty provide regular feedback regarding their quality. In one study high-lighting the value of feedback on medical documentation, percentage of documentation errors fell from the first to second months of a rotation following feedback.[36]

Did you know...

Medical students recorded data on teaching encounters, including learning and feedback activities, during an inpatient medicine rotation. Of the activities that occurred in the nearly 2,700 teaching encounters that were examined, receiving feedback on the written history and physical exam was next to last in terms of frequency of occurrence (frequency of 36%).[37]

Rule # 144 Assess your own write-up before submission.

This evaluation form should be used as a self-assessment tool. Your write-up should meet every single requirement.

	Below average	Average	Above average	Excellent
The write-up was turned in on time				
The write-up is legible and free of spelling errors/poor grammar				
The patient is clearly identified*				
The chief complaint is concise and stated in the patient's own words				
The HPI begins with an introductory statement that includes the patient's age, race, sex, and relevant past medical history				
The HPI is chronologically organized				
Each symptom is explored (onset, precipitating/palliative factors, quality, radiation, location, severity, temporal aspects)				
Pertinent positive information is included in the HPI				
Pertinent negative information is included in the HPI				
Past medical/surgical history, medications, allergies, social history, family history, and review of systems are included and complete				
Physical exam includes general appearance				
Physical exam includes vital signs				
Physical exam is presented in logical order				
All pertinent physical exam findings (positives and negatives) are included				
Breast exam in women is included				
GU/pelvic exam is included. If not performed, the reason is specified				

Rectal exam is performed				
Results of all test results are reported				
Problem list is complete				
Problem list is presented in descending order of importance				
An assessment and plan is given for all problems				
An adequate differential diagnosis is provided for each problem				
An adequate diagnostic and therapeutic plan is given for each problem				
Student is knowledgeable about illness or topic, including up-to-date literature				

*Your clerkship may ask you not to include the name, medical record number, or other identifying information on the write-up for purposes of patient confidentiality.

References

[1]O'Brien B, Cooke M, Irby D. Perceptions and attributions of third-year student struggles in clerkships: do students and clerkship directors agree? *Acad Med* 2007; 82(10): 970-8.

[2]Association of American Medical Colleges. Learning Objectives for Medical Student Education: Guidelines for Medical Schools (MSOP Report). Washington, DC: Association of American Medical Colleges; 1998.

[3]Gliatto P, Masters P, Karani R. Medical student documentation in the medical record: a liability? *Mt Sinai J Med* 2009; 76: 357-64.

[4]USMLE website. http://www.usmle.org/news/cse/step2csfaqs1103.htm. Accessed December 23, 2009.

[5]Kogan J, Shea J. Psychometric characteristics of a write-up assessment form in a medicine core clerkship. *Teach Learn Med* 2005; 17(2): 101-6.

[6]Parenti C, Harris I. Faculty evaluation of student performance: a step toward improving the process. *Med Teach* 1992; 14 (2-3): 185-8.

[7]University of Wisconsin Internal Medicine Clerkship. http://www.med.wisc.edu/education/md/curriculum/years-3-4/clerkships/internal-med/feedback-evaluation-and-grading/136. Accessed January 30, 2011.

[8]Hartzband P, Groopman J. Off the record – avoiding the pitfalls of going electronic. *N Engl J Med* 2008; 358(16): 1656-8.

[9]Thielke S, Hammond K, Helbig S. Copying and pasting of examinations within the electronic medical record. *Int J Med Inform* 2007; 76(Suppl 1): S122-8.

[10]Embi P, Yackel T, Logan J, Bowen J, Cooney T, Gorman P. Impacts of computerized physician documentation in a teaching hospital: perceptions of faculty and resident physicians. *J Am Med Inform Assoc* 2004; 11(4): 300-9.

[11]University of Florida Department of Medicine. http://www.medicine.ufl.edu/3rd_year_clerkship/responsibilities_expectations.asp. Accessed January 30, 2011.

[12]Sheppard J, Weidner L, Zakai S, Fountain-Polley S, Williams J. Ambiguous abbreviations: an audit of abbreviations in pediatric note keeping. *Arch Dis Child* 2008; 93(3): 204-6.

[13]Manzar S, Nair A, Govind P, Al-Khusaiby S. Use of abbreviations in daily progress notes. *Arch Dis Child Fetal Neonatal Ed* 2004; 89(4): F374.

[14]Kuhn I. Abbreviations and acronyms in healthcare: when shorter isn't sweeter. *Pediatr Nurs* 2007; 33(5): 392-8.

[15]Das-Purkayastha P, McLeod K, Canter R. Specialist medical abbreviations as a foreign language. *J R Soc Med* 2004; 97(9): 456.

[16]Joint Commission Official "Do Not Use" List of Abbreviations. http://www.jointcommission.org/Do_Not_Use_List_of_Abbreviations/. Published 2004. Accessed January 30, 2011.

[17]Institute for Safe Medication Practices List of Error-Prone Abbreviations, Symbols, and Dose Designations. http://www.ismp.org/tools/errorproneabbreviations.pdf. Accessed January 30, 2011.

[18]Carroll A, Tarczy-Hornoch P, O'Reilly E, Christakis D. Resident documentation discrepancies in a neonatal intensive care unit. *Pediatrics* 2003; 111: 976-80.

[19]Szauter K, Ainsworth M, Holden M, Mercado A. Do students do what they write and write what they do? The match between the patient encounter and patient note. *Acad Med* 2006; 81 (10 Suppl): S44-7.

[20]Sharma R, Kostis W, Wilson A, Cosgrove N, Hassett A, Moreyra A, Delneyo C, Kostis J. Questionable hospital chart documentation practices by physicians. *J Gen Intern Med* 2008; 23(11): 1865-70.

[21]Beers M, Munekata M, Storrie M. The accuracy of medication histories in the hospital medical records of elderly persons. *J Am Geriatr Soc* 1990; 38(11): 1183-7.

[22]Jaski M, Schwartzberg J, Guttman R, Noorani M. Medication review and documentation in physician office practice. *Eff Clin Pract* 2000; 3(1): 31-4.

[23]Tauber S. A complete initial patient history. What are the benefits? *American Institute of Personal Injury Physicians e-Journal.* http://aipip.org/a/10000/files/A%20Complete%20Initial%20Patient%20History.pdf. Accessed January 30, 2011.

[24]Worzala K, Rattner S, Boulet J, Majdan J, Berg D, Robeson M, Veloski J. Evaluation of the congruence between students' postencounter notes and standardized patients' checklists in a clinical skills examination. *Teach Learn Med* 2008; 20(1): 31-6.

[25]Cox J, Zitner D, Courtney K, MacDonald D, Paterson G, Cochrane B, Mathers J, Merry H, Flowerdew G, Johnstone D. Undocumented patient information: an impediment to quality of care. *Am J Med* 2003; 114(3): 211-6.

[26]McLeod P. Faculty assessment of case reports of medical students. *J Med Educ* 1987; 62(8): 673-7.

[27]Moran M, Wiser T, Nanda J, Gross H. Measuring medical residents' chart-documentation practices. *J Med Educ* 1988; 63(11): 859-65.

[28]Goldsmith H. The facts on the legibility of doctors' handwriting. *Med J Aust* 1976; 2(12): 2462-3.

[29]Berwick D, Winickoff D. The truth about doctor's handwriting: a prospective study. *BMJ* 1996; 313(7072): 1657-8.

[30]Schneider K, Murray C, Shadduck R, Meyers D. Legibility of doctors' handwriting is as good (or bad) as everyone else's. *Qual Saf Health Care* 2006; 15(6): 445.

[31]Hester D. Do you see what I see? Illegible handwriting can cause patient injuries. https://www.kyma.org/uploads/file/Patient_Safety/Physicians/Do_you_see.pdf. Accessed January 30, 2011.

[32]Zurad E. Don't be a target for a malpractice suit. *Fam Pract Manag* 2006; 13(6): 57-64.

[33]Kripalani S, LeFevre F, Phillips C, Basaviah W, Baker D. Deficits in communication and information transfer between hospital-based and primary care physicians: implications for patient safety and continuity of care. *JAMA* 2007; 297(8): 831-41.

[34]van Walraven C, Seth R, Austin P, Laupacis A. Effect of discharge summary availability during post-discharge visits on hospital readmission. *J Gen Intern Med* 2002; 17(3): 186-92.

[35]Louden K. Creating a better discharge summary. Is standardization the answer? *ACP Hospitalist* March 2009. http://www.acphospitalist.org/archives/2009/03/discharge.htm. Accessed January 22, 2011.

[36]Harchelroad F, Martin M, Kremen R, Murray K. Emergency department daily record review: a quality assurance system in a teaching hospital. *QRB Qual Rev Bull* 1988; 14(2): 45-9.

[37]Torre D, Simpson J, Elnicki D. Learning/feedback activities and high-quality teaching: perceptions of third-year medical students during an inpatient rotation. *Acad Med* 2005; 80(10): 950-4.

Chapter 17

The Outpatient Setting

The report "Medical Schools in the United States, 2008-2009," published by *JAMA*, evaluated how much time students spent in the ambulatory setting during required third year clerkships. The time ranged from 23% in surgery to 91% in family medicine.[1] Fifty-four schools had a separate ambulatory care clerkship, during which nearly the entire time was spent in the ambulatory setting. This data makes it clear that a substantial period of your third year will be spent in the outpatient setting.

Most students look forward to outpatient work. In the outpatient world, you'll experience medicine as it is practiced by most clinicians. You'll have the opportunity to develop your clinical skills in an environment far different from the inpatient setting. While one can argue that the skill set is similar, there are important differences, some of which present unique challenges.

Differences between the inpatient and outpatient setting	
Inpatient setting	**Outpatient setting**
Usually team concept (attending physician, resident, intern, students)	Generally you and your preceptor (often allows for more contact with faculty)
Follow up to 3-4 patients at a time	May see as many as 6 patients during a half-day clinic
Luxury of time	Time constraints
Opportunity to observe an illness over a period of days in the hospital	Contact with patient limited to one clinic day (i.e., patient may return for follow-up appointment after you have completed the rotation)
Expectation to carry out extensive and comprehensive evaluations of patients' complaints	Need to shorten and focus the history and physical exam

Develop treatment plan for the patient based on data gathered from comprehensive evaluation, including test results	Develop treatment plan for the patient based on data gathered from focused history and physical exam (often with no test results available)
Longer case presentations	Shorter case presentations a necessity due to other patients waiting to be seen
Call	No or minimal call
Weekend responsibilities	No weekend responsibilities
Longer hours	Better hours
Schedule often unpredictable	Schedule generally predictable

In this chapter, we offer recommendations to help you meet the challenges specific to outpatient medicine.

Rule # 145   Outpatient rotations are essential preparation for the USMLE Step 2 CS exam.

The USMLE Clinical Skills (USMLE Step 2 CS) exam is required for graduates of US medical schools. The exam simulates a typical day in the outpatient setting, lasting eight hours and requiring focused examinations of patients with a variety of presenting complaints. The absolute best way to prepare for this type of exam is to hone your skills as a physician in the outpatient setting.

Why is this exam required for graduates of US medical schools? The website www.usmle.org describes the need for a national standard, as medical schools differ in their teaching of clinical skills and their evaluations of those skills.[2] They state that: "During recent field trials, 20 percent of the fourth-year students who completed a survey said they had been observed interacting with a patient by a faculty member two or fewer times. One in 25 said they had never been observed by a faculty member."

The exam utilizes trained individuals who act as patients. The exam includes a total of twelve patient encounters, and students are given 15 minutes to examine each patient. During this time they must take a history, perform a focused physical examination, and communicate with the patient. They then have 10 minutes to document their findings in the patient note. The cases are chosen to represent the types of problems that would normally be encountered in medical practice. Just as in real life, therefore, the cases may suggest more than one diagnosis, and part of your skill lies in formulating and supporting a differential diagnosis.

Your grade will also be based on your ability to effectively communicate with the patient. The standardized patients are trained in the use of ratings skills to assess communication, interpersonal skills, and English-speaking skills. As in the clinic setting, don't ever be so caught up with the medical issues that you fail to communicate appropriately with your patient. You will also be tested on your documentation, including important positive and negative findings, your differential diagnosis, and your assessment and plan.

The exam is pass/fail, and further information on the exam format, grading, and examples of documentation may be found at www.usmle.org.

Rule # 146   Create your own orientation if one isn't offered.

Since many third year clerkships are exclusively or largely inpatient rotations, you may be relatively unfamiliar with the outpatient setting. The office setting is very different from the inpatient setting and many students find it difficult to move from one to another. Therefore, you should begin your outpatient work with an orientation.

Some preceptors recognize the importance of an orientation and have already developed one. Others may provide a sparse orientation, and you may need to gather the essential information yourself. Questions to ask your preceptor or the support staff include:

- Who will I be working with?
- What are the office hours?
- What is the dress code?
- Where should I park?
- Is there a space for me to work? Where should I keep my personal belongings?
- How does the patient schedule operate? How will I know which patients are assigned to me?
- What role would you like me to assume in patient care?
- How much time do I have to see an assigned patient?
- What parts of the physical exam can I do without you? What parts of the physical exam would you prefer we do together?
- What are the forms (radiology, lab request) that I need to become familiar with?
- Can you walk me through a typical patient chart? How is the chart organized? Where are charts kept?
- Would you like me to present the patient's case inside or outside the patient's room? Are there any differences in the way you would like me to present in these different settings?
- Would you like me to write or dictate patient notes?
- How do I order lab, imaging, and other tests?
- How do I schedule consultations?
- How do I schedule follow-up appointments?

- Can you show me a typical exam room? What instruments are available in the room for use? Where are supplies located (e.g., hemoccult cards, tongue blades)?
- Is there a computer that I can use? Who should I talk to regarding computer access?
- What resources, including textbooks and journals, are available?
- Would you like me to write prescriptions? If so, is there a particular way I should write them?
- If I have questions, whom should I contact?

Your preceptor may also ask you some questions, such as "Can you tell me what you hope to learn during this rotation?" She may also want to know about your previous clinical rotations, level of experience in the outpatient setting, career goals, and comfort level dealing with certain patients and patient problems. Sharing your goals is important. The American College of Physicians states that "explaining your agenda will help him or her teach to your needs."[3]

Tip # 46

I've seen many students rotate in an outpatient clinic and never bother to meet the nurses, medical assistants, and receptionists. In the outpatient setting, they are your team. They participate in patient care, help the clinic run efficiently, and can help you with your responsibilities. Make it a point to introduce yourself on the very first day of the rotation.

Did you know ...

In a study comparing the experiences of third-year students in the ambulatory versus inpatient setting, students in the ambulatory rotation "felt more like doctors, more responsible for patients, and more able to know and help their patients." They also reported better relationships with their teachers.[4]

Rule # 147   Clarify your responsibilities.

Depending on the field of medicine and your particular preceptor, your roles and responsibilities will vary widely. In some primary care settings, for example, you'll be given a great deal of responsibility. You may be asked to be an active participant in the care of patients assigned to you. This typically involves gathering relevant data from the patient's history and physical exam, organizing your thoughts, determining the likely diagnosis, developing a management plan, presenting the case to your preceptor, writing a clinic note, and following up on patient care issues. Unlike the inpatient setting in which time is generally not a constraint, in the outpatient setting you must complete all of this in a much shorter period of time.

In other clerkships, your role may be much more limited. You may even function primarily as an observer. Even if your responsibilities are limited, you should make it a point to ask your preceptor if there are any tasks that you may help with. This may include serving as a scribe, in which you write the note in the patient chart while the attending discusses care with the patient. You may write prescriptions as the attending outlines the plan of care with the patient, and then present them for signature. Even if your attending asks you to serve in a very limited capacity, you can still find ways to be helpful. Students can call for the nurse, obtain patient information material, or fill out lab requisition forms.

Rule # 148   Don't walk into the exam room unless you have some information about the patient or the reason for the visit.

In contrast to the inpatient setting, the time that you have to evaluate a patient's problem in the office will be limited. For this reason, the more you know about the patient before you walk into the exam room, the more you can accomplish. You must do all you can to adhere to the time constraints of the office in order to avoid putting strain on your preceptor's schedule. Keep in mind that while you're seeing your assigned patients, your preceptor will also be seeing patients.

Some preceptors assign specific patients to students. Assignments are often, but not always, made in advance. The day before clinic, ask the scheduling clerk for a list of patients assigned to you along with the reasons for their visit. You can then pull the patient's chart and learn about his active medical problems. It's far easier to do this the day before the visit when you have the luxury of time.

As you review the chart, make note of the following:

- What is the reason for the visit?

  For follow-up visits, determine which issues need to be addressed. Review of the previous clinic note will help.

- What active issues does the patient have?

  Many patients will have active issues that need to be reassessed at each appointment. Some of these problems may be in the process of evaluation, without an established diagnosis. An example would be anemia. With other problems pertaining to an established diagnosis, such as hypertension, the condition will need to be reassessed.

- What medications is the patient taking?

- What are the results of diagnostic tests (lab, x-ray)?

The process of reviewing a chart can take considerable time, especially at the beginning when you aren't familiar with the layout of the chart. As you become more familiar with its organization, your speed will increase and it may only take you 5-10 minutes to gather the key information.

Tip # 47

If you're having difficulty obtaining key information, ask your preceptor to orient you to each section of the chart. They can provide valuable tips on how to review a chart.

Before seeing the patient, your preceptor may also provide additional patient information that will help focus the visit. For example, you may be given a brief medical history and background, including the patient's current problems and concerns, and then asked to proceed with a directed evaluation.

Tip # 48

Before entering the patient's room, always have a patient care agenda. If the patient is presenting with a specific complaint, this will be the focus of your evaluation. However, in reviewing the chart, you may also note that the patient's blood pressure has been elevated at the last few clinic visits and that she's due for her screening colonoscopy. Your agenda may be to evaluate the patient's cough, check control of high blood pressure, and remind her to schedule her screening colonoscopy.

Rule # 149   Introduce yourself to the patient properly.

Because patients expect that they'll see their personal physician, it's best to have either the preceptor or a member of the office staff prepare the patient for your role in their care. Some preceptors will meet with the patient to request permission for student involvement in their care. Others may choose to have you accompany them into the patient's exam room while they make the request.

Some preceptors would rather have you introduce yourself to the patient. Dr. Kurth and colleagues at the Columbia University College of Physicians and Surgeons offer the following example of a good introduction:[5]

> Hello, Ms. J, I am SM, the medical student working with Dr. Y.
> With your permission, I will talk to you and examine you before
> Dr. Y comes in to see you.

It is always the patient's right to refuse such a request. Never take it personally. Also don't be surprised if a patient who agreed to a student evaluation later changes his mind. In these cases, don't argue. Simply respect the patient's wishes.

Did you know...

In a survey of over 1,000 patients visiting obstetrics and gynecology clinics, approximately 85% of patients would allow medical students to be involved in their care.[6]

You must make sure that the patient understands exactly who you are. Well-intentioned preceptors will sometimes introduce a student as "young physician" or "physician-in-training." It is very important that your patient understands that you are not a doctor but a medical student. There should be no ambiguity.

It also helps to inform the patient of your role in their care. You can simply explain to the patient that you will be performing their history and physical exam. Following this, you will return with your preceptor to complete the evaluation.

Rule # 150   Focus on the correct patient issues.

It's always best to ask the patient himself what prompted the visit to the clinic. You may already have been given a reason for the visit. It's surprising how often the given reasons vary from the actual reason.

Begin with "What brings you to the office today?" or "What concerns do you have today?" Many patients will visit the clinic with a specific complaint or symptom. Some will present to follow up on a particular issue. For example, a patient may be there for a blood pressure check after having his blood pressure medication adjusted at a previous visit. If the patient doesn't know the reason for the visit, the previous clinic note should help.

You should also ask what the patient believes is causing the problem, and what he thinks should be done about it. Patients often have expectations, and they may not share these unless you bring them up.

Outpatient primary care medicine provides a number of challenges. One of these is that patients often present with a number of concerns. In the short period of time that you have, it isn't possible to address all issues. Instead, you should aim to tackle two or three of the patient's problems. Which problems should be addressed at this visit? Let the severity of the problem and the importance the patient places on it guide you. For problems that aren't addressed, inform the patient that another appointment can be scheduled to address them.

After taking the history, excuse yourself while the patient changes into a gown. Return to the patient's room to perform the physical exam. In contrast to the inpatient setting where patients are new to the attending physician, most outpatients will have seen your preceptor in the past. Therefore, you usually won't be asked to perform a thorough physical exam, as you would in a newly hospitalized patient. Instead, you should perform a focused physical exam. If the patient is new to the clinic, however, a thorough examination may be necessary. Ask your preceptor.

Did you know...

In a videotaped analysis of histories performed by senior medical students, 24% of all students did not ascertain the patient's main problems.[7]

Rule # 151   Pay attention to key aspects of preventive care in the outpatient setting.

Physicians must remain current with preventive care guidelines. These guidelines change regularly as the results of ongoing research become available. Prior recommendations may be debunked, as in the utility of hormonal replacement therapy for post-menopausal women. Others recommendations are found to have utility, and become standard practice in specific populations, such as the administration of the pneumococcal vaccine to individuals $\geq$ 65 years.

Preventive care looms just as large in the management of chronic diseases. For patients with diabetes, part of the visit may be spent in titrating medication dosage to ensure optimal control of blood glucose. However, preventive care is a major component of diabetes management. Has the patient had their yearly eye exam? When was a urine test to check for microalbuminuria last performed?

Despite our knowledge of preventive care guidelines, implementation is a different story. Researchers from the Rand Corporation published their findings on implementation of recommended care for acute conditions, chronic conditions, and preventive care. They found that care for medical conditions varied widely. For example, recommended care in hypertension was provided only 64.7% of the time. In patients with diabetes, only 24% had received three or more glycosylated hemoglobin tests over a two-year period. Unfortunately, adherence to guidelines for preventive care was similarly poor. Only 54.9% of the patients studied received the recommended preventive care.[8]

In the inpatient setting, acute care is the entire focus. "Let's get this patient better and get this patient discharged." When students rotate in the outpatient primary care setting, they finally have the opportunity to focus on health maintenance. Do not overlook key aspects of patient health education and preventive care.

Rule # 152   Time constraints in an outpatient clinic are an unfortunate reality. Go above and beyond to ensure thorough and accurate documentation.

In the hospital setting, you have the time to complete a very thorough and accurate patient write-up. Time constraints in an outpatient clinic mean that your note must be written quickly. However, it must still be written with the same attention to detail and accuracy. Even among practicing physicians, proper documentation is an issue of concern. In one study of internists and pediatricians, documentation was 88% for compliance with screening guidelines, and only 61.6% for drug allergies.[9] For medical students, the clinic setting with its need for thoroughness and efficiency, along with speed, is a major challenge.

Rule # 153   Perform a thorough analysis of the data.

After performing the patient's history and physical examination, you are ready to evaluate the data. As you analyze the information, try to answer the following questions:

- What is the differential diagnosis?

    The differential diagnosis is a list of conditions that could account for a patient's symptom(s). Note that you won't always be required to develop a differential diagnosis. If the patient presents only for a blood pressure check following an adjustment in therapy, a differential diagnosis isn't needed.

- What is the most likely diagnosis?

    From the data you've collected, determine which one of the conditions in the differential diagnosis best accounts for the patient's symptom(s). Be able to offer support for your hypothesis. You should also be able to tell your preceptor why other conditions in the differential diagnosis are less likely.

- What tests are needed?

    Does any testing (lab, radiology) need to be ordered? You may wish to obtain tests to confirm the diagnosis, exclude other conditions in the differential diagnosis, or assess the severity of the patient's problem. You should be able to explain your rationale for ordering all tests.

- What is the treatment plan?

    Be able to explain the rationale for your management choices.

Did you know ...

In a recent study of the surgery clerkship, researchers found that students have greater opportunities to develop their critical thinking skills in the outpatient setting.[10] When compared to the inpatient setting, students in the clinic were more often the first to elicit the history (59.6 vs 4.3% of cases), perform the physical exam (70.2 vs 8.7% of cases), and generate the hypotheses (29.8 vs 2.2% of cases).

Rule # 154   Present succinctly.

After seeing the patient, you will present the case to your preceptor, either inside or outside the exam room. You must be brief, generally taking no more than a few minutes. One study found that teaching a medical student in an internal medicine outpatient clinic added 32.3 minutes to the clinic session.[11] Even without your presence, many preceptors are under considerable time constraints, with a highly scheduled clinic and with patients in the waiting room. Recognize that teaching adds to their time pressures, respect these time constraints, and present in an organized manner with only relevant patient information.

Tip # 49

In the inpatient setting, you are usually asked to make a thorough presentation. In the outpatient setting, however, time limitations require you to be as concise as possible. While you should strive to know everything you can about the patient, only present pertinent information.

If you're asked to present inside the exam room, you have additional considerations. It can be very difficult to present in front of the patient. Students often make the mistake of speaking about the patient as if they weren't there. In actuality, you should make every effort to include the patient in your discussion. Before you present, invite the patient to chime in during your presentation if the patient feels it's necessary. This way the patient can feel comfortable clarifying, correcting, or adding to the history as you relate it to your preceptor. You should also speak in such a way that the patient understands you. You should replace medical terms or jargon, including abbreviations and acronyms, with words that the patient can easily understand. It can be difficult to put this into practice, especially when you've been seasoned to present in a particular way during inpatient rotations. With delicate or complex issues, such as a possible diagnosis of cancer, you should bring this up with your preceptor before entering the room together. While you'll probably have questions stemming from your patient encounter, avoid asking esoteric or difficult questions in front of the patient.

Did you know...

Studies of resident outpatient clinics suggest that only 4-7 minutes are typically available for the case presentation and discussion.[12, 13] A poorly organized case presentation can consume much of this time. According to McGee, the case presentation should be less than 2 minutes long, and this requires that you prepare accordingly.[14]

Rule # 155   Outpatient presentations may be succinct, but they should still be formal.

You must adhere to the time constraints of the outpatient setting. In some clinics, that means very brief, focused presentations. However, don't take that as license to present in an unprofessional manner. Even though oral case presentations in the outpatient setting are brief affairs, they should still follow a specific, formal format.

"This is an older guy with a lot of AKs we need to treat."

Versus:

"This is a 76-year old Caucasian man with a history of multiple basal cell and squamous cell skin cancers. This is his six-month skin exam, and I performed a full body skin exam. I saw no lesions suspicious for skin can-cer. He has about twelve actinic keratoses on his hands and arms, and two on his nose. I have the liquid nitrogen ready to freeze those."

Especially given the tendency of most students to think that brief equates to sloppy, your well-structured presentations will stand out in comparison.

Rule # 156   Be prepared for your preceptor's questions.

After you present your case, your preceptor will ask questions. Some will be clarifying questions to ensure understanding of the patient's clinical presentation. Examples include "Does his chest pain worsen with deep breaths?" and "What's the dose of his lisinopril?" Note that these ques-tions are not asked to gauge your knowledge level.

Contrast this with probing questions, which are asked to assess your fund of knowledge and your understanding of the patient's medical prob-lems. Examples include:

- What do you think is going on with this patient?
- What findings support your diagnosis?
- What other conditions did you consider? Why are these conditions less likely?
- What test(s) should we obtain to confirm your diagnosis?
- How should we treat this patient?

Rule # 157   When presenting the patient, provide an assessment and plan.

Many students present the patient's history and physical exam and then just stop.

They deliberately avoid providing an assessment and plan. They feel they don't have enough experience or information to reach a correct diag-nosis, and don't want to be wrong. However, in order to develop your rea-soning and problem-solving skills, you should commit to a diagnosis, even if you feel you're going out on a limb. And if you don't provide an assessment, attendings will often prompt you with "What do you think is going on?"

A diagnosis is not enough, though. Most attendings will continue by asking how you reached your conclusion. Therefore, you should commit to a diagnosis and then provide evidence to support your impression. Don't worry if your preceptor doesn't agree with your assessment and plan. You're not expected to be right all the time. The fact that you took it upon yourself to offer an assessment and plan demonstrates initiative, a highly regarded quality.

Rule # 158   In many rotations, you are expected to follow up on those patients that you evaluated in clinic.

In most outpatient rotations, the expectation is that you will follow up on patients you saw in the clinic. After discussing the patient's case with the preceptor, the two of you will decide on a plan of action. A lab test or x-ray may be ordered. An issue may arise that requires research on your part. No matter what it is, it's your responsibility to follow through. For example, if a lab test is ordered, make a note of it and find out when the result will be available. When you do receive the result, determine what it means and report back to your preceptor.

Your follow-up responsibilities may include:

- Arranging for lab work or an imaging test
- Scheduling a follow-up appointment
- Writing or dictating a clinic note
- Educating the patient
- Calling the patient to assess response to therapy
- Updating the patient's problem list in the chart
- Updating the patient's medication list in the chart
- Arranging a referral to a specialist
- Scouring the literature to answer a question related to the evaluation or management of the patient's problem

Following through on these types of issues may not be a stated expectation of the rotation. However, it is still in your best interests to make this one of your responsibilities. You will benefit from the educational experience. In addition, preceptors are impressed with students who understand that the evaluation and management of patients does not simply end when the patient leaves the clinic.

Tip # 50

Your learning experience shouldn't end when the patient leaves the clinic. Follow through on all issues.

Rule # 159   Make effective use of your downtime.

In some rotations, students may encounter a great deal of downtime. This is particularly common when several students rotate in the clinic at the same time, and then have to wait their turn to present patients. Do not waste this downtime. Some students spend the time loitering in the hallway, talking about their plans for the weekend or the sports game from last night. Remember that conversations in the hallway can be overheard by patients in the examination rooms. They can also be heard by an attending walking by or busy in an exam room. Refrain from unprofessional behavior or casual conversation when in public areas.

Most students also somehow fail to realize that downtime can be an ideal time for learning about your patients. Unlike in the inpatient setting, you don't have the benefit of spending hours reading authoritative texts about your patient's case. Although you may only have a few minutes, that can be enough to significantly improve the quality of your patient presentation and ability to answer attending questions. In every rotation, you should carry a handbook or digital resource in your lab coat. Make sure you use it.

You can also use your downtime to review general topics, especially the evaluation and management of common problems seen in the clinic setting.

Type of clinic	Common symptoms or complaints
General internal medicine clinic[15]	Chest pain, fatigue, dizziness, headache, edema, back pain, dyspnea, insomnia, abdominal pain, numbness, impotence, weight loss, cough, and constipation
Family medicine clinic[16]	Abdominal pain, abnormal vaginal bleeding, chest pain, cough, dementia, depression, dizziness, dyspnea, dysuria, early pregnancy, headache, joint pain, leg swelling, low back pain, skin lesions, skin rashes, upper respiratory infections, vaginal discharge
Gynecology	Menorrhagia, polymenorrhea, intermenstrual bleeding, amenorrhea, oligomenorrhea, postcoital bleeding, dysmenorrhea, premenstrual syndrome, breast mass, nipple discharge, breast pain, contraception, dyspareunia, dysuria, menopause, pelvic mass, pelvic pain, vaginal discharge, urinary incontinence
Pediatrics[17]	Well infant exam, general medical exam, fever, skin rash, cough, sore throat, immunization, weight check, URI, earache, nasal congestion

Rule # 160　　Fully utilize electronic resources.

In some hospitals and clinics, particularly ones with electronic medical records, you may have computers in every room along with ready internet access. This means that in the span of just a few minutes, you can complete a preliminary literature search on just about any topic. Internet access means that you can do a Pubmed search, review information in UpToDate, read the chapter in Emedicine, or perform a Google search.

In many hospitals, you may also be able to access specialized databases or resources. In the Michael E. DeBakey VA Medical Center in Houston, you can access UpToDate, Lexi-Comp Online, and Micromedex, among others. Not familiar with these resources? You should be. These online resources are valuable tools in both inpatient and outpatient settings.

One of your first tasks as a clerk is to learn how to perform a literature search. Many medical center libraries will offer classes in how to maximize your use of Pubmed. You can also take the online tutorial at www.pubmed.org. You should learn how to perform the best possible search. This includes learning how to refine your search efforts. For example, typing in "sarcoidosis" pulls up nearly nineteen thousand references. In contrast, typing in "sarcoidosis and review" pulls up approximately two thousand. You should also learn what databases and journals your institution can access online, and from what computers. This allows you to pull up full-text articles from many journals. An excellent resource to help you navigate these tools is your librarian. I rarely see medical students speak to librarians, but they are experts in retrieving information efficiently. Also utilize the resources available in your pocket. Many students have access to PDA resources such as Epocrates, but don't use them as often as they should. In Chapter 9, The New Rotation, we describe a number of useful electronic resources.

Tip # 51

Learn the full extent of online resources available at your institution. Don't just rely on your resident's knowledge of what's available. Many medical center libraries, hospitals, and even outpatient clinics offer access to multiple databases and full-text journals.

REFERENCES

[1]Barzansky B, Etzel S. Medical schools in the United States, 2008-2009. *JAMA* 2009; 302(12): 1349-55.

[2]USMLE website. http://www.usmle.org/news/cse/step2csfaqs1103.htm. Accessed December 23, 2009.

[3]Steenburgh J. American College of Physicians Tips to Prepare for a Rotation in Outpatient Medicine. *ACP Observer* July-August 2003. http://www.acpinternist.org/archives/2003/07/outpatient.htm. Accessed January 23, 2011.

[4]Kalet A, Earp J, Kowlowitz V. How well do faculty evaluate the interviewing skills of medical students? *J Gen Intern Med* 1992; 7(5): 499-505.

[5]Kurth R, Irigoyen M, Schmidt H. A model to structure student learning in ambulatory care settings. *Acad Med* 1997; 72(7): 601-6.

[6]Mavis B, Vasilenko P, Schnuth R, Marshall J, Jeffs M. Medical students' involvement in outpatient clinical encounters: a survey of patients and their obstetricians-gynecologists. *Acad Med* 2006; 81(3): 290-6.

[7]Rutter D, Maguire G. History-taking for medical students. *Lancet* 1976; 2(7985): 558-60.

[8]McGlynn E, Asch S, Adams J, Keesey J, Hicks J, DeCristofaro A, Kerr E. The quality of health care delivered to adults in the United States. *N Engl J Med* 2003; 348(26): 2635-45.

[9]Soto C, Kleinman K, Simon S. Quality and correlates of medical record documentation in the ambulatory care setting. *BMC Health Serv Res* 2002; 2(1): 22.

[10]Boehler M, Schwind C, Dunnington G, Rogers D, Folse R. Medical student contact with patients on a surgery clerkship: is there a chance to learn? *J Am Coll Surg* 2002; 195(4): 539-42.

[11]Denton G, Durning S, Hemmer P, Pangaro L. A time and motion study of the effect of ambulatory medical students on the duration of general internal medicine clinics. *Teach Learn Med* 2005; 17(3): 285-9.

[12]Knudson M, Lawler F, Zweig S, Moreno C, Hosokawa M, Blake R. Analysis of resident and attending physician interactions in family medicine. *J Fam Pract* 1989; 28: 705-9.

[13]Williamson H, Glenn J, Spencer D, Reid J. The development of clinical independence: resident-attending physician interactions in an ambulatory setting. *J Fam Pract* 1988; 26: 60-4.

[14]McGee S, Irby D. Teaching in the outpatient clinic: practical tips. *J Gen Intern Med* 1997; 12(Suppl 2); S34-40.

[15]Kroenke K, Mangelsdorff A. Common symptoms in ambulatory care: incidence, evaluation, therapy, and outcome. *Am J Med* 1989; 86(3): 262-7.

[16]Duke University Family Medicine Clerkship. http://fmclerkship.mc.duke.edu/student/commprob.html. May 20, 2010. Accessed January 30, 2011.

[17]Serwint J, Thoma K, Dabrow S, Hunt L, Barratt M, Shope T, Darden P, et al. Comparing patients seen in pediatric resident continuity clinics and national ambulatory medical care survey practices: a study from the continuity research network. *Pediatrics* 2006; 118(3): e849-58.

Chapter 18

Evaluations

"Different doctors...achieve competency in remarkably similar ways, despite working in disparate fields. Primarily, they recognize and remember their mistakes and misjudgments, and incorporate those memories into their thinking. Studies show that expertise is largely acquired not only by sustained practice but by receiving feedback that helps you understand your technical errors and misguided decisions."

- By Jerome Groopman MD, author of *How Doctors Think*[1]

Feedback is a critical tool in medicine. Physicians utilize feedback from patients, from colleagues, and from their own observations of patient outcomes in order to improve patient care. In clerkships, the main purpose of formal evaluations is to provide valuable feedback that students can act upon to improve patient care.

Clerkship evaluations are also used to grade students. These grades, and comments on evaluation forms, are taken seriously by residency programs. In our companion book, *The Successful Match*, we review all the factors that form the basis of residency selection. The most important factor is grades in required clerkships. While the USMLE score is very important, it's a commonly held misconception that this one score is the most important factor in match success. The fact that grades in clerkships are most important overall makes sense. The number one goal of any residency program is to produce good doctors who provide outstanding patient care, and therefore reflect well on their training programs. Evaluations in core clerkships focus on those same attributes and the same overriding goal: outstanding patient care.

There is a growing body of literature devoted to the study of accurate evaluation. Evaluating a student's performance on a clinical rotation is challenging. In the basic sciences, the process is straightforward, as the evaluation is completely objective - what score did the student receive on the exam? In clinical rotations, subjective factors become much more important.

In this chapter, the focus is on the evaluation form, the factors used by faculty and residents to rate students, and the use of formal feedback. You'll learn the ways in which you can use this knowledge to improve your provision of patient care and increase your chances of clerkship success. You'll also learn about the inherent difficulties in subjective evaluations, and how you can ensure that these issues don't affect your evaluation.

Medical schools utilize a number of methodologies to evaluate students' clinical performance. These include end-of-clerkship written and oral examinations, objective structured clinical exams (OSCE), attendance at mandatory clerkship learning activities (lectures, rounds), review of required assignments (write-ups), and faculty/resident ratings. Of these methodologies, the latter is nearly ubiquitous throughout core clerkships done at U.S. medical schools.

The Liaison Committee on Medical Education (LCME) performed full accreditation surveys at 97 medical schools. As part of the survey, the LCME sought to determine how students were evaluated in clinical clerkships. The results showed that almost all clerkships rely on faculty and resident ratings as a method of evaluating student performance.

Percentage of 97 U.S. Medical Schools Using Faculty/ Resident Ratings for the Evaluation of Students in the Core Clinical Clerkships	
Clerkship	**% of medical schools**
Family Medicine	96.7
Internal Medicine	98.9
Obstetrics and Gynecology	96.9
Pediatrics	100.0
Psychiatry	96.9
Surgery	96.8

From LCME Medical Education Databases for 97 U.S. medical schools that underwent full accreditation surveys between July 1993 and June 1998. Also from Kassebaum DG, Eaglen RH. Shortcomings in the evaluation of students' clinical skills and behaviors in medical school. *Academic Medicine* 1999; 74 (7): 841-9.

Faculty and resident ratings usually account for a large percentage of a student's clerkship grade. Typically, 50 to 70% of a student's grade is based on these ratings. The following pages will help you understand all the factors that impact these ratings, and will help you maximize your chances of an outstanding evaluation.

Rule # 161   You must know, at the start of the rotation, exactly what your evaluators seek.

In a broad sense, you will be assessed in two areas – your clinical skills and your professional behavior. Evaluators will observe your day-to-day performance during patient care in order to draw conclusions about your abilities in these two areas. In particular, faculty members and residents will take note of your ability to take histories, perform physical examinations, present patient information, create patient write-ups, and interact with team members and patients.

From their observations of your work, your evaluators will rate you on these competencies. While all evaluators in a particular clerkship will be asked to complete the same evaluation form, the emphasis placed on the different competencies will vary.

Did you know ...

In an analysis of physician ratings of student clinical performance, residents and faculty were found to use different criteria to evaluate students.[2] Residents tended to place more value on a student's work ethic, teamwork, motivation, punctuality, interest in the specialty, and patient involvement. Faculty, on the other hand, placed more emphasis on a student's knowledge base and interest level. In another study, faculty reported that medical knowledge and problem-solving abilities were most important for the purposes of clerkship grading.[3]

Even among evaluators at the same training level, there are differences in the standards used to evaluate clinical performance. The following study highlighted these differences.

Did you know ...

In a study of over 200 faculty internists, participants watched a videotape of a resident performing a work-up of a new patient.[4] Immediately following the viewing, the faculty members rated the clinical skills of the resident. They also evaluated the overall clinical performance of the resident. There was significant disagreement between the raters. With one resident, for example, 5% of the faculty participants rated the overall clinical performance as unsatisfactory. However, this same resident's overall performance was rated as superior by 5% of the rater group. The performance was rated marginal by 26%, while 64% rated it as satisfactory. A similar result was noted with a second resident. Based on these results, investigators concluded that evaluators base their ratings on different criteria and standards. Evaluators may also assign different weights to the criteria that they use for evaluation.

Rule # 162   Specific faculty and resident comments are important.

The Medical Student Performance Evaluation or MSPE, formerly known as the Dean's letter, is an important component of the residency application. It summarizes an applicant's performance and accomplishments during medical school. Typically created in the summer and fall of the student's fourth year by one of the Deans or his designee, the MSPE is used by residency programs to aid them in the resident selection process.

Although the MSPE contains information about preclinical performance and extracurricular activities, the focus tends to be on clerkship performance. In addition to providing residency programs with the overall clerkship grade, narrative information from clerkships is included. Where does this information come from? On evaluation forms, there is usually a section in which evaluators are asked to comment on a student's clinical performance. Comments about professionalism, knowledge, communication skills with other health care professionals, clinical reasoning, and clinical judgment are most common.[5]

While comments are generally positive, evaluators may also include negative comments. Since comments made by faculty and residents are often taken verbatim from these evaluations and placed in the MSPE, you have to ensure your best effort in all rotations. Don't let your dislike of a specialty or a particular attending affect how hard you work or how well you work with others.

> *"Stacy rotated on our Obstetrics service, where she received a grade of Pass. She is interested in a future career in dermatology, and in evaluating her work ethic, we found that lifestyle issues did appear to be of importance to her."*

Such comments may sink your chances of matching into the residency program of your choice, or even your field of choice.

When reading the comments of an evaluator, you may at times notice a lack of correlation between the evaluator's comments and his rating of your performance. Comments may be quite positive, but not reflected in the numerical ratings. Why does this happen? First, an evaluator may not feel comfortable writing anything negative in the comments section. Second, an evaluator may place a higher value on factors that he didn't discuss in the comments section. You may be described in the comments section as "hard-working," a valued attribute. If the evaluator judged your problem-solving ability to be average, though, and gives that section more weight than work ethic, your ratings will be lower overall.

Did you know ...

While MSPE comments are generally positive, negative comments <u>are</u> included. In an analysis of nearly 300 MSPEs, negative comments included:[6]

"His most annoying attribute, he failed to show appropriate respect for his colleagues."

"She did not turn in write-ups on time and was felt by many to be defensive in the face of constructive criticism."

Rule # 163   Review, in detail, your clerkship evaluation form.

Clerkships will usually provide students with a copy of the evaluation form. This form is often included as part of the orientation material. If not, it may be on the clerkship's website. If you can't locate it anywhere, ask the clerkship director for a copy.

Evaluate this form early in the rotation. Your goal is to know the criteria on which you will be evaluated. This requires a thorough review.

The typical clerkship evaluation form consists of a number of general categories. These categories may include the following or variations of the following:[7]

- Eliciting a history
- Physical examination
- Interpretation and synthesis
- Technical skills
- Medical knowledge
- Oral presentation
- Written presentation
- Relationship to other health care providers
- Communication with patients and families
- Professional behavior
- House officer potential

Next to each category is a rating scale, which is usually numeric. For example, an evaluator may be asked to rate the student's relationship with patients on a scale of one to five, with five being the highest score. To guide evaluators, clerkship directors often place written descriptors of what constitutes high, middle, and low scores. On the Baylor College of Medicine "Evaluation of Student Performance" form, for example, the highest mark for "relationship with patients" is given to the student that has the patient's "full confidence" and "works exceptionally well with difficult patients." These written descriptors are important, and indicate the specific types of behavior required for the highest ratings.

The Baylor evaluation form asks evaluators to rate students in the category of patient-specific fund of knowledge. In this category, the form clearly states that the highest marks should be given to the student who "assimilates and applies relevant literature." There are a variety of ways in which students can demonstrate use of the literature. Examples include sharing a journal article with the team or listing references from the literature in a write-up. When students don't show me any signs that they're assimilating and applying relevant literature, I bring this to their attention at their mid-rotation feedback meeting.

These students are surprised to learn that they therefore can't receive the highest rating in this area. While all of them had seen the evaluation form, they had either missed or hadn't internalized this important point. My advice is to read your evaluation form carefully at the start of your rotation and then revisit it several times. Also consider filling out the form yourself as a self-assessment tool. This exercise may provide some insight into your progress towards meeting the clerkship's goals.

Tip # 52

As soon as you start a new clerkship, study the evaluation form. Familiarize yourself with the criteria on which you'll be evaluated. What descriptors are used to describe top performance in each category?

Rule # 164   Formal evaluations of your performance may be submitted by a number of individuals.

At most schools, residents and attending physicians are asked to complete evaluations of your performance. Although less common, other members of the healthcare team, including interns and nurses, may also be asked to provide evaluation information. At the start of the clerkship, determine which team members will be formally evaluating you. As obvious as this may seem, many students overlook this important detail.

Tip # 53

Are evaluations of your clinical performance weighted differently at your school? In other words, do attending physician evaluations carry more weight than resident evaluations?

Did you know...

Some clerkships use a multisource or 360° feedback evaluation system. In this system, students are also evaluated by other members of the healthcare team (beyond the attending physician and residents), including nurses and social workers. This evaluation system is thought to be more revealing in certain areas, such as professionalism, interpersonal skills, and communication. The Department of Anesthesiology at the University of Toledo writes that "in the 360-degree system of evaluations, information relating to your professionalism may be obtained from anyone you deal with in the course of your clerkship."[8]

Did you know...

Clerkships may use medical student peer evaluation, where classmates rate one another's performance in different areas. Peer evaluation is thought to provide greater insight into cooperative learning and interpersonal skills.[9]

Did you know...

Research has shown that patients and family members may be a valuable source of information about medical student performance. In one study, parents of hospitalized children evaluated medical students involved in their child's care. Although most comments were positive, critical comments were also received. The critical narratives focused most often on communication and confidence.[10]

Rule # 165   **Team members can and will talk to one another about your performance.**

Even if you learn that a team member has no formal input into your evaluation, realize that those with input can, and often do, seek the opinions of other team members. Attendings will often approach interns and residents to supplement their own assessments. This is a problem for students who consciously perform at a high level for those with input, but at a lower level for everyone else.

Did you know...

Faculty often receive information about students' performance from residents.[5] 66% received input about interpersonal/communication skills with other health care professionals. 56% received input about surgical/medical knowledge. 44% received input about clinical reasoning/clinical judgment, professionalism/dependability, and interpersonal skills with patients.

Did you know...

Directors from the different clerkships within an institution meet regularly, most often monthly. In one study, nearly half of the clerkship directors surveyed reported that these meetings "are the venue to discuss not only students who are in academic difficulty ('struggling') but also students' performance in general during clerkships." In other words, directors from other clerkships may hear of your performance prior to your rotation.[11]

Rule # 166   **The write-up and oral case presentation are critical components of your evaluation.**

Ideally, your evaluators will base their ratings on direct observation of your work. The evaluation of your ability to take a history and perform a physical exam should be based on direct observation. The literature has shown, however, that faculty members often don't observe students during a history and physical. How then do faculty rate students in these areas? In my opinion, if a faculty member doesn't have sufficient data to rate a student in a particular area due to lack of observation, he should refrain from evaluating a student in that area. Most evaluation forms provide the option "not observed."

While some mark "not observed," others will proceed to rate you based on inferences made from their interactions with you during rounds. In particular, the quality of your oral case presentations and write-ups will be used to draw conclusions about your skill in taking a history and performing a physical exam. If your evaluator feels that your oral case presentation and write-up on a particular patient was complete, he may conclude that your history and physical exam was complete as well. This conclusion may or may not be true.

Did you know ...

The AAMC asked over 13,000 graduating medical students in 2009 if they agreed with this statement: A faculty member personally observed me taking a history during the clerkship. Over 30% of students disagreed with the statement for the obstetrics/gynecology (32.7%) and surgery clerkships (37.4%).[12]

Did you know ...

In a study of students at the University of Virginia School of Medicine performed at the end of their third year, 51% reported never having a faculty member observe them while taking a history.[13] 81% had never been observed performing a complete physical examination.

Did you know ...

In one study, five of the nine faculty participants rated a student's ability to take a history and physical exam from factors other than direct observation.[5] They wrote that "in the clinic setting, for example, if a student presents a patient to an attending and is verbally facile, succinctly describing a focused history and physical examination, the inference may be drawn that the student expeditiously obtained the relevant history and performed an appropriate physical examination."

Rule # 167   **Direct observation of the history and physical examination is considered an important evaluation tool. Ascertain expectations and prepare accordingly.**

In recent years, the importance of direct observation has received considerable attention. Clerkships now strongly encourage evaluators to observe their students performing a history and physical examination. If your supervisor wishes to observe, ascertain expectations before the observed patient encounter. If you're unsure of his expectations, refer to the recommendations below. You should follow these recommendations even when not observed.

During an observed history...

- Begin your patient encounter by greeting the patient and family member(s) if present. Make good eye contact while shaking hands.
- Introduce yourself properly as a medical student, explain your role in the patient's care, and obtain consent to proceed with the history and physical exam.
- Inquire about the patient's physical comfort, and respond to any emotions the patient expresses.
- Sit with your body position bent forward slightly.
- Start the interview with the question, "Could you tell me why you came to the hospital?"
- Listen to the patient's story carefully. Avoid taking extensive notes while the patient is speaking.
- Let the patient speak without interrupting. Encourage the patient to continue by nodding, saying "uh-huh," or "please go on."
- Initially, ask open questions to encourage the patient to elaborate. As the interview progresses, ask closed questions to further characterize the patient's symptom(s).
- Avoid the use of medical jargon. Instead use common language the patient can understand.
- If the patient shows emotion, acknowledge and encourage the patient to discuss how he is feeling.
- Periodically summarize the information to ensure that you've understood correctly.
- Toward the end of the interview, ask the patient what he thinks is causing the illness. Ask the patient about his concerns and expectations.

During an observed physical exam...

- Begin by asking the patient for permission to proceed with the physical examination.

- Before laying your hands on the patient, wash your hands with soap and water.

- Prepare the patient for the different parts of the exam by informing him what you plan to do.

- Respect the patient's privacy. Do not expose any more of the patient than is absolutely necessary.

- Provide the patient with feedback during the exam ("your heart sounds fine").

- Be attentive to the patient's comfort during all aspects of the exam.

- If the patient asks a question during the exam, either answer the question or inform the patient that you will address it when the exam is complete.

- At the end, summarize the key findings.

- Complete the physical exam with a statement that informs the patient of what will happen next.

Rule # 168   Pay close attention to both intended and unintended feedback.

One of the most common complaints students have about their rotation experience is the lack of feedback. Many team members can and should do a better job of providing students with feedback. However, you can learn a lot about your performance by observing your colleagues and how they respond to you.

Many attendings and residents dislike giving negative feedback. Therefore, they may give you a lower evaluation without specifying the reasons. Students who pay close attention to nonverbal behaviors can pick up on dissatisfaction or disapproval before it is ever voiced, and even if it is never voiced.

Did you know ...

To highlight the importance of reading those around you, consider the results of a study that determined how attendings respond to students and residents who behave in a manner that conveys a negative attitude toward a patient.[14] Three types of problematic behaviors were identified. These included showing disrespect for patients, cutting corners, and outright hostility or rudeness. It was noted that attendings often did not respond to these behaviors. When they did, they often responded subtly with nonverbal gestures such as rigid posture, failing to smile, or remaining silent.

Rule # 169   Learn the skills of self-assessment, but don't rely on them exclusively.

As a physician you will have few, if any, formal evaluations of your performance. Therefore, you will need to rely on your self-assessment skills. Unfortunately, studies have demonstrated that the self-assessment skills of medical students are lacking. Students need to improve in this area, and you can begin by asking yourself the following questions:

- What did I learn?
- Was I an engaged listener during rounds?
- Did I ask enough questions?
- Was I on time? dependable? enthusiastic?
- What questions was I unable to answer?
- What feedback did I receive about my oral case presentation, write-up, progress note, etc.?

Even though educators emphasize the importance of self-assessment, several studies have cast doubt on the accuracy of students' skills in this area. In a study examining the accuracy of self-assessment among 130 medical students, students were asked to complete a form at the end of their anesthesiology rotation.[15] Their self-assessed grades were then compared to their teachers' evaluations. The results showed that only 4.6% were in general agreement. In another study, 47 medical students were asked to assess themselves at the end of their Obstetrics/Gynecology rotation in the following areas:[16]

- Fund of knowledge
- Personal attitude
- Clinical problem-solving skills
- Written/verbal skills
- Technical skills

These self-assessments were then compared to their final clerkship grades in each of these areas. The results demonstrated poor agreement between students' self-assessment and teacher assessment in the areas of global fund of knowledge, personal attitudes, and clinical problem-solving skills.

The results of these studies suggest that students' self-assessment during a clerkship is not accurate in predicting how residents and faculty will evaluate them. Therefore, students can't rely on self-assessment alone. They should solicit feedback to more accurately determine their own strengths and weaknesses.

Rule # 170   If a mid-rotation feedback meeting isn't scheduled, then you should request it.

The mid-rotation feedback meeting is an important one, and one that you should have with every team member that supervises you. At the mid-point of the rotation, you need to be informed of your progress in meeting expectations.

Did you know ...

The LCME requires clerkships to provide mid-rotation feedback for all students on core rotations.[17]

During this meeting, you and your supervisor can discuss your experience to date. You need to learn about your strengths as well as your weaknesses. You may be surprised. As disconcerting as it may be to learn that you're falling short of expectations, it's far better to learn about this now than at the end of the clerkship. With half of the rotation remaining, you can work with your supervisor to develop a plan for improvement. While students often don't have a clear idea of what they need to do to improve, you can ask for specific recommendations.

Rule # 171   Complete the rotation by meeting with your attending.

Before leaving a clerkship you should have a face-to-face final meeting with your attending. During this meeting, you will hear his thoughts regarding your clinical performance, along with suggestions for improvement. Although clerkships usually require these meetings, attendings don't always initiate them. If so, request one. "Dr. Parsi, since Friday's my last day, would it be possible for us to meet to discuss our month together and any suggestions you might have for me?" In order to learn and improve during your next clerkship, it is essential that you have such meetings before moving on to your next rotation.

During this meeting, you should receive a verbal assessment of your performance. Your main goal is to process the information so that you can improve your future performance. If you're not sure what actions you can take, you should ask for specific recommendations. If your attending has been particularly impressed with your performance, you may wish to ask for a letter of recommendation. Although some students hesitate, there's no rule that says you have to wait until the start of the residency application process.

These meetings can also have unintended consequences. There is some data to suggest that face-to-face discussion can lead to grade inflation. Two ward evaluation systems were compared at the University of Michigan Medical School.[18] In the old system, faculty filled out an evaluation form after the student had completed the rotation. It was rare for a faculty member to have a face-to-face discussion with the student to discuss the evaluation. In the new system, faculty were asked to fill out the same evaluation form but also had face-to-face final meetings with students. Significant grade inflation was found with the new system. The average grade increased from 5.11 ± 0.11 to 5.62 ± 0.07, with a 5 equaling high pass and 6 equaling honors.

Rule # 172   Elicit feedback from the resident and intern.

You know the importance of meeting with the attending to obtain feedback on your performance. It's equally important to meet with your intern and resident. You typically work much more closely with the intern and resident than with the attending. Having worked up patients with you, they'll be able to comment on your ability to perform a history and physical exam. They have also observed your performance of simple procedures such as phlebotomy and can evaluate your proficiency in these areas.

A formal one-on-one feedback session should take place halfway through the rotation. Ask about the areas in which you are doing well and the areas that need improvement. Your rotation should end with another feedback meeting. If your intern and resident don't initiate these meetings, you should.

Did you know ...

In one study, the teaching behaviors of fourteen internal medicine residents were observed during work rounds.[19] Residents offered feedback to team members in only 11% of 158 patient encounters.

Rule # 173   Seek specific feedback.

Consider the following statements made by attendings to their students:

"Your presentation was too long."

"Your progress note is too disorganized."

"Your write-up needs to be more detailed."

All are examples of feedback, but note that the comments aren't specific. What part of the presentation was too long? Is there a particular section of the write-up that requires more detail? Without specific feedback, it can be difficult to determine what changes need to be made.

When you ask for feedback, make your request as specific as possible. Too often, students ask general questions such as "How am I doing?" or "How do you find my progress notes?" Attendings often respond to these general questions with general responses. "You're doing just fine." By asking specific questions, you increase your chances of receiving useful feedback.

Rule # 174   Learn how to receive feedback, especially when negative.

Feedback is an important component of growth. Dealing with positive feedback is fairly easy - we all like to hear about things we're doing well. Negative feedback is more of an issue for students. Some individuals have a difficult time handling negative feedback. They may become defensive, shift the blame elsewhere, or deny that any problem exists. Some students view any suggestions for improvement as a personal attack. These responses give the impression that you aren't receptive to feedback and are unwilling to alter your behavior.

There are correct ways to react to and respond to negative feedback. Always allow the person to finish before you respond. As obvious as this seems, you'd be surprised how often students won't let an evaluator finish a negative statement. Especially with negative feedback, you need to stay in control of your emotions, because you may experience feelings of shame, embarrassment, frustration, or anger. After unfavorable feedback, students have been known to react in all sorts of ways, including outbursts of anger and crying.

If you disagree, your goal is to determine why the attending feels differently. Negative feedback is not a personal attack, but rather one individual's opinion of your performance. After listening, ask for clarification if any items are unclear. Summarize what has been said before you respond, which is a good way to make sure you've interpreted the feedback correctly. If you have erred, take responsibility for the mistake, take action to correct the situation, and inform your attending that it won't happen again. If you think the feedback is unfair or unfounded, you can, of course, express your opinion and defend yourself. Do so in a professional and collegial manner.

Tip # 54

Attending physicians commonly sandwich their feedback, starting with positives, followed by areas needing improvement, and ending with positives. With this approach, students sometimes only hear the positives. To avoid this, always summarize the feedback you receive so that you are clear on the positives as well as the areas needing improvement.

Did you know…

How you respond to feedback gives others a sense of your professionalism. Being defensive or resistant to advice/criticism, showing an unwillingness to consider a change in behavior, and refusing to acknowledge self as a cause of failure are all behaviors that indicate a lack of learner professionalism.[20]

Rule # 175   Act on feedback.

With some feedback, students aren't sure how to proceed. The attending may inform you that your oral case presentations on newly admitted patients are taking up too much time during rounds. How do you shorten your presentation? Do you shorten the history of present illness, the review of systems, or some other section? Start by asking the individual who identified the problem. In this situation, the attending probably has a solution, or at least some suggestions. As you make changes, check back to see if you're progressing satisfactorily.

Tip # 55

It's never too late to make changes. If you've performed poorly overall or in some specific regard, don't assume that you can't change the way others view you and your abilities. Recognize that things can improve and consistently demonstrate that they have improved.

Rule # 176   You must learn, and manage whenever possible, those factors that can cloud your evaluation.

The clinical evaluation of students during rotations is far from perfect. Evaluators can be affected by a variety of factors, some of which can lead to ratings that are lower than the student deserves. These sources of bias are shown in the following table.

Rating error	Description
Central tendency	The evaluator rates everyone as average regardless of performance because of laziness or the desire not to appear too harsh or lenient. It can also occur when the evaluator has difficulty rating a student accurately because he has observed the student infrequently or briefly.
Severity bias	The evaluator is extremely harsh in his assessment regardless of performance ("hawk").
Horn effect	The student is rated lower across the board because of one factor that is particularly bothersome to the evaluator. A student may be above average in working with others, paying attention to detail, and fund of knowledge, but since they're seen as overly quiet, the performance is rated lower.
Recency bias	The student is rated lower because his most recent clinical performance was suboptimal (over-emphasis on recent performance). With recency bias, an evaluator fails to take into account the entire period of evaluation.
Primacy bias	The student is rated lower because his early performance was suboptimal (over-emphasis on early performance). The evaluator is not able to get past the student's bad start.
Contrast effect	Rather than comparing the student's performance against the expectations, goals, and objectives of the clerkship, the student is compared with the occasional student who far exceeds the highest standards. This can lead to a lower rating than the student deserves.

To guard against these errors, evaluators ideally should be trained on how to complete evaluation forms properly. Unfortunately, schools don't often offer this training and, even when they do, evaluators may not take advantage of the opportunity. As a result, rating errors can and do occur. This isn't because of malice. Evaluators are simply unaware that they're making these errors. What can you do to avoid a rating error?

- Work with your evaluators as closely as you can, letting them observe you as you complete your tasks and fulfill your responsibilities. If your evaluators have observed you frequently, they are less likely to rate you as average (provided that you perform at a high level). Average ratings sometimes result when students are observed infrequently.

- Finish your rotation on a high note. As obvious as this seems, for some students it can be difficult to put into practice. Why? Because as the rotation draws to a close, students naturally start spending more time preparing for the end-of-clerkship exam and less time reading about their patients. Don't lose sight of the fact that your evaluation will be completed either at the end of the rotation or soon after the rotation ends. Your performance at the end of the rotation will be fresh in the minds of your evaluators. Your work early in the rotation may not be remembered as well.

- Don't underestimate the importance of making a good first impression. With every task you complete, strive to do your best work right from the start. This is especially true for your oral case presentations and write-ups. If you start off impressively, you may be seen as a student who is further along than most.

Even if you follow these recommendations, you can't guarantee that a rating error won't occur. Clerkship directors realize that rating errors can occur and make attempts to overcome the effects of these tendencies. In many rotations, clerkship directors will solicit multiple evaluations from those that supervise your work. When a number of evaluations are obtained, assessments can be averaged, leading to a more accurate assessment of your performance. This will mitigate the effect of any one person's rating error.

Did you know ...

At a study performed at five medical schools, 107 surgery faculty members each evaluated four or more students.[21] A total of 1482 ratings were obtained. From these ratings, the investigators were able to determine that 14% of the raters were significantly more stringent. Stringent raters were shown to rank students with true clinical ability at the 50th percentile at the 23rd percentile or lower.

Rule # 177   You may benefit from a rating error.

While rating errors may lower your evaluation unfairly, you may also benefit from them.

Rating error	Description
Halo effect	The student's performance is rated higher across the board because the evaluator is particularly impressed with one aspect of the student's performance. A student's high level of enthusiasm may lead an evaluator to rate other aspects of his performance just as well, even if the student is mediocre in these areas.
Leniency bias	The evaluator is extremely lenient in his assessment regardless of performance ("dove"). This tends to happen with students who are especially well liked by evaluators or when evaluators feel uncomfortable giving low ratings.
"Similar To Me" bias	The student is rated higher because the evaluator and student share something in common (e.g., alma mater, friend, personality, style, values).
Recency bias	The student is rated higher because his most recent clinical performance was significantly better than his previous performance (over-emphasis on recent performance). For example, a previously lazy, disinterested student picks up his work, energy level, and enthusiasm during the last week of the rotation, leading to higher ratings.

If you haven't performed as well as you would have liked during the first half of a rotation, don't assume that you can't receive a good evaluation. Since evaluation forms are completed either at the end of the rotation or soon after the rotation ends, evaluators can be influenced by what happens toward the end of a rotation. Finish the rotation on a high note.

Did you know ...

At a study performed at five medical schools, 107 surgery faculty members each evaluated four or more students.[21] A total of 1482 ratings were obtained. From these ratings, the investigators were able to determine that 13% of the raters were significantly more lenient. Lenient raters were shown to rank students with true clinical ability at the 50th percentile at the 76th percentile or higher.

Don't underestimate the "likability" factor. Your interpersonal skills, your communication skills, and your ability to interact well with team members can all influence your final evaluation.

Did you know ...

In a survey of LCME accredited schools, 48% of Internal Medicine clerkship directors felt that grade inflation did exist.[22] Among the factors that directors felt contributed to grade inflation was "a tendency to reward one aspect of a student's skills, that is, interpersonal skills, over skills in such areas as problem solving and history and physical examination..."

Did you know...

How much can likability influence your ratings? Consider the results of two studies. In one study, faculty were asked to view videotaped student case presentations in an effort to determine what effects personal characteristics have on the ratings of student performance.[23] This study demonstrated that personal characteristics could significantly influence the ratings. In another study, faculty observed students interviewing standardized patients on videotape.[24] Two nationally recognized experts were also asked to do the same. When compared with the experts, it was shown that likability was a significant factor that influenced faculty ratings.

Interpersonal skills can and do influence the assessment of student performance. Don't ignore this aspect of your performance. We discuss in other sections recommendations for enhancing communication and rapport with patients and team members.

Rule # 179   The rotation's not over until the evaluations are in.

Sarah did well on her rotation, frequently receiving strong positive feedback from her attending Dr. Bauer. She was confident that she would receive a great clinical evaluation. Several weeks later, though, she was disappointed to receive a high pass. The clerkship director informed her that while she met the criteria for honors based on her exam score, the overall grade fell just short of honors, due to her average on clinical evaluations. She learned that out of all her evaluators, only Dr. Bauer didn't submit an evaluation, probably impacting her final grade.

As a student, this may seem far-fetched. Unfortunately, this scenario plays itself out all too frequently. Clerkship directors will tell you how difficult it is for them to get faculty and residents to not only complete and submit clinical evaluations, but also to do so on time. As one clerkship director told me, "It's the bane of my existence."

> **Did you know ...**
>
> In a survey of U.S. and Canadian deans for student affairs, survey participants described a variety of problems with the clinical evaluation system, including tardy submission of clerkship evaluation forms.[25] Over 30% of evaluation forms were turned in more than 2 months late.

Rather than taking a passive attitude, you should be proactive. Some rotations encourage students to give evaluation forms directly to residents and faculty several days before the clerkship ends. The idea is that residents and faculty will find it harder to resist a request to complete an evaluation when it comes directly from the student. If your clerkship has such a policy, approach your evaluators at least a week before the rotation's end, hand them the evaluation form, and schedule a day and a time to discuss your overall performance.

If your clerkship sends clinical evaluation forms directly to evaluators, you can still encourage them to complete and submit these forms. To begin with, set up a final meeting to discuss your overall clinical performance. Often this will spur evaluators to complete the evaluation as a way to organize their thoughts and prepare for the meeting.

Rule # 180   One poor clinical evaluation must be taken in context.

As upsetting as an unfavorable evaluation can be, it is just one component used to determine your clerkship grade. Evaluations are typically gathered from a number of individuals who have supervised your work. The unfavorable evaluation may be just one of a handful. If the others are glowing, it may have little effect on your grade.

If you disagree with your clerkship grade, schools will usually allow you to appeal. Most schools have a policy in place that guides students through the process. Since guidelines for appealing a grade differ, you should familiarize yourself with the process at your own school.

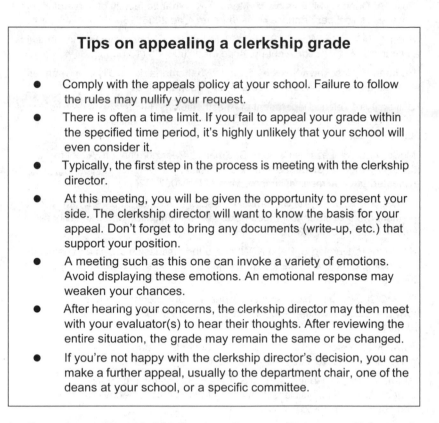

Tips on appealing a clerkship grade

- Comply with the appeals policy at your school. Failure to follow the rules may nullify your request.

- There is often a time limit. If you fail to appeal your grade within the specified time period, it's highly unlikely that your school will even consider it.

- Typically, the first step in the process is meeting with the clerkship director.

- At this meeting, you will be given the opportunity to present your side. The clerkship director will want to know the basis for your appeal. Don't forget to bring any documents (write-up, etc.) that support your position.

- A meeting such as this one can invoke a variety of emotions. Avoid displaying these emotions. An emotional response may weaken your chances.

- After hearing your concerns, the clerkship director may then meet with your evaluator(s) to hear their thoughts. After reviewing the entire situation, the grade may remain the same or be changed.

- If you're not happy with the clerkship director's decision, you can make a further appeal, usually to the department chair, one of the deans at your school, or a specific committee.

In discussions with clerkship directors, it seems that successful appeals are the exception rather than the rule. However, if you feel that an error has been made, you should certainly consider it. It is possible, for example, for the clerkship to make a mathematical error in the calculation of your final grade.

References

[1]Groopman J. *How doctors think?* New York; Houghton Mifflin Company: 2007.

[2]Metheny W. Limitations of physician ratings in the assessment of student clinical performance in an obstetrics and gynecology clerkship. *Obstet Gynecol* 1991; 78(1): 136-41.

[3]Wimmers P, Kanter S, Splinter T, Schmidt H. Is clinical competence perceived differently for student daily performance on the wards versus clerkship grading? *Adv Health Sci Educ* 2008; 13: 693-707.

[4]Noel G, Herbers J, Caplow M, Cooper G, Pangaro L, Harvey J. How well do internal medicine faculty members evaluate the clinical skills of residents? *Ann Intern Med* 1992; 117(9): 757-65.

[5]Pulito A, Donnelly M, Plymale M, Mentzer R. What do faculty observe of medical students' clinical performance? *Teach Learn Med* 2006; 18(2): 99-104.

[6]Shea J, O'Grady E, Wagner B, Morris J, Morrison G. Professionalism in clerkships: an analysis of MSPE commentary. *Acad Med* 2008; 83 (10 Suppl): S1-4.

[7]Hoffman K, Hosokawa M, Donaldson J. What criteria do faculty use when rating students as potential house officers. *Med Teach* 2009; 31: e412-7.

[8]University of Toledo Department of Anesthesiology. http://www.utoledo.edu/med/depts/anesthesiology/clerkship/clerkship_info.html. Updated January 14, 2011. Accessed January 30, 2011.

[9]McCormack W, Lazarus C, Stern D, Small P. Peer nomination. A tool for identifying medical student exemplars in clinical competence and caring, evaluated at three medical schools. *Acad Med* 2007; 82(11): 1033-9.

[10]Liu G, Harris M, Keyton S, Frankel R. Use of unstructured parent narratives to evaluate medical student competencies in communication and professionalism. *Ambul Pediatr* 2007; 7(3): 207-13.

[11]Hemmer P, Durning S, Papp K. What are the discussion topics and usefulness of clerkship directors' meetings within medical schools? A report from the CDIM 2007 national survey. *Acad Med* 2010; 85(12): 1855-61.

[12]AAMC 2009 GQ Medical School Graduation Questionnaire. https://www.aamc.org/download/90054/data/gqfinalreport2009.pdf. Accessed January 30, 2011.

[13]Howley L, Wilson W. Direct observation of students during clerkship rotations: a multiyear descriptive study. *Acad Med* 2004; 79(3): 276-80.

[14]Burack J, Irby D, Carline J, Root R, Larson E. Teaching compassion and respect. Attending physicians' responses to problematic behaviors. *J Gen Intern Med* 1999; 14(1): 49-55.

[15]Sclabassi S, Woelfel S. Development of self-assessment skills in medical students. *Med Educ* 1984; 18(4): 226-31.

[16]Weiss P, Koller C, Hess L, Wasser T. How do medical students self-assessments compare with their final clerkship grades. *Med Teach* 2005; 27(5): 445-9.

[17]Guidebook for Clerkship Directors 3rd edition. http://www.allianceforclinicaleducation.org/publications/publications.htm. Accessed January 30, 2011.

[18]Coletti L. Difficulty with negative feedback: face-to-face evaluation of junior medical student clinical performance results in grade inflation. *J Surg Res* 2000; 90(1): 82-7.

[19]Wilkerson I, Lesky L, Medio F. The resident as teacher during work rounds. *J Med Educ* 1986; 61(10): 823-9.

[20]Hicks P, Cox S, Espey E. Goepfert A, Bienstock J, Erickson S, Hammoud M, Katz N, Krueger P, Neutens J, Peskin E, Puscheck E. To the point: medical education reviews – dealing with student difficulties in the clinical setting. *Am J Obstet Gynecol* 2005; 193(6): 1915-22.

[21]Littlefield J, DaRosa D, Anderson K, Bell R, Nicholas G, Wolfson P. Accuracy of surgery clerkship performance raters. *Acad Med* 1991; 66 (9 Suppl): S16-8.

[22]Speer A, Solomon D, Fincher R. Grade inflation in internal medicine clerkships: results of a national survey. *Teach Learn Med* 2000; 12(3): 112-6.

[23]Wigton R. The effects of student personal characteristics on the evaluation of clinical performance. *J Med Educ* 1980; 55(5): 423-7.

[24]Kalet A, Earp J, Kowlowitz V. How well do faculty evaluate the interviewing skills of medical students? *J Gen Intern Med* 1992; 7(5): 499-505.

[25]Hunt D. Functional and dysfunctional characteristics of the prevailing model of clinical evaluation systems in North American medical schools. *Acad Med* 1992; 67(4): 254-9.

Chapter 19

The Written Exam

Most, if not all, of your third year clerkships will end with a written examination. Full accreditation surveys of U.S. medical schools done by the Liaison Committee on Medical Education (LCME) found that the written exam was the second most common method of student evaluation in core clinical clerkships, just behind faculty/resident ratings of student performance.

For many years, the faculty at each school was responsible for the development of the written exam. In recent years, however, an increasing number of clerkships have adopted the National Board of Medical Examiners (NBME) subject examination as their end-of-clerkship exam. In a survey of medical schools, the NBME sought to determine the percentage of clinical clerkships using NBME subject examinations.

Percentage of Medical Schools Using NBME Subject Examinations for the Evaluation of Students During 2007 - 2008	
Clerkship	**% of medical schools**
Family Medicine	49%
Internal Medicine	93%
Obstetrics and Gynecology	97%
Pediatrics	84%
Psychiatry	87%
Surgery	92%
From National Board of Medical Examiners 2008 Clinical Clerkship Directors Survey	

Clerkships use written exams to assess students' factual knowledge and their ability to apply it. The commonly used NBME subject examinations are carefully constructed to ensure their reliability, validity, and objectivity. Because these exams are easy to administer and they provide data comparing performance to national norms, they've been adopted by many clerkships nationwide.

These are difficult exams. While medical students are almost uniformly good test takers, clerkships pose challenges that can affect your performance. In this chapter, we offer practical and specific strategies that will help you maximize your exam performance.

Exam preparation involves three main facets: the hands-on process of patient care, didactic lectures, and extensive reading. Providing care for your patients, learning from their real-life examples of typical medical histories and physical examination findings, and having those experiences reinforced and strengthened by teaching from your residents and attending is an invaluable learning experience. A number of studies have shown that student performance on NBME subject examinations improves with increasing clerkship experience.[1, 2, 3, 4]

Extensive reading is important. When in-depth reading about each of your patients is done correctly, it can be very effective. In this chapter, you'll learn the questions that should guide your reading on each patient. We also provide concrete recommendations for taking the exam, including a review of the possible formats, and a review of the NBME website to determine the content of each exam.

Before the exam

Rule # 181   The written exam may significantly impact your grade.

The weight that the written examination score carries in the determination of the overall clerkship grade varies from clerkship to clerkship, even at the same school. Typically, the written exam accounts for 20 to 40% of a student's clerkship grade.

Median Contribution of the Written Examination to a Student's Grade	
Family Medicine	20.0%
Internal Medicine	25.0%
Obstetrics and Gynecology	40.0%
Pediatrics	25.0%
Psychiatry	33.3%
Surgery	30.0%
From LCME Medical Education Databases for 97 U.S. medical schools that underwent full accreditation surveys between July 1993 and June 1998. Also from Kassebaum DG, Eaglen RH. Shortcomings in the evaluation of students' clinical skills and behaviors in medical school. *Academic Medicine* 1999; 74: 841-9.	

While evaluations of your clinical performance are generally more important than your written exam score, it's important that you understand your
clerkship's grading policy. Some important points to consider:

- In most rotations, a superb performance on the written exam won't
  make up for a poor performance on the wards.

- Most clerkships require a passing score on the exam to pass the
  rotation. According to the NBME, the average minimum passing score
  ranges from 53 in psychiatry to 62 in medicine.

- A passing exam score may not be sufficient to achieve a clerkship
  grade of honors, even with outstanding clinical evaluations. In some
  rotations, you must exceed a certain exam score or percentile to be
  considered for an overall clerkship grade of honors.

- If you fail the exam, you'll usually have to retake it. In some cases,
  students are asked to repeat the entire clerkship.

Did you know ...

Performance on the NBME internal medicine exam has been shown to
have some predictive value in identifying students at risk of performing
poorly on the USMLE Step 2 exam.[5] In another study, a significant
independent correlation was found between the NBME obstetrics/
gynecology subject exam and USMLE Step 2 score.[6] Failing the subject
exam increased the likelihood of USMLE step 2 failure fivefold.

Did you know ...

In a survey of internal medicine clerkship directors, 89% of clerkships
permitted students to retake the exam after a failed first attempt.[7]
However, after passing the retake, the highest overall clerkship grade that
the student could achieve was pass (62%).

Rule # 182   Exam preparation begins on Day 1 of the rotation.

Studying for the written exam should begin on Day # 1 of the rotation,
especially with short rotations that may last only a few weeks. With longer
clerkships, it can be tempting to delay exam preparation. However, clerkship days often start early and end late, leaving students with little time to
study. In the basic sciences, students get used to coasting in the first few
weeks, and then doing their heavy studying closer to exam time. Clinical
rotations don't allow for that type of preparation, as the workload is heavy
throughout the rotation. An early start to preparation is the key to not only
getting through the material, but also in providing the time needed to
properly review the subject matter.

Tip # 56

One of the best ways to prepare for the exam is to read actively about your patients. A particularly effective approach is to read about each problem on the patient's problem list. Then, for each problem, ask yourself:

What are the symptoms of the disease?
What are the signs of the disease?
What is the differential diagnosis?
How are these diagnoses differentiated from one another?
How do you work-up or evaluate the disease?
What test(s) are available to confirm the diagnosis?
What are the treatment options?
What is the prognosis?
What is the pathogenesis?

Rule # 183   Some of the best exam preparation comes from real world patient care.

Providing care for your patients, learning from their real-life examples of typical medical histories and physical examination findings, and having those experiences reinforced and strengthened by teaching from your residents and attendings is an invaluable learning experience. In a study of over 1,800 students from 17 U.S. medical schools, caring for more patients per day was associated with higher NBME internal medicine exam scores. Most clerkship directors felt that students should follow 3-4 patients at a time.[8]

Did you know...

A number of studies have shown that student performance on NBME subject examinations improves with increasing clerkship experience.[1, 2, 3, 4] This gives students taking the exam at the end of the third year an advantage, especially over students who take it early in the year.

Rule # 184   Didactic lectures may be valuable tools for exam preparation.

Several studies have shown that lecture attendance may affect NBME exam performance. When researchers compared exam performance between students who did or did not have a clerkship lecture series, NBME scores in internal medicine were about one half of a standard deviation higher in students who had a lecture series.[9] Another study showed that failure to attend clerkship lectures was associated with poorer performance on the exam.[10] While association does not prove causation, and lecture attendance may instead serve as a marker for more motivated students, the results are suggestive.

Rule # 185   Review the format and content of the exam.

At the start of the rotation, find out if your exam will be an essay, multiple choice, or standardized exam. If your clerkship uses the NBME subject examination, take the time to review the content of the exam at www.nbme.org. At their website, the NBME has made available the content of each subject examination, including the percentage of questions that will come from different areas. If your clerkship uses its own exam, refer to the orientation syllabus for information about exam content.

Clerkships often recommend that students use comprehensive textbooks such as *Harrison's Principles of Medicine, Cecil's Textbook of Medicine,* or *Nelson's Textbook of Pediatrics* as their primary resource. Because of their length and level of detail, these books are not ideal for exam preparation. It's better to use these books for patient-directed reading and to rely on shorter books for exam prep. You'll find that opinions vary widely among students regarding "the book" you should use. Solicit input from a number of colleagues, review the recommended titles, and select one that you feel is a good fit for you and your learning style.

Rule # 186   Set a schedule for exam preparation.

Savvy students create a schedule to help them stay on track. Create a reasonable schedule – one that doesn't force you to do too much on a daily basis but that does allow for coverage of all topics before the exam. If a busy day prevents you from reading about your scheduled topic, your schedule should afford you enough flexibility to catch up on a subsequent day.

Take advantage of downtime during the day. Since you never know when you'll have some extra minutes, it's best to be prepared for these blocks of time by having reading material handy. At the end of the day, these short blocks of time add up. Many students complete their scheduled reading during the workday while waiting for a lecture to begin, waiting for rounds to begin, or while on the bus ride home.

Tip # 57

Carry with you copies of the chapters you're scheduled to read. They're easier to carry than the book itself.

During the exam

Rule # 187   Pace yourself.

Students are given two hours and thirty minutes to complete an NBME subject examination consisting of 100 questions. Essentially, you have a minute and a half per question. While this at first appears reasonable, many students have had difficulty answering all questions in the time allotted.

What can you do to make sure you finish in time? It isn't practical to time yourself as you read and answer every question. Instead, determine where you need to be at one quarter, one half, and three quarters of the time allotted to finish. Don't rely on the proctor — you may or may not receive updates on how much time you have left.

Rule # 188   Read the question before you read the
clinical vignette.

The NBME states that questions on clinical science subject examinations are "framed in the context of clinical vignettes." These vignettes are often long and students have to read a considerable amount of information before they reach the actual question. It's better to read the question before the vignette. This helps you focus on the pertinent information in the vignette. As you consider the answer choices, read each and every option. Many students err by picking the first choice that seems like the best answer. Instead, consider each option carefully.

Rule # 189   If you don't know the answer, move on.
Avoid rumination.

NBME subject examination questions tend to be as difficult as USMLE Step 2 questions. On such a difficult exam, you'll come across questions to which you don't know the answer. Make an educated guess and then move on to the next question. Frustration or discouragement will only affect your concentration. I recommend that you:

- Not spend too much time on a difficult question. This cuts down on the time you have for the remaining questions. You don't want to miss easy questions located at the end of the exam because you spent too much time on questions at the beginning.

- Make an educated guess rather than leaving it blank. Unanswered questions tend to weigh on your mind. Will you have enough time to return to them? Preoccupation can affect your performance on the rest of the exam.

Tip # 58

Leave some time to review questions that gave you difficulty. Information you read in one question might jog your memory or provide a clue to help you answer a previous question.

Tip # 59

There is no penalty for guessing on the NBME subject examination. Answer all questions.

References

[1]Manley M, Heiss G. Timing bias in the psychiatry examination of the National Board of Medical Examiners. *Acad Psych* 2006; 30: 116-9.

[2]Reteguiz J, Crosson J. Clerkship order and performance on Family Medicine and Internal Medicine National Board of Medical Examiners exams. *Fam Med* 2002; 34: 604-8.

[3]Hampton H, Collins B, Perry K, Meydrech E, Wiser W, Morrison J. Order of rotation in third year clerkships: influence on academic performance. *J Reprod Med* 1996; 41: 337-40.

[4]Cho J, Belmont J, Cho C. Correcting the bias of clerkship timing on academic performance. *Arch Pediatr Adolesc Med* 1998; 152: 1015-8.

[5]Ripkey D, Case S, Swanson D. Identifying students at risk for poor performance on the USMLE Step 2. *Acad Med* 1999; 74 (10 Suppl): S45-8.

[6]Ogunyemi D, Taylor-Harris D. Factors that correlate with the U.S. Medical Licensure Examination Step-2 scores in a diverse medical student population. *J Natl Med Assoc* 2005; 97(9): 1258-62.

[7]Torre D, Papp K, Elnicki M, Durning S. Clerkship directors' practices with respect to preparing students for and using the National Board of Medical Examiners Subject Exam in medicine: results of a United States and Canadian Survey. *Acad Med* 2009; 84(7): 867-71.

[8]Griffith C, Wilson J, Haist S, Albritton T, Bognar B, Cohen S, Hoesley C, Fagan M, Ferenchick G, Pryor O, Friedman E, Harrell H, Hemmer P, Houghton B, Kovach R, Lambert D, Loftus T, Painter T, Udden M, Watkins R, Wong R. Internal medicine clerkship characteristics associated with enhanced student examination performance. *Acad Med* 2009; 84(7): 895-901.

[9]Magarian G. Influence of a medicine clerkship conference series on students' acquisition of knowledge. *Acad Med* 1993; 68(12): 923-6.

[10]Riggs J, Blanco J. Is there a relation between student lecture attendance and clinical science subject examination score? *Obstet Gynecol* 1994; 84(2): 311-3.

Chapter 20

Rotation Success

"Just when you start to catch on, you're thrown in to a new situation with new people, new problems, new patients, and new locations. It's back to square one."

- From *Surviving Medical School* by Robert Coombs[1]

"Going into third year my preceptor gave me no expectations, no rules, nothing except for, "here we go, follow me." You don't know what his expectations are. Then you wonder, as far as being assessed, how is that going to work out?"

- From "Perceptions and Attributions of Third-Year
Student Struggles in Clerkships,"
published in *Academic Medicine*[2]

Providing excellent patient care is your number one goal in medical school. Receiving recognition for that excellence is a related topic, and one that encompasses additional factors. You never just want to be the medical student on the team. You want to be recognized as a vital member of the health care team, making significant contributions to the care of your patients.

In order to succeed on a rotation, you need to learn how to quickly adapt to a new culture and new responsibilities. You have to hone your communication skills and establish relationships with every member of your new team. These interpersonal skills are critical for the most effective patient care, and you will be graded on them. Lastly, you need to strengthen certain characteristics that signal outstanding medical students. Many of these traits are the same that patients will use to evaluate your skills and effectiveness.

Quickly becoming effective in a new setting is always challenging. Transitioning between clerkships is even more so. In the outside world, you may start a new job, have a few weeks to settle in and get used to new responsibilities, and then have a few months to get used to the culture of your organization. In clerkships, this process is compressed dramatically. You may have only a few days to learn an entirely new set of responsibilities, along with learning how things work on this particular rotation and with your particular team. How well you adapt to these constantly shifting responsibilities and teams plays a major role in your chances for rotation success. In this chapter, we provide some practical techniques for maximizing your effectiveness during these transitions.

Every day on every rotation provides an opportunity to live your values and demonstrate your character. Integrity. Credibility. Enthusiasm. Initiative. How can you convey these essential physician characteristics? Evaluating a student on these qualities is a highly subjective matter, and yet patients and attendings must do so regularly. In this chapter we provide the results of research studies that have looked at medical professionals and these essential qualities. We also provide advice on conveying these subjective traits.

Rule # 190   Before you begin a rotation, speak with the students who have recently completed the rotation.

Classmates who have recently completed a rotation are a valuable source of information. Your goal is to learn how to maximize the learning opportunities presented by the rotation, and how to excel during the rotation. You need the answers to the following:

- Describe what you did during a typical day.
- What are the must-have books?
- What things did you find most difficult during the rotation?
- What would you have done differently?
- Who will be evaluating me?
- What is the exam format?

Rule # 191   Read the clerkship orientation information before the rotation starts.

Clerkships usually send students information several weeks before the start of the rotation. They may include forms for parking, computer access, and name badges. You may be asked to complete and return these forms prior to the start of the rotation. Failure to do so means that you'll be dealing with these issues on the first day of the rotation, while your colleagues are off and running.

If you're sent orientation information, then read it prior to the first day of the rotation. If you haven't received any information, turn to your clerkship's website, where detailed information may be available. At the very least, you need to know when and where to report, and if driving, where to park.

Tip # 60

A new clerkship is like a new job. There is a job description which discusses the requirements of the clerkship and your responsibilities as a student. Take the time to read this information.

Rule # 192   The clinical evaluation counts much more than the exam.

Students just starting clinical rotations often don't realize that the grading system is dramatically different from that used during the basic science years. During the basic science years, your course grade was based on objective findings. In other words, it depended solely on your exam performance. In your clinical rotations, the bulk of your grade will be based on clinical evaluations submitted to the clerkship director by your attending physician and residents. While most clerkships end with exams, these exams typically count much less in the determination of your overall clerkship grade.

Tip # 61

Although you will still have an exam at the end of the clerkship, it generally counts much less than your clinical evaluation. Don't focus so much on the exam that you let your clinical evaluation suffer.

Rule # 193   Don't miss any of the critical information during the clerkship orientation.

Clerkships typically begin with an orientation, in which the clerkship director provides an overview. The director will use the orientation to set the tone for the rotation, discuss her educational philosophy, inform you of the clerkship's expectations regarding student performance and attitudes, and convey other key aspects of the rotation. They will typically discuss these aspects of the clerkship:

- Course goals and objectives
- Overall course management and leadership
- Course policies and procedures, including hours of duty, overnight call policy, number of patients admitted on call nights, number of patients to follow at any given time, and guidelines for the written and oral presentation of newly admitted patients
- Student responsibilities, including required assignments and deadlines
- Attendance requirements
- Lecture/conference schedule
- Professionalism policy
- Recommended/required reading
- Learning resources
- Test/examinations
- Grading/evaluation process
- Whom to notify in the event of an emergency

A considerable amount of information will be presented. If necessary, take notes. Many students have run into trouble because they missed important details. I still remember one student who performed at an honors level but received a final clerkship grade of pass. She didn't realize that her write-up had to be submitted to the clerkship director for review by a certain date.

You should also, carefully, obtain information about the evaluation process. Be careful when doing so, as a perceived preoccupation with grades will reflect poorly. Find out who your evaluators will be, when this evaluation will take place, and what qualities will be evaluated.

Rule # 194   Focus on all of the important elements of the job, not just the obvious ones.

Some students are focused exclusively on learning how to perform patient care tasks. These include admitting patients, writing daily progress notes, presenting patients, and performing procedures. While your team members are observing your progress in these areas, they're concerned with many more aspects of patient care that are involved in becoming a competent, and hopefully outstanding, physician.

These additional concerns are not directly related to task performance. They include your ability to work effectively with other team members, your ability to learn new subject material, your communication skills with patients and the medical team, and your overall work ethic. When team members are asked about what impresses them most about new students, the ability to perform tasks is much lower on the list. Ranked much higher are skills in patient communication, ability to learn the rules of the rotation quickly, to get along with the team, and to display the proper attitude and work ethic. Note that these are not skills related to task performance, but rather so-called "soft" skills centered on your ability to communicate and interact successfully with others.

Rule # 195   If you must, make the right kind of mistakes.

As a new student, your work, behavior, and actions will be closely watched. Under such scrutiny, you may wonder how it's possible to avoid mistakes. It's not. Realize that you will make mistakes. Your goal is to make the right mistakes.

What are the "right" mistakes? These are the mistakes that are made naturally in the process of learning. For example, if you've never written a daily progress note, you'll probably make mistakes your first time. Contrast this with more serious mistakes, such as those that call into question the strength of your character. You never want your honesty, integrity, sense of responsibility, or reliability called into question.

Whenever you make a mistake, learn from it, own up to it, and take corrective action so that it doesn't happen again. Operate with the philosophy that while mistakes may occur, the same mistake won't occur twice.

Did you know ...

Errors made by students have been divided into two types.[3] The first type is technical or judgmental errors. These errors are to be expected as part of the learning process and are the result of inexperience or lack of knowledge. The second type of mistake has to do with professionalism or lack thereof. Examples include arguing with other healthcare professionals, failing to establish rapport with patients, and dishonesty.

Rule # 196   Effective relationships are the foundation of an effective team.

Your team is a group working towards a common goal - the delivery of outstanding patient care. The success of the team and yourself depends on how well your group works together. As simple as this seems, it's easy to lose track of the team concept, especially in the first few days. Unless you build good relationships with team members, rotation success will be elusive.

In the early days of a new rotation, many students are overwhelmed, and feel that their time is best spent in the library or secluded in the conference room. However, it's difficult to become a top performer if you don't place an emphasis on establishing rapport with your team members. That's why it's important to take the time to develop these relationships, especially in the early days of a new rotation. If opportunities to spend time with the team present themselves, take advantage of them. Go to lunch with the team. Take a coffee break with them. These are ideal times to learn about your team members.

Rule # 197   Anticipate, rather than react.

Edgar and his team admit Mrs. Motumbo, a patient with pyelonephritis. After a full evaluation, intravenous antibiotics are ordered. Edgar completes his work, heads home, and retires for the night. The next day, however, the patient's symptoms have not changed despite 24 hours of antibiotic therapy. During rounds, the attending turns to Edgar and asks, "What do you suggest we do now?" "I'm really not sure. The intravenous antibiotics should have worked. Maybe we just need more time?"

This is a common scenario. However, when admitting any patient and reading about their issues, you should always anticipate the possible outcomes. After starting treatment, there are only three possible outcomes: the patient's condition will be better, the same, or worse. You should always plan in advance on the course of action required with these different outcomes.

You should approach rounds by anticipating issues on the team's other patients as well. Most students approach attending rounds with the "let me play it by ear" attitude. They react to situations as they arise in rounds. Students who anticipate can better prepare. If your intern admits a patient with diabetic ketoacidosis, he will present the patient during rounds the following day. The attending is likely to discuss this topic. Although the patient isn't yours, anticipating the discussion and reading about the condition means that you can contribute to the discussion. You can ask intelligent questions and respond intelligently to any questions.

Rule # 198   The rules of the rotation may outline what's expected of students. Exceed those expectations.

Team A was on call and getting slammed with new patient admissions. Julie had finally finished her work evaluating two new patients.

Niko, her resident, asked "Can you help us evaluate and write orders on this next patient with pyelonephritis? I really want to get the antibiotics started."

"I've already worked up two patients, and the clerkship director made it clear that we were only required to pick up two patients on call."

"I realize that, Julie, but we could really use your help."

"All right, I'll do it" replied Julie abruptly.

As in this true story, some students plan to adhere to the bare minimum of requirements. In fact, many students do only what they need to do to get by. They operate with the idea that if they do something beyond what they are asked or expected to do, it should result in some immediate, tangible return. If you, in an effort to be helpful, retrieved all of the patients' films from the file room, you expect a show of immediate gratitude. This may not happen. The long-term returns, however, may include enhanced patient care, more teaching, better teaching, gratitude, and a more favorable evaluation.

Rule # 199   Always maintain the highest level of integrity.

In your efforts to be a successful student, you will often have opportunities to choose paths that may compromise your ethics and values. While such paths may lead to some success, they don't make you a better physician, your ultimate and overriding goal. The guilt and regret you will experience just serve to highlight this important fact. Always maintain your integrity.

Opportunities to compromise your integrity arise almost on a daily basis. A student is asked to order a serum TSH level, but forgets to do so. The student only remembers when asked during the next day's rounds. Not wanting to look bad, he says the result isn't back yet, knowing fully the test was never ordered. Such situations arise frequently, and many students choose to lie rather than admit the truth. The correct way to handle this situation is to admit the mistake, apologize, assure the attending it won't happen again, and then proceed to correct the situation.

Did you know ...

In a survey of students who admitted to cheating during the clinical years of medical school, reported examples included "recording tasks not performed" and "lying about having ordered tests."[4]

Did you know ...

In a study performed at the University of New Mexico School of Medicine, students were asked whether certain behaviors were ethical or unethical.[5] Survey participants were also asked if they had heard of or witnessed these behaviors on the part of their student colleagues. 21% had personal knowledge of students "reporting a pelvic examination as 'normal' during rounds when it had been inadvertently omitted from the physical examination." 35% had personal knowledge of students "reporting a lab test or x-ray as 'normal' when in actual fact there had been no attempt to obtain the information."

Rule # 200   Maintain your credibility.

Your credibility boils down to this- do you keep your word? Students run into trouble when they say things they don't mean or make promises they don't keep. In every interaction with your team, you have the opportunity to establish your credibility. If you tell your intern that you'll finish the patient's progress note by 10:30 AM, then do so. You can establish your credibility by consistently saying what you mean and doing what you say.

Did you know ...

Questionnaires were sent to the deans of student affairs at U.S. and Canadian medical schools, inquiring about the use of noncognitive criteria for student evaluation. Of the noncognitive criteria cited, honesty was mentioned most often, followed by professional behavior, dedication to learning, appearance, and respect for others.[6]

Did you know …

In a survey of interns and residents in a university-based internal medicine residency program, researchers sought to determine the frequency and type of unprofessional behavior among students, residents, and faculty over a one-year period.[7] Unprofessional behaviors that were noted included breaching patient confidentiality in public places, documenting history and physical examinations not actually performed, lying to patients, and signing others' names.

Being credible also involves the willingness to admit to mistakes. The credible student admits the error in a straightforward manner rather than ignoring, minimizing, or covering it up. If need be, she apologizes for the error, without offering justification. By taking responsibility, she demonstrates strength of character. She then corrects the mistake right away or, if not possible, takes action to improve the situation.

Credibility is something that is earned and requires effort to maintain. As many students have learned, it is easily destroyed, and once destroyed, can be difficult to restore.

Rule # 201   Take initiative.

Initiative is a characteristic that all successful students possess. Without initiative as a driving force, you yourself would not have reached this point today. Students with initiative are prized by their teammates because they get things done. During clinical rotations, opportunities to demonstrate initiative arise every day. The best way is to begin a task and follow it through to completion. The task may be assigned or one that you seek out yourself. Examples include volunteering to perform a procedure or give a talk.

You don't have to wait to be asked. Make it a point to recognize tasks that need to be completed. Identify the opportunity, inform your team members that you will take responsibility for it, and then proceed to get it done. "I know Mr. Sapolsky has been hesitant to get the bone marrow biopsy done. I went to the library and pulled some patient information booklets. Would it be alright if I sat down with him and went over the information?"

Tip # 62

Look for opportunities to demonstrate initiative. Don't wait for other team members to invite you to observe a procedure or perform one. If a procedure is to be performed, ask if you can do it. If not, ask if you can observe. Better yet, ask if you can help get everything ready for the procedure.

Did you know…

Initiative has been defined as "motivation, willingness to conduct patient care without prompting." In an analysis of comments written by faculty on medical student clerkship evaluation forms, 50% of students had a comment in the category of "initiative."[8] This is an example of a negative comment in this category:

A little uninvolved in the flow of patient care initially in the rotation, but toward the end was more active in coming to the OR.

Written comments placed in the evaluation form may not only affect your clerkship evaluation, but may also find their way into your Medical Student Performance Evaluation (Dean's letter), an important component of your residency application.

Did you know…

In the document "The Obstetrics and Gynecology Clerkship: Your Guide to Success," the Association of Professors of Gynecology and Obstetrics encourage students to "take initiative. 'How can I help out? I'll write the note on that patient' goes a long way to make the team function better and gives the residents more time to teach you."[9] Among other ways to show initiative is to "teach the team. Volunteer to help the team by reading about topics in depth and by sharing what you have learned with the group."

Rule # 202   The best physicians have a passion for learning.

Some students demonstrate a passion for learning. It doesn't matter what rotation they're on. They are excited to be learning about this particular field and are thrilled to have the chance to finally take care of real-life patients with these diseases. In the article "What does it mean to be a physician?" Dr. Whitcomb states that one of the essential attributes of a physician is that they must be inquisitive.[10] This attribute "contributes in an important way to the quality of care provided by physicians by ensuring that they continue to acquire the knowledge and skills they will need to meet their professional responsibilities as the nature of medicine changes during their careers." As a medical student, not every rotation will interest you to the same degree. The best students, though, recognize that every aspect of medicine is important to their education. They display this passion for learning on every rotation by working hard and reading extensively. As you gain more experience, you'll learn that every field of medicine may have future relevance in your work as a physician. Every field may also have a personal impact on the health of your own family and friends.

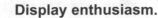

Display enthusiasm.

ıt is enthusiasm? One measure of its importance is the fre-
ᴡhich the word "enthusiasm" appears on clerkship websites.
In their Orientation to the Surgery Clerkship document, the University of
Virginia Health System writes that "most of the evaluation that occurs
from the interaction between the faculty and residents with the student as
far as grades are concerned has to do with the **enthusiasm**, interest, and
energy displayed by the student on the wards and not by their exact fund
of knowledge during the clerkship." At the website for the University of
Washington School of Medicine Department of Obstetrics and Gynecology Education and Training, it is stated that "preparation, interest, **enthusiasm**, and availability will maximize your opportunity to have one-on-
one interaction with faculty and staff, to develop problem-solving techniques, and to participate in hands-on activities in the wards, clinics, and
operating suites."

As one attending remarked, "if a student takes her education seriously, gives me her complete attention, values rounds, and essentially
carries an attitude that there is nothing else she would rather be doing,"
she is demonstrating enthusiasm. Attendings measure enthusiasm and
interest in many ways. They take note of how students speak, how they
sit, their facial expressions, their body language, and their questions.

Tip # 63

Displaying enthusiasm regularly can have a "halo effect" on your work.
Team members may tend to view all aspects of your work in a more
positive light.

Rule # 204   Smile.

When you begin a new rotation, your team will know nothing about your
character and abilities. Your goal is to appear confident and friendly, and
to quickly build rapport with patients and team members. A smile is one
of the most basic techniques for doing so.

Did you know …

Researchers observed the nonverbal behavior of 36 Harvard medical
students while they interviewed a patient or parent during their pediatrics
clerkship.[11] This analysis was compared with the final clerkship grade to
determine if nonverbal behavior was predictive of grade. They found that
the "profile of the highly evaluated student-physician, irrespective of
gender, was that of an individual who showed greater smiling..."

Rule # 205   As a future physician, every field of medicine is important and worth learning about.

In evaluating students, there are some who are clearly focused and determined to become the best physicians possible. They are clearly driven to learn as much about medicine as possible in order to provide the best patient care. They bring that sense of determination to every rotation. I can clearly remember several students who exhibited this trait. One was a prior nurse, going into primary care, who carried his dermatology handbook in clinic and read about every patient he saw. Another was applying to neurosurgery, and he also came to clinic clearly committed to learning as much about dermatology as possible.

I've also seen the opposite and can clearly remember a number of students who are only focused on their chosen specialty. They're going into radiology, could care less about this rotation, and spend the time between patients chatting about the baseball game last night.

You will often encounter rotations that you don't like or find meaningless. You may like the team members but could care less about the specialty. This attitude will affect your working relationships, and you'll miss out on valuable learning opportunities. As I tell students rotating in the dermatology clerkship, it really doesn't matter what field of medicine they choose. Everyone, eventually, will have a dermatology question, either for themselves, a patient, or a friend at a party. As a physician, some knowledge of every field of medicine may ultimately prove helpful.

Your attending will also be evaluating your performance, and that evaluation has considerable bearing on your overall clerkship grade. This grade will be part of your transcript. The attending physician's comments may find their way, often word for word, into your Dean's letter. "Stacy rotated on our Obstetrics service, where she received a grade of Pass. She is interested in a future career in dermatology, and in evaluating her work ethic, we found that lifestyle issues did appear to be of importance to her." Such a grade, and such a comment, will definitely have the potential to weaken your residency application.

Rule # 206   Be confident, not arrogant.

The most successful students project confidence. However, there's a fine line between self-confidence and arrogance. How can you be certain you're projecting the correct attitude?

While the confident student believes in herself, the arrogant student considers herself superior. The confident student is not afraid to admit a mistake, while the arrogant student never does. There are many more examples.

Of course, in the end, it is those around you who decide. If you ever receive feedback that suggests that you are overconfident, cocky, or arrogant, take it seriously. Make inquiries to find out what it is about your manner, language, or attitude that gives this impression.

Did you know ...

In one report, arrogance was one of the top 10 examples of unprofessional behavior.[12] Others include:

Dishonesty
Arrogance and disrespectfulness
Prejudices
Negative interactions with colleagues
Lack of accountability for medical errors
No or lack of commitment to lifelong learning
Lack of due diligence (ie., carelessness, laziness, and not following
  through)
Personal excesses (ie., substance abuse, gambling, and reckless
  behavior)
Sexual misconduct

References

[1]Coombs R. *Surviving medical school.* Thousand Oaks, California; Sage Publications: 1998.

[2]O'Brien B, Cooke M, Irby D. Perceptions and attributions of third-year student struggles in clerkships: do students and clerkship directors agree? *Acad Med* 2007; 82(10): 970-8.

[3]Bosk C. *Forgive and remember: managing medical failure.* Chicago; University of Chicago Press: 1979.

[4]Dans P. Self-reported cheated by students at one medical school. *Acad Med* 1996; 71(1 Suppl): S70-72.

[5]Anderson R, Obenshain S. Cheating by students: findings, reflections, and remedies. *Acad Med* 1994; 69(5): 323-32.

[6]Miller G, Frank D, Franks R, Getto C. Noncognitive criteria for assessing students in North American medical schools. *Acad Med* 1989; 64(1): 42-5.

[7]Shea J, Bellini L, Reynolds E. Assessing and changing unprofessional behavior among faculty, residents, and students. *Acad Med* 2000; 75(5): 512.

[8]Frohna A, Stern D. The nature of qualitative comments in evaluating professionalism. *Med Educ* 2005; 39(8): 763-8.

[9]The Obstetrics and Gynecology Clerkship: Your Guide to Success," the Association of Professors of Gynecology and Obstetrics. http://www.apgo.org/binary/Clerkship%20Primer%20Online%20Version.pdf. Accessed January 20, 2011.

[10]Whitcomb M. "What does it mean to be a physician?" *Acad Med* 2007; 82: 917-8.

[11]Rosenblum N, Wetzel M, Platt O, Daniels S, Crawford J, Rosenthal R. Predicting medical student success in a clinical clerkship by rating students' nonverbal behavior. *Arch Pediatr Adolesc Med* 1994; 148(2): 213-9.

[12]Hicks P, Cox S, Especy E, Goepfert A, Bienstock J, Erickson S, Hammoud M, Katz N, Krueger P, Neutens J, Peskin E, Puscheck E. To the point: medical education reviews – dealing with student difficulties in the clinical setting. *Am Obstet Gynecol* 2005; 193(6): 1915-22.

Attendings

Have the physical exam skills of physicians deteriorated over the years? It's widely believed that they have, thought to be partly related to an increased dependence on lab testing and radiologic imaging. This loss of skills may also be related to clinical skills training in medical school and residency. According to Dr. Sal Mangione, director of the physical diagnosis curriculum at Jefferson Medical College, too little time is spent during medical school learning these skills. "Surveys have indicated that less than 16% of attending time may be spent at the patient's side."[1]

These issues have real consequences. In one eye-opening study, over 300 internal medicine residents were tested on cardiac auscultatory skills.[2] They listened to 12 prerecorded cardiac events. It was found that their proficiency was poor, with mean identification rates of only 22% in American residents.

Clinical clerkships are a critical time in your education. If you want to become proficient in exam skills, you have to learn now. These aren't skills you can learn from reading a textbook. You need to evaluate patients with these findings, and you need to have a teacher who can demonstrate these findings. You need to be able to ask questions freely in order to learn all the finer points of physical exam skills. This isn't something you can easily do as a resident, and certainly not as a board-certified physician. If you don't know how to measure jugular venous pressure by the end of medical school, you may never learn.

In this chapter, the focus is on the attending. The attending physician is the leader of the team. His or her primary goal is to ensure that the patients assigned to the team receive the best possible care. The attending is also responsible for providing a solid educational experience for the resident, intern, and medical students.

If you wish to succeed as a physician, you have to learn everything you can during clinical clerkships. Your attending enhances your education in many ways. Starting with the basics of modeling and teaching skills in history-taking and physical exam, to the complexities of disease management, your attending is vital to your education. There's a reason why medicine is one of the few professions that still utilizes an apprenticeship type of training model. There are many skills that you can't learn in the classroom, or from textbooks, or from online courses. You need to have real-world experience with a teacher.

Attendings may also have significant influence over your future career. They are responsible for clerkship evaluations, and these are considered by many program directors to be the best indicators of potential for residency success. In order to be an outstanding physician, you must provide outstanding patient care. However, you typically won't be observed by the attending during direct patient care. Your interactions will often be limited to attending rounds. Since the attending has a great deal of control over your final grade, your excellence in patient care must be conveyed by other methods. These involve being well read on your patients' problems, delivering solid oral patient presentations, turning in thoughtful and thorough patient write-ups, and giving outstanding talks. In this chapter, we discuss general rules on how to interact with attendings, how to maximize your medical education, and how to convey your excellence in patient care. We discuss the rules that govern oral patient presentations, patient write-ups, talks, and rounds in other chapters.

Tip # 64

The relationship you have with your attending physician has a significant impact on your clerkship grade. Treat your attending as you would someone who has significant influence over your future - because right now, she does.

Did you know...

In a survey of over 300 attending physicians, respondents were asked to name "the one value/attitude they try to pass on" to learners.[3] Nearly 50% of physicians placed the highest priority on attitudes and values related to caring (e.g., empathy, compassion, concern, caring, understanding, and consideration).

Rule # 207   Strategize and plan to work with the best attendings.

There are many compelling reasons to seek out great teachers. You'll be working long, tiring hours with your team. An inspiring attending can motivate you to do your best work. Dedicated attendings work hard to help students excel with their oral case presentations and write-ups, skills that are transferable to all rotations. Excellent clinical teachers can improve students' clinical skills. These skills may include, among others, data gathering, an appreciation of physical findings through bedside teaching, formulation of differential diagnoses, or therapeutic decisions. In short, it behooves you to do everything possible to seek out attendings known to be great teachers.

Did you know ...

At the University of Michigan Medical School, researchers determined that "attending faculty's clinical teaching ability has a positive and significant effect on medical students' learning."[4] They found that ratings of teaching ability were strong predictors of students' performance on the end-of-clerkship NBME subject examination.

Did you know...

Researchers at the Medical University of South Carolina found that "students with attendings who received poor teaching evaluations performed more poorly on OSCE data-gathering stations than did students with attendings rated as average or good."[5] Students who worked with attending physicians with higher teaching evaluation scores were found to score higher on the NBME surgery subject examination.

One to two months before your clerkship begins, call the clerkship office for a list of attendings on service during your rotation. At many schools, attendings are evaluated by their students, and in some cases these evaluations are available for review. If your school permits, take advantage of the opportunity, making note of well regarded teachers. Contact the clerkship office to see if you can be placed on one of these teams. Make sure you call early enough, before team assignments are made. Don't be surprised, though, if the clerkship is not receptive to your request. Some rotations make it a policy not to accept student requests for team assignments.

Rule # 208   Maintain a written file of your accomplishments throughout the rotation.

As you progress through the rotation, keep track of your successes. Make an actual written list and a file of your accomplishments. For example, if your attending has written glowing remarks on your write-up, file it carefully. If your talk was particularly well received by the attending, jot down her comments, what she specifically liked about your presentation, and the subject of your talk. If your patient wrote you a thank-you letter, place it in your file.

If you later decide to ask the attending for a letter of recommendation, you'll have a record of these accomplishments that you can provide. Remember that attendings work with many students. As the months pass, specific memories may fade. While the attending may remember that you excelled, she may have forgotten the details. The strongest letters of recommendation are those that provide evidence to support their claims. "Aleks is a very compassionate and dedicated student. One of our patients wrote a very heartfelt letter attesting to these qualities."

Tip # 64

In a survey of internal medicine clerkship directors, respondents were asked about factors important in rating letters of recommendation. "Most important was the depth of understanding of the applicant, with 72% rating the category as essential..."[6] Since this is such an important feature of letters of recommendation, make it as easy as possible for the attending to write a glowing letter that demonstrates this depth.

Rule # 209   Active participation during rounds is necessary for rotation success.

Your interaction with the attending will mainly take place during attending rounds. It's important that you participate and contribute to the discussion. Some students don't participate at all, while others participate minimally.

Did you know ...

Teaching rounds were observed in a core clerkship at the University of Illinois. Analysis of these teaching sessions showed that medical students often functioned as a passive audience. In teaching rounds, students talked only 4% of the time.[7]

There are many reasons for this lack of participation. For some students, it's a matter of shyness, timidity, or insecurity. Others don't participate because they're bored, fatigued, or simply indifferent to the topics under discussion. Lack of knowledge, frustration with the rotation experience, dislike of the specialty, cultural norms, and a history of passivity in group teaching sessions are other reasons that impede participation. Most often, though, lack of participation stems from fear of criticism or embarrassment.

Students often hesitate to participate because they feel they have nothing profound to say. You are not expected to offer a breakthrough suggestion or profound comment every time you open your mouth. You are, however, expected to be an active and enthusiastic participant. If you talk to students who have completed a rotation or two, many will describe the same scenario: they wanted to make a suggestion, but didn't want to look dumb, so they kept quiet. Instead, another team member expressed the same intelligent thought and stole their thunder.

Asking questions is one way to demonstrate interest in the subject matter. In addition, attendings expect students to ask them questions. They welcome questions because they often stimulate discussion that can enrich the entire team's educational experience. If you're nervous about speaking up, you can develop a list of potential questions before rounds. You can develop this list as you read about your patients' problems.

Another concern is that of taking valuable time away from necessary tasks. If the attending is feeling time pressured, she may choose to answer questions after rounds, or during the next day's rounds.

Lastly, many team rooms are not conducive to teaching. If you're seated in a corner of the room, you may send a nonverbal message that you aren't interested in participating. If you've been assigned to a workstation in the corner, plan on moving to a better location. Reinforce your message that you want to learn and be involved.

Tips on increasing participation during attending rounds

- Do your homework. You'll feel more comfortable participating if you have prepared for rounds.

- Sit where you will be noticed, preferably between two team members who are active participants.

- Establish good relationships with team members. If you're comfortable with everyone, you're more likely to share your thoughts.

Rule # 210   Listen actively during rounds.

Rounds aren't always fascinating. Sometimes they're downright boring. Many students tend to focus on what interests them during rounds, such as discussions regarding their own patients. They may tune out the rest.

Attendings can pick up on this disinterest pretty easily. Body language cues can be very detrimental to a student's perceived level of interest. Attendings assume that you're not interested if you are:

- Looking through papers or working on the computer (unless it pertains to rounds)
- Slouched in your seat or repeatedly shifting position
- Talking to others
- Sitting with your feet up on the table or chair
- Doodling, playing with your hair, tapping or clicking your pen, drumming your fingers, tapping your feet, or twisting paperclips

I'm guessing you're thinking that you wouldn't be caught doing any of these. Most students, however, have no awareness of these habits.

Enter rounds with the proper attitude and motivation, recognizing that all of the discussion is ultimately relevant to your education. Students who are active listeners maintain an interested expression, make eye contact with the attending, and nod their head occasionally while listening. They may take notes to help them focus on the material being presented. They also ask questions which demonstrate their interest.

Occasionally, they may paraphrase by saying "If I understand you correctly …" or "So what you are saying is…"

Tip # 65

Students fall asleep during attending rounds all the time. Don't think it won't happen to you. The combination of fatigue, long hours, lack of sleep, and boredom can easily cause you to nod off. Actively taking notes can help.

Rule # 211   Prepare for an attending physician's talk.

On occasion, an attending will give a talk to the team. In some cases, this will be announced in advance. If you learn that the attending will be speaking on a particular topic, then read about that topic in advance. You'll become more familiar with the subject matter and you'll gain much more from the talk. If the talk is interactive and the attending asks questions, your preparation will help you field them.

Rule # 212   Greet your team members.

Early in my career, I was surprised how infrequently my team members, including students, would greet me when I arrived for attending rounds. Upon entering the team's conference room, I would usually find students, interns, and residents busily working. It was a rare team member who would stop what he was doing to acknowledge me with a smile, friendly gesture, or a greeting.

It is common for attendings to visit the team outside of rounds. The attending may simply want to be available to answer any questions or check on the progress of a patient. Irrespective of the reason for the visit, make it a point to acknowledge his presence. Don't be the student who just keeps his head down and continues to work until the attending physician leaves.

Rule # 213   Say thank you.

Your attending will be involved in your training, supporting you in different ways and offering feedback essential to your growth. Let your attending know how much you appreciate her help by saying "thank you." You don't need to wait until the end of the rotation.

As studies have demonstrated, working with an excellent clinical teacher can improve a student's overall performance in the rotation. If you have found that your attending was particularly helpful, you can reinforce the specific behavior by showing your appreciation and thereby increasing the chance that it will be repeated. "Dr. Huang, I really found it helpful when you went over the cardiac exam with me at the patient's bedside. Thank you for taking the time to do so."

Rule # 214   Don't be labeled a "difficult" student.

By the time third year draws to a close, some of your classmates will be labeled "difficult" students. Shortly put, that's not a label you want.

What makes a student "difficult?" Researchers studied how faculty members evaluate student performance in small group settings.[8] Three types of interaction problems were identified:

- Non-participating, quiet, and passive student
- Disruptive student who is sarcastic, disrespectful, or interrupts discussions
- Student who tries to take over the group and control it

Tip # 66

Even one instance of unreasonable behavior, particularly if it's offensive, can taint all your prior positive performance. It can be difficult or even impossible to recover from a disrespectful comment, racist remark, or deceptive act.

In a study looking at problem behaviors in medical students, teachers were asked to review a list of 21 types of "problem" students.[9] Residents and attendings were asked to comment on how frequently they encountered a particular problem type and the level of difficulty the problem posed for them. Frequent problems included:

- Bright with poor interpersonal skills
- Excessively shy, non-assertive
- Poor integration skills
- Over-eager
- Cannot focus on what is important
- Disorganized
- Disinterested
- A poor fund of knowledge

Of these frequent problems, two were consistently identified as the most troubling for teachers - students who were bright but had poor interpersonal skills and students who displayed excessively shy, non-assertive behavior. Of the problems that were less frequent, teachers were most troubled by students who could not be trusted, had psychiatric or substance abuse problems, or were manipulative. Note that attendings and residents have relatively more difficulty dealing with non-cognitive, or personality problems, than cognitive problems such as poor fund of knowledge.

Did you know...

In a survey of 83 clerkship directors of internal medicine at U.S. medical schools, struggling students were defined as "those at risk of receiving a grade of less than pass because of problems with knowledge, clinical skills, professionalism, or a combination of these items." Nearly all clerkship directors reported having students who struggled during the core internal medicine clerkship. At some schools, 15% of students were identified as struggling each year.[10]

Rule # 215   Many medical students are shy. Work to ensure that this does not impact your evaluation.

While not often discussed in medical school, it is a fact of life that personality traits may impact subjective evaluations. On wards, there are excellent students whose evaluations suffer because they are shy. Many attendings find it difficult to evaluate the shy student, and may draw erroneous conclusions. Is the student quiet because of his personality? Or is the student quiet because he lacks interest, motivation, or knowledge? Such students need to make a conscious effort to participate and be heard.

Did you know ...

In a study evaluating problem students, clerkship coordinators, clinical faculty members, and residents were asked to identify the frequency with which certain problem types were encountered.[11] Among 21 types of problem students, the "excessively shy, nonassertive" student was the second most frequently encountered problem type in obstetrics and gynecology, the fourth in surgery, and the fifth in internal medicine, pediatrics, and psychiatry.

Did you know ...

The Myers-Briggs type inventory (MBTI), a personality inventory, was administered to medical students during their obstetrics/gynecology clerkship.[12] The purpose was to determine if a student's personality characteristics could influence the results of performance evaluations. Researchers found a significant positive correlation between MBTI extraversion and clinical evaluations, suggesting that personality characteristics may influence evaluation of clinical performance.

Did you know ...

Researchers surveyed nearly 2,000 medical students to measure their degree of reticence.[13] Examples of reticence statements used in the study along with the percentage of students agreeing with the statement are as follows:

- I do not readily respond to questions from residents and attendings because I am uncomfortable speaking out (19%).
- I am uncomfortable responding to questions because I'm not always sure I'm right (47.9%).
- I do not always ask questions because I am afraid people will think my questions are foolish (38.7%).
- Out of respect for my superiors, I prefer not to challenge or openly question their decisions (59.7%).

Rule # 216   Demonstrate diplomacy.

Dr. Greco took Albert aside halfway through the rotation to ask him about his rotation experience.

"Is there anything I can do to make your experience better?"

"What about shorter rounds?" replied Albert.

Another true story. To thrive in a team environment, you must use tact and sensitivity when dealing with your fellow team members. This isn't kindergarten, but you should still always consider others' feelings before speaking or acting. Review any online physician discussion forum, and you'll realize how many physicians don't, or won't, follow this rule.

Tip # 67

If your attending physician asks you how the rotation is going, be positive, unless of course you have a major concern. Answer with a "I'm really enjoying learning about...," or "I really appreciate all the teaching."

Rule # 217   Don't let your dislike of an attending physician affect your rotation performance or working relationship.

Most of the time, you don't get to choose your attending. Therefore, be ready to encounter attendings with a variety of personalities and work styles. Be ready to encounter individuals whom you don't like or with whom you find it difficult to work.

This won't be the last time you'll have to work with someone you don't like. In our professional lives, there are many times when we have to work with or deal with such people. Learning how to do so is a valuable skill. First and foremost, always remain polite, courteous, and respectful.

Liking someone is not a prerequisite for displaying professionalism. Ask yourself what you can learn from your attending. You can still learn useful facets of medicine from attendings you don't like. Lastly, evaluate your interactions. You will encounter similar personalities in the future, and you need to learn the best way to work with such individuals.

However, certain behaviors are never acceptable in any individual, and certainly not from an individual in a position of authority. If you experience harassment, discrimination, or are the target of derogatory comments, you need to speak to the clerkship director or the dean's office.

References

[1]Kelly C. Good diagnostic skills should begin at the bedside. *ACP Internist.* February 2001. http://www.acpinternist.org/archives/2001/02/diagnostics.htm. Accessed January 30, 2011.

[2]Mangione S. Cardiac auscultatory skills of physicians-in-training: a comparison of three English-speaking countries. *Am J Med* 2001; 110(3): 210-6.

[3]Wright S, Carrese J. Which values do attending physicians try to pass on to house officers? *Med Educ* 2001; 35(10): 941-5.

[4]Stern D, Williams B, Gill A, Gruppen L, Woolliscroft J, Grum C. Is there relationship between attending physicans' and residents' teaching skills and students' examination scores? *Acad Med* 2000; 75(11): 1144-6.

[5]Blue A, Griffith C, Wilson J, Sloan D, Schwartz R. Surgical teaching quality makes a difference. *Am J Surg* 1999; 177(1): 86-9.

[6]DeZee K, Thomas M, Mintz M, Durning S. Letters of recommendation: rating, writing, and reading by clerkship directors of internal medicine. *Teach Learn Med* 2009; 21(2): 153-8.

[7]Foley R, Smilansky J, Yonke A. Teacher-student interaction in a medical clerkship. *J Med Educ* 1979; 54(8): 622-6.

[8]Blue A, Elam C, Fosson S, Bonaminio G. Faculty members' expectations of student behavior in the small-group setting. *Med Educ Online* [serial online] 1998; 3:5.

[9]Hunt D, Caroline J, Tonesk X, Yergan J, Siever M, Loebel J. Types of problem students encountered by clinical teachers on clerkships. *Med Educ* 1989; 23: 14-8.

[10]Frellsen S, Baker E, Papp K, Durning S. Medical school policies regarding struggling medical students during the internal medicine clerkships: results of a national survey. *Acad Med* 2008; 83(9): 876-81.

[11]Tonesk X, Buchanan R. An AAMC pilot study by 10 medical schools of clinical evaluation of students. *J Med Educ* 1987; 62(9): 707-18.

[12]Davis K, Banken J. Personality type and clinical evaluations in an obstetrics/ gynecology medical student clerkship. *Am J Obstet Gynecol* 2003; 193(5): 1807-10.

[13]Lee K, Vaishnavi S, Lau S, Andriole D, Jeffe D. "Making the grade:" noncognitive predictors of medical students' clinical clerkship grades. *J Natl Med Assoc* 2007; 99(10): 1138-50.

Chapter 22

Working as a Team

As an intern on call, I was assigned a patient in the ER with presumed bacterial meningitis. Our team evaluated the patient and wrote orders at record speed, and the patient was sent to the floor quickly. On my way to evaluate another patient, I stopped by the patient's room. Despite my stat orders, two hours later the IV antibiotics still weren't hanging. Somewhere in the chain between the written orders, the pharmacy, the technician delivering the antibiotics, and the nursing staff, this patient, for whom literally every hour counted, still hadn't received his lifesaving medication.

It takes a team of health care professionals working together effectively to provide the best patient care. While you'll round with your intern, resident, and attending, the patient care team is much more extensive. This team also includes nurses, social workers, pharmacists, physical therapists, other physicians, and other professionals. Your success as a physician depends on maximizing the combined efforts of each of these health care professionals.

As a third year student, you'll spend most of your time with the intern and resident. Every patient on the team is assigned to an intern, who functions as the patient's primary caregiver. When issues arise during the patient's hospitalization, the intern is usually the first to be notified by the nurse. Among other activities, they order tests, write progress notes, call consultants, write orders, and perform procedures. Residents supervise interns, and are responsible for conducting work rounds.

Learning how to maximize the efforts of an entire team of health care professionals will provide concrete benefits to your patients. Patient care is always a collaborative effort, and the most successful physicians live by this daily.

Rule # 218   Patient care is always a team project.

Physicians never care for patients alone. In order to deliver quality care to your patients, you will rely on a team of caregivers. This team may include nurses, social workers, pharmacists, physical therapists, and other physicians. Your success as a physician depends on how well you work with members of your team.

Your introduction to this team approach will occur during your clinical years of medical school. From the first day of your new rotation, you are part of a team. Your nuclear team typically consists of an attending physician, resident, interns, and students. You will also be a part of a larger team that includes other healthcare professionals. Even though every person on the team has different roles and responsibilities, you all share the same goal – to provide your patients with the best care possible. Dedicated students look out for the best interests of the team rather than themselves. This involves determining the needs of your team by being observant and making inquiries. Learn about their standards for high quality work, the best way you can support them, and how you can increase their efficiency.

Did you know ...

In a study in which interviews were conducted with residents and attending physicians to ascertain the behaviors that make students "good" or "bad" clerks, it was learned that supervisors viewed behavior as positive when students acted "for the sake of patient care, for the sake of their own learning, or for the sake of their own team."[1] Behavior was considered negative if students were thought to be shirking responsibility or "acting for the sake of appearance."

Rule # 219　　　**Collaborative care leads to improved patient outcomes. Some doctors pay lip service to this concept. The most effective doctors live by it.**

Evidence is accumulating that effective collaboration between all members of the health care team leads to improved patient outcomes. In response to this growing literature, organizations, including the Institute of Medicine and Accreditation Council for Graduate Medical Education, have urged medical schools to educate students about the roles of non-physician providers.

Educators from Johns Hopkins School of Medicine described a course in which medical students were exposed to non-physician hospital providers and staff, including nursing, pharmacy, social work, rehabilitation therapy, and home care. As part of the course, students worked a full shift with a preceptor in each of these disciplines. Feedback from participating students showed that students gained a deeper understanding of the roles of non-physician providers and how their services complement that of physicians. The authors wrote that the experience "empowered students to collaborate more actively with the non-physician colleagues, whom they would encounter in their careers, to provide coordinated patient care."[2]

When physicians work together with all members of the hospital team, including nurses, pharmacists, social workers, home care workers and others, patients experience concrete benefits, including a lower risk of death. In a study done in the intensive care unit, Knaus found that greater interaction of staff in different disciplines was associated with lower patient mortality.[3] In a study of surgical patients, relational coordination across disciplines was associated with reduced pain and shorter length of stays among total hip and knee arthroplasty patients.[4]

Rule # 220 **Your nursing colleagues are trained professionals. Learn how to work with them to improve patient outcomes.**

Research has shown that collaborative relationships between physicians and nurses in particular lead to improved patient outcomes.[5] Unfortunately, the relationship between these two groups is often suboptimal. This may be due to misconceptions among medical students about the responsibilities and capabilities of nurses. Registered nurses, or RNs, typically have either a BSN [Bachelor of Science in Nursing] or an ADN [associate degree in nursing], which require four years of study or two years of study, respectively. In a study at a university teaching hospital, third year medical students were found to interact with residents the best and nurses the worst, while nurses were found to interact with nurses the best and students the worst. The authors concluded that the "quality of interaction between medical students and nurses during third-year clinical rotations is poor, which suggests that medical students are not receiving the sorts of educational experiences that promote optimal physician-nurse collaboration."[6]

Similar results have been found with respect to physicians and nurses with regards to communication. In one study of randomly selected hospitalized patients, nurses and physicians were interviewed.[7] Nurses reported communicating with physicians only 50% of the time. Participants were also asked about the plan of care. The authors wrote that "there was no agreement between nurses and physicians on planned tests or procedures for the day in 25% and 11% of instances, respectively. There was no agreement between the nurses and physicians on planned medication changes for the day in 42% of instances."

Did you know...

In focus groups with nurses and physicians, study participants were asked to reflect on effective and ineffective interprofessional communication.[8] Common themes of effective communication were found, and both groups are encouraged to practice these behaviors:

- Deliver clear and precise messages
- Collaborate to solve problems
- Show support and appreciation
- Maintain mutual respect
- Have an authentic understanding of the unique professional role

Several themes of ineffective communication were also noted. Among these were derision (humiliation, making others feel incompetent) and dependence on electronic systems. One participant stated "electronic medical records...put physicians in this sort of fantasy. I had expected things to happen because it was...in the computer, but it goes a long way to have verbal communication and also follow up on the things that had happened."

Rule # 221   Optimize your teamwork with the intern and resident.

As a student, you have the ability to aid your intern and resident in many ways.

- Understand their goals and priorities, and anticipate their needs
- Keep them informed of any new developments with your patients.
- Pay attention to what makes their lives more difficult. Volunteer to help in these areas.
- When the opportunity arises, offer praise. If your intern is going above and beyond in his teaching role, let the attending know.

Tip # 68

Your team members are not your friends. They can be your friends later. During the rotation, consider them your supervisors. Treat them as you would any other person who has considerable influence over your grade and career - because right now, they do.

Did you know...

Your team members want you to be as involved as possible. To keep you involved, they need you to be easily accessible. They only have a short time in which to reach you before they take care of any issues on their own. Keep your resident and intern informed of where you will be at all times, check with them before you leave for a conference, and respond to pages quickly. This avoids the "Where have you been?" or "I've been looking all over for you."

Did you know ...

Although it's more common than one would imagine, don't date team members. It has the potential to affect your performance, and if you receive recognition for your work, others may attribute it to the relationship rather than your skills. In a study of 154 residents at hospitals affiliated with the Brown University Medical School, over 25% reported that a supervisor had dated a fellow trainee.[9] Over 7% had been asked on a date by a supervisor.

Rule # 222　　**Maximize your medical education. Learn how to obtain the best teaching from your resident and intern.**

If you are fortunate, you will be on a team where the resident and intern enjoy teaching and make it a priority. Even with the best teachers, the amount of teaching you receive will vary from day to day depending on the workload. On some days, the team will be so busy they hardly have time to breathe, let alone teach. On other days, the workload may be lighter, allowing for more teaching.

What can you do if you aren't receiving enough teaching? Avoid the unproductive responses of whining or escalating frustration. Instead, consider the following:

- The best way to increase teaching is to help create some time in the resident's day for teaching. Offer to help your residents, even with tasks not involving your patients. This will free up time for teaching and demonstrate that you are a team player. Residents often reward such students with increased teaching.

- Determine your residents' interests and strengths. If your resident is particularly strong in ECG interpretation, then bring him your patient's ECG and engage him in a discussion about interpretation.

- Be visible and accessible. You never know when a lull in the action might occur. The resident might take advantage of this time to teach, but if he can't find you, the opportunity may quickly be lost.

- Express your appreciation. After a teaching session, always thank your resident. Your goal is to reinforce the behavior by showing your appreciation.

Students often don't realize how much teaching they do receive. They tend to think of teaching only in the traditional sense: a block of time is set aside and a prepared talk on a particular topic is given. On the wards, teaching often doesn't occur in this form. Examples of teaching:

- An intern instructing the student on how to organize patient data
- An intern reviewing the student's progress note and suggesting ways in which the note can be improved
- An intern showing the student how to prioritize, use time wisely, and accomplish work efficiently
- A resident demonstrating a procedure and then supervising the student

Rule # 223   No work is beneath you.

As a student, it sometimes seems as though all you ever do is grunt work. No one would argue that tasks such as filling out forms, calling for laboratory test results, or pulling radiology films are exciting. Students often label this menial work "scut" or "scut work." The Wikipedia dictionary defines scut as "menial work, especially in the medical profession, to describe the work that medical students are required to do for residents and attending physicians."

In the American Medical Student Association (AMSA) document titled "Principles regarding wellness of medical students and housestaff," AMSA maintains "that the performance of repetitive scut work, past the point where such work is a learning experience, is an infringement upon the medical student's educational time and should not be required of the student." Note that AMSA states that scut work does have educational value. This important point is often forgotten by students. Even mundane tasks have learning value. Since you'll be performing these tasks as an intern, an introduction to it now will teach you how to manage your time.

While most students don't have any problem doing this work for their own patients, doing it too often for other patients may be an issue. While some residents don't scut their students at all, others have a reputation for it. If you're asked to perform occasional scut work for another patient, embrace the opportunity with the same level of enthusiasm and professionalism you bring to other aspects of the rotation. Team players are often rewarded with increased teaching, chances to participate in procedures, and other exciting opportunities.

What should you do if the scut work is excessive or inappropriate? One option would be to simply comply with the requests. Many students would choose this option, declining to make it an issue for fear that it might affect their clerkship grade. Another option would be to bring it up directly with your resident. You may prefer to discuss it first, however, with a more neutral party such as your mentor or clerkship director.

Rule # 224   Conflict is an unavoidable aspect of the practice of medicine. Learn how to handle it properly.

Stress among medical students, not surprisingly, is common, and the issue has been studied by researchers. Lloyd and Gartrell found frequent stressful interactions between students and their attending and residents during the junior year of medical school.[10] Researchers at the University of Illinois College of Medicine examined the nature of conflict situations that students encountered.[11] They found that conflict situations were common, occurring, on average, every other day. While one would assume that stressful interactions would decrease as students become more familiar with the clinical arena, the literature doesn't support this assumption. Researchers found that while some stresses did decrease as the junior year progressed, stresses due to conflict with superiors and peers did not.[12]

The results of these studies demonstrate that conflict is common. The question is not if you will experience conflict, but rather when. What types of conflict situations might occur? In the University of Illinois study, the majority of the conflict situations (57/99) involved problems with residents, attending physicians, or others in positions of authority. The nature of these situations varied considerably and included problems as minor as asking for clarification of a responsibility or making small talk, to as major as handling public criticism.

Most minor conflicts have no lasting impact, and you can just move on. However, significant conflict may occur. While students tend to retreat from such situations, avoidance generally doesn't lead to resolution, and in some cases may worsen it.

The preferred method of handling major conflict is to address the issue directly and quickly with the other person, with a face to face meeting. Arrange a proper time and location for this meeting. It shouldn't take place in a public area, such as the hallway.

Conflict often arises from miscommunication, incorrect assumptions or incomplete information. Listen closely and choose your words carefully. Remember that your goals are to resolve conflict by finding a fair solution. Since you'll continue to work with this individual, you must do what you can to preserve the relationship.

If you can't reach a resolution, then you may need to discuss the issue with your clerkship director. If you sense that you'll need to, then you should begin documenting your problems. Keep a daily diary of events, with a record of the date and time of any incidents, a factual description of the behavior, names of witnesses, impact of the behavior on patient care, and the effects of any actions taken to resolve the problem.

Tip # 69

You should not be harassed, discriminated against, or belittled. Unfortunately, the literature shows that such behavior does occur. Should you experience such behavior, discuss it with the clerkship director. Often, students don't bring these issues to light, which prevents the clerkship director from taking corrective action.

Rule # 225   **Toxic colleagues are common in medicine. (For examples, peruse any online medical discussion forum.) Plan on how you'll handle these individuals.**

While most medical students are collegial, some are difficult to work with because of their competitiveness. These students may use a variety of underhanded and unscrupulous tactics in an effort to shine, while diminishing their colleagues. Examples of such toxic behaviors include lying, cheating, blaming their mistakes on fellow students, rounding on other students' patients, or writing progress notes on other patients without permission.

What do you do if you find yourself in this type of situation? First and foremost, maintain your own professionalism. Don't pursue a similar approach, which may damage your reputation and erode your self-respect. Meet with your colleague to discuss the situation, and choose your words carefully. "We've had a good working relationship but, over the last few days, I've noticed that something has changed. Yesterday, during rounds, I felt that you …" As you discuss the situation, emphasize cooperation rather than competition. Some students will respond with a change in their behavior, while others won't. You may need to involve other team members, especially if your colleague's behavior is interfering with your ability to work or is damaging your reputation. If you must meet with a supervisor, present the facts of the situation, how it has affected your ability to do your work, and what you have done to resolve it. End with "I would like to get your thoughts on what else I can do." As a final note, remember that most evaluation forms ask evaluators to rate students on how well they interact with their peers.

Tip # 70

When dealing with an overly competitive student colleague, consider his past actions. If his behavior is out of the ordinary, it may be because of extenuating circumstances. Illness, family issues, and other stressors can cause otherwise decent people to behave in negative ways.

Tip # 71

Assume that everyone you work with, including students, has the ability to influence your grade. Never make a classmate look bad in an effort to make yourself look better.

References

[1]Lavine E, Regehr G, Garwood K, Ginsbury S. The role of attribution to clerk factors and contextual factors in supervisors' perceptions of clerks' behaviors. *Teach Learn Med* 2004; 16(4): 317-22.

[2]Pathak S, Holzmueller C, Haller K, Pronovost P. A mile in their shoes: interdisciplinary education at the Johns Hopkins University School of Medicine. *Am J Med Qual* 2010; 1-6.

[3]Knaus W, Draper E, Wagner D, Zimmerman J. An evaluation of outcome from intensive care in major medical centers. *Ann Intern Med* 1986; 104: 410-8.

[4]Gittell J, Fairfield K, Bierbaum B, et al. Impact of relational coordination on quality of care, postoperative pain and functioning, and length of stay: a nine-hospital study of surgical patients. *Med Care* 2000; 38: 807-19.

[5]Baggs J, Schmitt M, Mushlin A, Mitchell P, Eldredge D, Oakes D, Hutson A. Association between nurse-physician collaboration and patient outcomes in three intensive care units. *Crit Care Med* 1999; 27: 1991-8.

[6]Nadolski G, Bell M, Brewer B, Frankel R, Cushing H, Brokaw J. Evaluating the quality of interaction between medical students and nurses in a large teaching hospital. *BMC Med Educ* 2006; 6: 23.

[7]O'Leary K, Thompson J, Landler M, Kulkarni N, Haviley C, Hahn K, Jeon J, Wayne D, Baker D, Williams M. Patterns of nurse-physician communication and agreement on the plan of care. *Qual Saf Health Care* 2010; 19(3): 195-9.

[8]Robinson F, Gorman G, Slimmer L, Yudkowsky R. Perceptions of effective and ineffective nurse-physician communication in hospitals. *Nurs Forum* 2010; 45(3): 206-16.

[9]Recupero P, Cooney M, Rayner C, Heru A, Price M. Supervisor-trainee relationship boundaries in medical education. *Med Teach* 2005; 27(6): 484-8.

[10]Lloyd C, Gartrell N. A further assessment of medical school stress. *J Med Educ* 1983; 58(12): 964-7.

[11]Spiegel D, Smolen R, Jonas C. Interpersonal conflicts involving students in clinical medical education. *J Med Educ* 1985; 60(11): 819-29.

[12]Linn B, Zeppa R. Stress in junior medical students: relationship to personality and performance. *J Med Educ* 1984; 59(1): 7-12.

Chapter 23

Giving Talks

The typical medical student talk, which we've sat through many times, usually follows this script:

Introduction: "The subject of my talk is pulmonary embolism."
Content: unrealistically extensive overview of a massive topic based on major texts
Conclusion: "Well, I guess that's all I have."

It's easy to make that talk significantly more impressive and memorable.

Introduction: *"Substantial and unacceptable."* Those were the words of Dr. Kenneth Moser, referring to the morbidity and mortality rate of venous thromboembolism ...[1] A major issue in reducing these high rates is enhancing early diagnosis. In my talk today, I'll review recent advances in diagnostic techniques of pulmonary embolism."

Content: in-depth review of a focused topic including recent medical literature

Conclusion: "As the recent literature has shown, the diagnosis of pulmonary embolism may clearly be challenging. As in the case of our patient Mr. Smith, however, a combination of diagnostic methods leads to improved sensitivity."

Being asked to give a talk is a common, yet anxiety-provoking, medical student experience. Medical students are often asked to give a talk to the team, usually pertaining to an issue that arises during rounds. Some students face anxiety and dread just at the thought of giving a talk. However, preparing and presenting a talk is a great opportunity to demonstrate your knowledge and grasp of clinical issues, and can definitely impress the team. While you can't control what an attending might ask during rounds, you do have complete control over your talk. With sufficient preparation and practice, you should be able to deliver an outstanding talk.

In this chapter, you'll learn specific recommendations to improve the quality and impact of your talks. You'll learn how to choose a topic and perform an audience analysis. You'll read a number of introductory and concluding statements that can be incorporated into any talk. You'll learn how to reduce anxiety and how to respond to audience questions. You'll also learn about specific recommendations that can enhance the quality of your speaking and your audiovisual aids.

Rule # 226   Be the first to volunteer to give the talk.

During attending rounds, an issue may arise that requires further research. Sometimes an attending will turn to the team and ask "Who wants to give us a talk about this subject?" As team members pointedly try to avoid the attending's gaze, the request is often met with silence. This isn't surprising. Most residents, interns, and students would rather not prepare and give a talk, if they had the choice. This reflects poorly on the entire team.

If the attending asks for a volunteer, you should be the first person to raise your hand. This is yet another opportunity to demonstrate your enthusiasm and initiative. You may not like the thought of giving a talk. However, as you'll see in the remainder of this chapter, with adequate preparation you can deliver an outstanding presentation.

Rule # 227   Choose the correct topic.

In most cases, the attending will assign the topic. However, if you're allowed to choose the subject, carefully consider the following:

- It's always better to choose a topic that you already know something about. If you recently cared for a patient with asthma, speak about some aspect of asthma. If in your last rotation you spoke about pulmonary embolism, speak about it again if it pertains to your current rotation.

- Choose a topic that you have an interest in.

- Make sure that your topic will be of interest to your audience.

- Make sure that you can discuss the topic in the time you've been given. In some cases, you may have been assigned a broad topic, such as lung cancer. It's hard to do justice to such a topic unless you've been given considerable time to speak. Instead, ask the attending if there's a specific aspect of the topic you may focus on. If he leaves it up to you, pick an aspect of the topic that would be relevant to your audience, such as the therapy of metastatic lung cancer.

Did you know...

In a study of medical student talks, Yale students were asked to present a 30-minute talk on a topic of their choice during the Internal Medicine Clerkship.[2] At the orientation, students were informed to avoid overviews or large topics. As an example, rather than talking about pneumonia, students were asked to focus on a particular aspect of pneumonia. Despite this recommendation, faculty evaluations noted that 35% of presentations were too broadly focused.

Rule # 228   If you'll be giving a talk, find out when.

In the student's mind, a 10-minute formal presentation requires at least two weeks of preparation. The attending feels otherwise, and asks for it two days later. The message: never assume that you know what your attending is thinking. When assigned a talk, ask when you are expected to give it.

Realize also that talks aren't always given on the specified date. A patient issue may consume more time than expected during rounds. While you prepared extensively, and would just like to give your talk and get it out of the way, there's not much you can do except be ready to give the talk on another day.

Tip # 72

Some attendings will give students a vague deadline. "There's no rush with the talk." Knowing when you're expected to give the talk is important information, so at least try to get a time frame. Above all, don't view a vague deadline as a license to procrastinate.

If just a few days remain before the end of the rotation and nobody mentions the talk you were assigned some time ago, you need to bring it up. Never leave a clerkship without finishing any project, including an assigned talk. If you don't bring it up, the attending may assume that you just didn't prepare.

The Urology Department at Virginia Commonwealth University reminds students to deliver their talk on the final day of the rotation even if it requires some degree of assertiveness. "Topics should be chosen by the conclusion of week one and the presentation should occur on the final day of the rotation unless otherwise requested. Students may not be 'reminded' regarding this requirement; however, they are encouraged to be assertive and make sure they are given dedicated time to present their work."[3]

Rule # 229   Find out how much time is allotted for your presentation.

You can't prepare for a talk unless you know how much time you have to speak. If the talk is a requirement of the clerkship, time limits may be defined in the orientation materials. For talks assigned by your attending, always ask about time limits. Your attending has a preconceived notion as to how much time your talk should take. A talk that lasts longer takes away from the completion of other tasks during rounds. One that is too short will prompt the attending to wonder how much effort you expended researching your topic.

Never take up more than the allotted time. As described in an article on presentations, "many speakers who have not adequately prepared their talk go beyond their time limit. The result is often an annoyed chairman, an irritated audience ..."[4] Exceeding the allotted time may also have a negative effect on your grade. The Department of Emergency Medicine at Maimonides Medical Center stresses to students that "the presentation should last roughly 20 minutes. Due to the large number of students giving presentations, exceeding the 20 minute allotted time frame may reflect negatively upon your grade."[5]

Rule # 230   Get to work.

After being assigned a talk, students do one of two things. They either begin working or they put it off. Most students choose the latter.

Students procrastinate mainly because of fear. They worry that they'll sound uncertain or unknowledgeable, or are scared to be the center of attention. These concerns may be stronger for new clerks, who haven't yet given a talk in the clinical setting. You can alleviate these fears by preparing for your talk as soon as it's assigned. With adequate preparation, you can polish your talk and gain confidence in your ability to deliver it well.

Rule # 231   You can't give a talk unless you know your audience.

Since you'll usually give talks to your team, you will know your audience beforehand. Keep in mind that this is a mixed audience. The team consists of members at different educational levels. Always take into account the knowledge level of your audience, which allows you to develop a talk that suits the needs of all listeners.

If you're assigned to speak before an unfamiliar audience, ask for information beforehand. During my psychiatry clerkship, the attending asked me to give a talk on obesity during psychiatry grand rounds. Having never attended psychiatry grand rounds, I was completely unfamiliar with the group. Only after finding out about the audience was I able to prepare a talk tailored to their needs and at a level that was appropriate for their educational background and expectations. Since many of the attendees were psychiatry faculty, I prepared a talk that took into account their knowledge and experience. If the group consisted only of fellow students, I would have prepared a very different talk.

Your audience analysis should yield answers to the following questions:

- How many people will be in the audience?
- How familiar is the audience with the subject?
- What is the educational background of the audience?
- What does the audience expect from me?
- How can I provide information relevant to their specialty?
- What would I like the audience to do with the information I present?
- What materials do I want to leave with the audience?
- What questions might audience members ask?

Students who carefully consider the composition and background of their audience are more likely to deliver a talk that meets the needs of their listeners.

Tip # 73

Careful consideration of your audience is the key to developing content that is appropriate. In her article "Presenting with precision," Happell wrote that "it is extremely frustrating to attend a presentation, confident that you are likely to learn something new, only to be exposed to basic information and knowledge that is readily available."[6]

Rule # 232   You cannot prepare an outstanding presentation unless you fully understand the purpose of the talk.

For most talks, your general purpose will be to inform. You also need to determine the specific purpose of your talk. You can do so by considering the needs of your audience and establishing goals and objectives. Without a specific purpose in mind, you run the danger of preparing a vague and disorganized talk.

When developing a purpose statement, be specific. Consider these purpose statements:

I want my listeners to know how to manage an acute gout attack.

I want my listeners to be able to specify at least three types of medications that can be used to manage an acute gout attack.

The latter statement is clearly more specific. It's much easier to develop a focused talk when you have a specific purpose statement.

Rule # 233   Strong introductions are critical.

Start your talk with an introduction that leaves your audience eager to hear what else you have to say. You only have one chance to make a strong first impression. When you fail to grab their attention, it can be difficult to capture it later. For this reason, plan your introduction carefully. Too often, students begin their talk with one of the following types of statements:

I'm talking today about …

The subject of my talk is …

You should include the topic and purpose of your talk in the introduction. However, rather than using a bland statement to open the talk, begin with an intro that will stir interest.

- **Ask a rhetorical question**

We all realize that pulmonary embolism is a major cause of death. Did you know that the diagnosis of pulmonary embolism is missed in approximately 400,000 patients per year? And that's just in the United States ...

- **Make a bold statement or share a startling statistic**

In the United States, 650,000 people are diagnosed with pulmonary embolism every year, with over 200,000 deaths.

- **Use a historical reference**

160 years have passed since Virchow's classic paper on thrombosis and hemostasis was published and we, of course, continue to use the principles of Virchow's triad in the diagnosis and management of patients with pulmonary embolism. From historical reports, Virchow was small in stature but possessed a quick wit. He was known to be sarcastic, particularly when he dealt with incompetence or inattention. Yet he could also be generous and friendly, recognizing those who had made significant contributions. If he were alive today, he would perhaps be impressed with the progress that has been made in the diagnosis and management of pulmonary embolism, but he might also berate us for not making more progress. After all, pulmonary embolism remains a major cause of death in the United States ...

- **Provide a thought-provoking quote**

"Substantial and unacceptable." Those were the words of Dr. Kenneth Moser, referring to the morbidity and mortality rate of venous thromboembolism ...[1]

- **Tell a brief story**

If you've ever seen a patient die suddenly of a massive pulmonary embolism, it's not something that you will ever forget ...

Tip # 74

Since the audience's attention is best at the start of a talk, create an attention-grabbing opening that will keep them interested in the remainder of your talk.

Rule # 234   Utilize the correct resources.

Do not use handbooks as your primary source of information. Instead turn to larger, more authoritative texts as well as the recent literature. While the information in your handbooks may suffice for your fellow students, remember that your audience will also consist of an intern, resident, and attending.

If you have difficulty finding data, seek the assistance of the research librarian. Research librarians are wonderful yet underutilized resources. They don't have all the answers, but they generally have a good idea of how to help you find the information you seek.

Did you know...

Your choice of resources may have bearing on how your talk is received or evaluated. For example, the University of North Carolina Department of Obstetrics & Gynecology requires students to give an oral presentation, which accounts for 5% of the total clerkship grade. The Department writes that "you will be evaluated on your use of resources, knowledge base and presentation style."[7]

Rule # 235   Your goal is to educate, not overload.

Before you even organize your talk, you have to first select material for your presentation. The real trick is determining what not to use. Your research will usually yield more material than you have time to talk about. You need to avoid information overload, as there is definitely a limit to what your audience can handle in a finite period of time. Happell writes that "there is a tendency for inexperienced presenters to over-do the content in their presentation. It is easy to feel that every little piece of information is vital, but we know from experience that even the most interesting topic becomes hard to follow when we feel we are bombarded."[6]

How do you know what to include and what to discard? When you're not sure, ask yourself if the information supports your purpose. Discard that which is irrelevant. As Starver and Shellenbarger stated in their article on presentations, "it is tempting to include lots of information about the topic, but be sure that it clearly fits the purpose of the presentation."[8]

Tip # 75

One of the most common mistakes students make is presenting too much information. Every point you make should support your talk's specific purpose. If it doesn't, cut it out.

Rule # 236   Make sure your data is accurate.

During your talk, you will present data that support your ideas. Your data must be accurate and relevant. Review all data several times. Nothing will damage your credibility more than passing along inaccurate information. Even one inaccurate fact can call into question the accuracy of your entire talk. With statistics, make sure that the information is up to date. Presenting statistics that are years old when more recent information is available will damage your credibility as well.

Rule # 237   Practice correctly.

When practicing, strive to simulate the actual experience as closely as you can. Whenever possible, practice in the room in which you'll actually speak. If this isn't possible, pick a room that closely resembles the real location of your talk. Doing so allows you the opportunity to become comfortable with the environment.

As you practice, don't just go over your talk in your head. There is a difference between going over a talk in your head and actually delivering it. For this reason, stand in the proper spot, imagine an audience in front of you, and rehearse your talk. Use your notes exactly as you plan to during the actual talk. If you'll be using audiovisual equipment, practice with the equipment.

Tip # 76

As you rehearse your talk, time yourself to ensure that your presentation fits within the allotted time. If you run over, delete material rather than increasing your pace.

You can learn a lot about how you'll appear by videotaping yourself. This is a valuable yet underutilized way of improving performance. Play it back so that you can see and hear yourself as others will. Students are often surprised by what they learn from a videotape of their performance. Annoying habits that usually aren't self-evident will be obvious during this type of review. Learn about these habits during a practice session when you still have the opportunity to correct them.

Tip # 77

If you'll be using audiovisual equipment, realize that problems often occur. The computer may crash. A bulb in the projector may burn out. Unfortunately, problems aren't always correctable. You must be able to continue your talk if an equipment failure can't be corrected.

Rule # 238   Do not, under any circumstances, read your talk word for word.

Many students write out their talk and then proceed to read it word for word. This is among the most common errors students make when giving a talk. It almost always leads to a monotonous delivery, a surefire way of boring your audience. It's also impossible to maintain eye contact with your audience save for an occasional upward glance, which diminishes credibility.

Tip # 78

Talks that are read are boring. They lack spontaneity and rhythm. Think about the best speakers at your medical school. How many of them read their talks word for word? Keep in mind the words of Edwards who wrote that "... natural rhythm of telling a story with its pauses and eye-to-eye contact with the audience is lost when the talk is read."[9]

Rather than reading your talk word for word, we recommend that you use note cards with no more than ten words on each card. You can use these words as a reminder of the points you wish to make and then proceed to formulate sentences to express these points. You might worry that this seems like a risky method, but you will be practicing with these note cards. With sufficient practice, you'll become comfortable developing sentences using the cues you have on the card. As you grow less dependent on your notes, consider memorizing your introduction, which allows for a great first impression.

If you can speak without detailed notes, you will enhance your image. Since so many students read their talks, attendings are impressed with students who can give a talk using a paucity of notes. This type of student comes across as brighter, confident, and more articulate.

Tip # 79

When quoting an article or conveying detailed statistics, it's better to refer to your notes. You don't ever want to misquote or pass along inaccurate data.

Tip # 80

Should you memorize your talk? It's a risky option. What if you draw a blank? Even if you don't, you're more likely to come across as robotic and stiff rather than natural and enthusiastic.

Rule # 239   Avoid-the-monotone.

Too often, students speak with the same force, pitch, and pace, leading to a monotonous delivery. Speaking in a droning monotone bores listeners. It also suggests a lack of interest in the topic.

Is this the impression you wish to convey? Of course not. However, this is precisely the impression that many students leave. You may be very interested in the subject matter. However, that does you no good if the force, pitch, and pace of your speech suggests otherwise.

Rule # 240   Utilize gestures appropriately.

Students commonly remain seated during talks given to a small group, such as their team. In the seated position, students generally place their hands underneath the table. This robs them of the ability to gesture. It has been found that voice patterns often follow hand movements. When hands are kept under the table, it can hamper your ability to vary inflection. Gesturing, if done appropriately, can help you speak with inflection, leading to a more powerful talk.

For this reason, we recommend that you give your talk while standing. Don't keep your hands in your pockets or clinging to a lectern. Instead, have them in front of your body with your palms open. In this position, you are able to effectively gesture.

Avoid gestures that indicate nervousness or a lack of confidence. These include:

- Keeping your hands in your pockets
- Gripping the lectern or audiovisual equipment
- Playing with keys or coins in your pocket
- Rocking back and forth or from side to side
- Rubbing the back of your neck
- Playing with your hair
- Clenching your fists constantly
- Pacing back and forth
- Fidgeting with clothes or jewelry

If you still choose to give your talk while seated, don't forget to lean forward in your chair, a gesture that conveys enthusiasm and confidence.

Since we're usually unaware of how we gesture, it is useful to take note of your movements while standing in front of a mirror and practicing. You can also review your gestures on videotape or solicit feedback from others after they watch you rehearse. Take note of any inappropriate gestures and make a conscious effort to eliminate them during practice.

Tip # 81

Only 7% of a speaker's message is felt to be obtained through actual spoken words.[10] 55% is conveyed through nonverbal communication, while 38% is transmitted through vocal tone.

Rule # 241　　　Don't use fillers.

Fillers are sounds like "um" and "er" that find their way into talks when speakers are thinking about what to say next. The use of fillers suggests that you lack knowledge or are unsure of your information. "The speaker's voice, tone, and inflection are powerful tools for attracting an audience ... Speakers are advised to refrain from speaking in a low, monotonous style and from taking long breaks with fillers such as 'uh...uh...'"[3]

Most students don't even realize that they use fillers. If you record your presentation and listen to it, you can determine if fillers are a problem for you. If so, practice replacing these fillers with short pauses.

Rule # 242　　　Speak at the proper pace.

You need to speak at a speed that allows your audience to understand what you're saying. Talks lead to a great deal of anxiety for most students. In students who normally speak at a reasonable pace, this anxiety can cause them to speak at a faster speed with few, if any, pauses. The effect can be poor enunciation with garbled words and sentences. "Too many ideas presented too quickly will not be understood, even to the most well-informed and intelligent audience."[9]

You must make a conscious effort to slow down so that your listeners can follow you. Accomplished speakers will also pause periodically to allow their listeners to fully process what they've said. You should aim to do the same. In their article on lecturing, Brown and Manogue wrote that lecturers, to improve clarity, should "speak clearly, use pauses, and don't go too fast ... Whilst these suggestions may seem common sense, observation of lectures suggest that they are not common practice."[11]

Did you know...

In a study of emergency medicine residents at the University of Toronto, faculty and peers completed feedback forms following resident presentations. In an analysis of these forms, researchers found that "slowing down" and "use appropriate volume" were frequently mentioned feedback statements (15% frequency).[12]

Rule # 243 Utilize the techniques of professional speakers to handle anxiety.

Some surveys have demonstrated that public speaking is the number one fear, ranked ahead of even the fear of death. Anxiety affects everyone, even the best speakers. However, the best speakers are able to channel that nervous energy into a better performance.

The following table suggests several methods that can combat anxiety. Just before the presentation, take several deep breaths, stand tall, make eye contact with your audience, and smile.

Ways to relieve anxiety before giving a talk	
Method	**Description**
Adjust your attitude	How you view the talk will have a large bearing on the anxiety that comes from it. Those who view it as a task to avoid may develop greater anxiety than those who see it as an opportunity to improve skills in communication.
Ensure adequate preparation and practice	The best way to lessen speech anxiety is to give yourself sufficient time to prepare and practice the talk.
Don't overestimate the talk's importance	A talk typically accounts for only a small percentage of the clerkship grade.
Use positive self-talk	"I know my topic, have prepared well for the presentation, and am confident that it will go well."
Visualize success	Athletes and actors, as well as public speakers, use the techniques of visualization. Visualize yourself, with full detail, delivering a well-received presentation

Did you know...

Too much anxiety is a problem, especially if it's apparent to the audience. However, studies have shown that speakers generally report a higher level of anxiety than what an audience can perceive.[13] In other words, audiences aren't very accurate in detecting a speaker's level of anxiety.

Rule # 244   Don't end with a whimper.

Some students conclude their talk by mumbling "I guess that's about all I have," or "I think I've gone over everything." These statements completely lack impact. Others even close with an apology. "I'm sorry I wasn't able to find more," "I'm sorry I couldn't get the projector to work," or "I'm sorry the talk went so long". In ending your talk, do not mumble and do not ever apologize. The conclusion is also no place for bringing up new points or rambling on and on. Students who don't take the time to think about their conclusion end up closing with a whimper rather than a bang.

To conclude in a way that leaves the audience with a lasting, powerful impression, begin with a phrase that tells your audience that you are wrapping up your talk. Examples include:

In concluding, I want to …

Let me leave you with …

As a final thought …

To wrap up my talk …

Since most of your talks will be informative presentations, it's reasonable to close by briefly summarizing your main points. After doing so, end your speech with an interesting closer, perhaps a quote or rhetorical question. Since a talk is often assigned when a team member raises an issue pertaining to a patient, one effective way to conclude is to apply your information to that specific issue. "As the recent literature has shown, the diagnosis of pulmonary embolism may clearly be challenging. As in the case of Mr. Smith, however, a combination of diagnostic methods leads to improved sensitivity." To leave your audience with a strong, final impression, avoid reading your conclusion. Instead, know it well enough that you can deliver the conclusion with few, if any, notes.

Tip # 82
Avoid the all-too-common abrupt or awkward conclusion. Instead, use a strong conclusion to leave your audience with a favorable impression.

Rule # 245   Eye contact is a critical component of delivery.

If you can't maintain eye contact with your listeners, it will be difficult to keep them absorbed in what you're saying. Too often, students make no eye contact whatsoever, reading their talk word for word from their detailed notes. Even when students try to present without reading, they often look elsewhere - at the floor, ceiling, table, or audiovisual material.

As you give your talk, make eye contact with your listeners. This keeps audience members interested, and helps you come across as more credible and confident. Looking into people's eyes while delivering a talk can be difficult for some students. If you find this unnerving, you don't actually need to look into people's eyes. Instead, focus on another part of the face such as the forehead, nose, or mouth. Your listeners won't know the difference.

As you make eye contact, don't be surprised if a team member isn't paying attention. You may notice your audience nodding off, as your audience, sadly but expectedly, is often a tired group. Don't be thrown off track if a pager goes off or if team members are engaging in conversation. As distracting as any of these may be, you can't let it affect your presentation.

Rule # 246   Pay attention to feedback.

It's very easy to be overwhelmed by the task of providing great content and ensuring an effective delivery. Most students are single-mindedly focused on giving a great presentation. However, you need to be alert to audience feedback. During a presentation, this takes the form of nonverbal cues, such as body language cues that indicate total boredom. While it's easier to process such feedback when you're an experienced speaker, such cues should be a warning sign. You may need to work on eye contact, or vary your volume, pitch, or pace of delivery.

Rule # 247   Project enthusiasm.

It would be great if you were only asked to speak about topics that you love. As a student, that just isn't going to happen every time. And speaking as an audience member, there is nothing more boring than listening to a talk where even the speaker isn't interested. It is imperative, therefore, that you learn to project enthusiasm about your subject material.

Tip # 83

As one attending physician once remarked to me, "There are no dull subjects, only dull presentations." If you don't have natural enthusiasm for a topic, find a way. Fake it if you must.

Did you know...

In a study of emergency medicine residents at the University of Toronto, faculty and peers completed feedback forms following resident presentations. In an analysis of these forms, researchers found that "being engaging and enthusiastic" was one of five top faculty themes.[12]

Rule # 248   Visual aids enhance presentations.

Studies on learning styles have clearly identified distinct preferences. Some individuals are visual learners, while others describe themselves as aural learners. Some learn better by seeing, others by hearing, but a talk that meets the needs of both learning styles will have the most impact. Whenever possible, then, you should incorporate visual aids.

Obviously, there are situations where this won't be possible. If the attending has asked you to give a quick 2-minute "blurb" on a topic while standing in the hallway between patient rooms, the short duration and location of the talk clearly preclude the use of visual aids. For longer talks that take place in an environment more conducive to the use of visual aids, there are compelling reasons to do so. Visual aids, if done well, can enhance your talk, making your presentation more interesting and enjoyable. Effective use of audiovisual aids can:

- reinforce your statements
- help you direct the audience's attention
- help your audience comprehend your ideas and points
- make you appear more credible and professional
- lead you to deliver a more memorable talk

Although a variety of visual aids are available, students most often use slides, PowerPoint projection, or overhead transparencies. All are useful presentation tools, but only when utilized well. While good visual aids can certainly complement your talk, bad ones can damage your talk. Below are some tips for PowerPoint presentations.

PowerPoint Do's and Don'ts

- Don't read the text.
- Use a font color that contrasts with the background color.
- Use the same background color throughout the presentation (medium blue is popular).
- Maintain consistency by using the same symbols and typefaces.
- Don't use full sentences. A good rule is to keep each line no more than 6-7 words.
- Don't place too many points on each slide (less is more).
- Use at least 18-font size (be sure that people in the back row can read the information).
- Avoid fancy fonts. Instead, choose a standard font like Arial or Times New Roman.
- Don't capitalize entire words unless necessary.
- Proofread your text for spelling, repeated words, and grammatical errors.
- Avoid overly complex tables, charts, graphs, or diagrams.

Should you provide your audience with a handout? In most cases, yes. Handouts can help the audience follow your train of thought. Most listeners appreciate written material that they can refer to later. The fact that you produced a handout will also give your audience some idea of the effort you put into the talk.

As you prepare the handout, pay careful attention to its presentation. Its appearance is a reflection of you. If it appears unprofessional, your listeners may form a negative impression of you and what you have to say, even before you open your mouth. As always, proofread your work to avoid misspelled words and grammatical errors.

You can either provide the audience with the handout before or after your talk. The disadvantage of handing it out at the start is that your listeners may pay more attention to the handout than to you. With complex subjects, however, you may find it preferable to have the audience follow your thought process.

Did you know ...

Cleveland Clinic researchers sought to determine which features of a lecture were most important to attendees.[14] Features found to be important included:

- Clarity and readability of slides
- Relevance of lecture material to the participants
- Presenter's ability to identify key issues
- Presenter's ability to engage the participants
- Ability to present material clearly and with animation

Rule # 249   Don't be afraid to say "I don't know."

At the conclusion of your talk, you should invite questions from your listeners. While few students end their talk with such a statement, it is important to do so. Many students would rather avoid questions, because they fear they won't know the answer. This is natural, and is a concern for experienced speakers as well. However, experienced speakers will prepare for the question and answer period by anticipating questions. They then proceed to develop responses to these questions, providing for more polished replies. You can do the same.

You can begin the question and answer period of your talk by simply asking the audience, "Do you have any questions?" When asked a question in front of a large group, you should rephrase the question before answering it. "Can you clarify the research methods used in the study on statins and inflammation?" "Certainly. The question refers to the research methods used in the study on statins and inflammation. In this particular study..." This technique ensures that everyone has heard the question and also provides additional time to formulate an answer.

While you are expected to be well read about the subject of your talk, you are not expected to have all the answers. In the event that you are asked a question for which you don't have an answer, you can opt to say "I don't know, but I will find out." Another option is to defer the question to your attending. "Dr. Chen, in your experience with pulmonary embolism, how would you handle this situation?" Avoid at all costs an attempt to bluff or to provide inaccurate information.

Tips for answering questions at the end of a talk

- Let your listeners know early in the talk when you will answer questions.
- Encourage questions by asking "Do you have any questions?"
- Listen carefully to the question to make sure you understand it.
- Make eye contact with the questioner while the question is being asked.
- Repeat the question, especially in a large group, to make sure it has been heard.
- Make eye contact with the audience as you answer the question.
- If you don't know the answer, don't bluff or lie. You also need not apologize.
- Consider deferring the question to an expert, if one is in the room.

Rule # 250   Feedback, feedback, feedback.

Hopefully, team members will offer you specific feedback after your talk. However, most feedback tends to be vague and short on the specifics that you need to improve your performance during future talks. To make the most of this experience, you must solicit specific feedback. Examples of questions you might ask:

- Was the introduction interesting?
- Was the topic and purpose of my talk clear?
- Did you feel that I made eye contact throughout the talk?
- Did I appropriately gesture? Did my gesturing enhance or detract from my talk's message?
- Was I able to maintain your interest?
- Did I come across as enthusiastic?
- Was the talk well-organized?
- Do you have any other suggestions for improvement?

Take team members' suggestions seriously. Determine how you will use this information to improve future talks. What specific steps will you take to improve in these areas? You'll have the chance to listen and appreciate some great speakers during your career. However, nobody starts out at that level. Speaking well is a learned skill.

Tip # 74

You can also solicit feedback during your practice sessions. Have a trusted colleague or friend listen to your talk. The constructive criticism you receive may be invaluable. If you've been given information as to how your talk will be evaluated, solicit feedback on these particular areas.

References

[1]Moser KM: Venous thromboembolism. *Am Rev Respir Dis* 1990 Jan; 141(1): 235-49.

[2]Kernan W, Quagliarello V, Green M. Student faculty rounds: a peer-mediated learning activity for internal medicine clerkships. *Med Teach* 27(2): 140-4.

[3]Virginia Commonwealth University Urology Department. http://www.vcu.edu/urology/m3m4_syllabus.pdf. Accessed January 30, 2011.

[4]Hoffman M, Mittelman M. Presentations at professional meetings: notes, suggestions and tips for speakers. *Eur J Int Med* 2004; 15(6): 358-63.

[5]Maimonides Medical Center Department of Emergency Medicine. http://webcache.googleusercontent.com/search?q=cache:tus61P3oVXUJ:www.maimonidesmed.org/workfiles/GMEresidency/Emergency/ORIENT~1.DOC+giving+presentations+in+clerkships&cd=1&hl=en&ct=clnk&gl=us. Accessed December 4, 2009.

[6]Happell B. Presenting with precision: preparing and delivering a polished conference presentation. *Nurse Res* 2009; 16(3): 45-56.

[7]University of North Carolina Department of Obstetrics and Gynecology. http://www.med.unc.edu/obgclerk/grading. Accessed January 30, 2011.

[8]Starver K, Shellenbarger R. Professional presentations made simple. *Clin Nurs Spec* 2004; 18(1): 16-20.

[9]Edwards M, McMasters K, Acland R, Papp K, Garrision R. Oral presentations for surgical meetings. *J Surg Res* 1997; 68(1): 87-90.

[10]Mehrabian A, Ferris S. Inference of attitudes from nonverbal communication in two channels. *Journal of Consulting Psychology* 1967; 31(3): 248-58.

[11]Brown G, Manogue M. Refreshing lecturing: a guide for lecturers. *Med Teach* 2001; 23(3): 231-44.

[12]Sherbino J, Bandiera G. Improving communication skills: feedback from faculty and residents. *Acad Emerg Med* 2006; 13(4): 467-70.

[13]Behnke R, Sawyer C, King P. The communication of public speaking anxiety. *Communication Education* 1986; 36(2): 138-41.

[14]Copeland H, Longworth D, Hewson M, Stoller J. Successful lecturing: a prospective study to validate attributes of the effective medical lecture. *J Gen Intern Med* 2000; 15(6): 366-71.

An excerpt from the best-selling book, *The Successful Match: 200 Rules to Succeed in the Residency Match...*

The Application

What does it take to match successfully? What does it take to match into the specialty and program of your choice?

In the 2007 Match, over 40% of all U.S. senior applicants failed to match at the program of their choice. In competitive fields such as dermatology and plastic surgery, over 37% of U.S. senior applicants failed to match at all.

Percentage of U.S. senior applicants who failed to match in 2007	
Specialty	**% of U.S. seniors failing to match**
Dermatology	38.8%
Plastic surgery	37.5%
Urology	31.3%*
Ophthalmology	30.7%*
Neurological surgery	28.3%*
Orthopedic surgery	19.7%
Otolaryngology	18.4%
Radiation oncology	18.4%
Diagnostic radiology	9.2%
*All applicants (U.S. seniors + other applicants) From www.nrmp.org, www.sfmatch.org, www.auanet.org	

The numbers are significantly worse for osteopathic and international medical graduates:

- 28.4% of the 1,900 osteopathic students and graduates who participated in the 2008 Match failed to match at all.
- 55% of the 10,300 international medical graduates who participated in the 2008 Match failed to match at all.

Did you know ...

Applicants who fail to match may participate in the Scramble. During the Scramble, applicants try to secure a first-year residency position in a program that failed to fill during the Match. In 2008, over 12,000 applicants scrambled for one of only 1,300 positions.

What does it actually take to match successfully? The issue is a hotly debated one, and surveys of students, reviews of student discussion forums, and discussions with academic faculty all find sharp divisions on the topic. In the following 400 plus pages, we answer the question of what it takes to match successfully. We also provide specific evidence-based advice to maximize your chances of a successful match.

Our recommendations are based on data from a full spectrum of sources. We present evidence obtained from scientific study and published in the academic medical literature. The results of these studies can provide a powerful impetus for specific actions. We present anecdotal data and advice that have been published in the literature and obtained from online sources. We also take an insider's look at the entire process of residency selection based on our experiences, the experiences of our colleagues in the world of academic medicine, and the experiences of students and residents with whom we have worked.

Who actually chooses the residents? We review the data on the decision makers. What do these decision makers care about? We review the data on the criteria that matter to them. How can you convince them that you would be the right resident for their program? We provide concrete, practical recommendations based on this data. At every step of the process, our recommendations are meant to maximize the impact of your application.

In Chapter 2, starting on page 21, we present specialty-specific data. Given the high failure to match rates for certain specialties, is there any literature available to applicants to guide them through the residency application process? For each specialty, we present the results of those studies. For example, in radiology, a 2006 survey of residency program directors obtained data from 77 directors on the criteria that programs use to select their residents (Otero). Which criteria did these directors rank as most important in deciding whom to interview? Which selection factors were most important in determining an applicant's place on the program's rank order list? What were the mean United States Medical Licensing Examination (USMLE) Step 1 scores among matched and unmatched U.S. seniors? What percentage of U.S. seniors who matched were members of the Alpha Omega Alpha Honor Medical Society (AOA)? This evidence-based information is critical to developing an application strategy that maximizes your chances of a successful match.

We review each component of the application in comprehensive detail in the following chapters. Each single component of your application can be created, modified, or influenced in order to significantly strengthen your overall candidacy. We devote the next 400 plus pages of this book to showing you, in detail, exactly how to do so.

Letters of Recommendation

Letters of recommendation are a critical component of the residency application. Since you won't be directly writing these letters yourself, it may seem as if you have no control over their content. In reality, you wield more influence than you realize. In our chapter on letters of recommendation, we detail the steps that you can take in order to have the best possible letters written on your behalf. These steps include choosing the correct letter writers and asking in the correct manner. We also discuss the type of information to provide, and the manner in which to provide it, in order to highlight those qualities that you hope your letter writer will emphasize.

The purpose of these letters is to emphasize that you have the professional qualifications needed to excel. The letters should also demonstrate that you have the personal qualities to succeed as a resident and, later, as a practicing physician. Since these letters are written by those who know you and the quality of your work, they offer programs a personalized view. In contrast to your transcript and USMLE scores, they supply programs with qualitative, rather than quantitative, information about your cognitive and non-cognitive characteristics.

What do the faculty members reviewing applications look for in a letter of recommendation? The first item noted is the writer of the letter. In a survey of program directors in four specialties (internal medicine, pediatrics, family medicine, and surgery), it was learned that a candidate's likelihood of being considered was enhanced if there was a connection or relationship between the writer and residency program director (Villanueva). "In cases where there was both a connection between the faculty members and in-depth knowledge of the student (i.e., personal knowledge), the likelihood was that the student's application would be noted." In a survey of 109 program directors of orthopedic surgery residency programs, 54% of directors agreed that the most important aspect of a letter was that it was written by someone they knew (Bernstein).

In another study, the academic rank of the writer was found to be an important factor influencing the reviewer's ranking of the letter, with 48% of the reviewers rating it as important (Greenburg). A survey of physical medicine and rehabilitation (PM&R) program directors asked respondents to rate the importance of letters of recommendation in selecting residents (DeLisa). The study showed that the "most important letters of recommendation were from a PM&R faculty member in the respondent's department, followed by the Dean's letter, and the PM&R chairman's letter." Next in importance were letters from a PM&R faculty member in a department other than the respondents' followed by a clinical faculty member in another specialty. The University of Texas-Houston Medical School Career Counseling Catalog gives this advice: "letters of recommendation from private physicians or part-time faculty, and letters from residents are generally discounted."

For international medical graduates (IMGs), this issue becomes even more important. A survey of 102 directors of internal medicine residency programs sought to determine the most important predictors of performance for IMGs (Gayed). When rating the importance of 22 selection criteria, the lowest rated criterion was letters of recommendation from a foreign country, with 93% of program directors feeling that such letters were useless.

What else do the faculty members reviewing applications look for in a letter of recommendation? They seek evidence of an applicant's strengths and skills. Most applicants assume that their letter writers know what to say and what information to provide in a letter to substantiate their recommendation. However, that is a dangerous assumption. In an analysis of 116 recommendation letters received by the radiology residency program at the University of Iowa Hospitals and Clinics (O'Halloran), reviewers noted the following:

- 10% were missing information about an applicant's cognitive knowledge
- 35% had no information about an applicant's clinical judgment
- 3% did not discuss an applicant's work habits
- 17% did not comment on the applicant's motivation
- 32% were lacking information about interpersonal communication skills

In another review of recommendation letters sent during the 1999 application season to the Department of Surgery at Southern Illinois University, writers infrequently commented on psychomotor skills such as "easily performed minor procedures at the bedside," "good eye-hand coordination in the OR," "could suture well," and so on (Fortune).

Our chapter on letters of recommendation, starting on page 159, reviews strategies to locate letter writers who will be most helpful to your candidacy. We review how to identify these writers and how to approach them. Most importantly, we describe the type of evidence you can provide to the writer and the professional manner in which to provide it. Your letter writers want to write the best letter possible, and you can do much more than you realize to make this a reality.

Read more of the first chapter at www.TheSuccessfulMatch.com

Clinician's Guide to Laboratory Medicine: Pocket

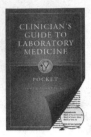

By Samir P. Desai, MD

ISBN # 9780972556187

In caring for patients, medical students and residents routinely order and interpret a wide variety of diagnostic tests. Unfortunately, many students have received no formal instruction in lab test ordering or interpretation. Not surprisingly, students are often unsure of the next step in the evaluation of an abnormal lab test.

The end result may be unnecessary additional testing, increasing the costs to the medical system. Even worse, misinterpretation of tests may significantly impact patient care, increasing morbidity and mortality due to missed or erroneous diagnoses.

In this book, you will find practical approaches to lab test interpretation. It includes differential diagnoses, step-by-step approaches, and algorithms, all designed to answer your lab test questions in a flash. See why so many consider it a "must-have" book.

"In our Medicine Clerkship, the Clinician's Guide to Laboratory Medicine has quickly become one of the two most popular paperback books. Our students have praised the algorithms, tables, and ease of pursuit of clinical problems through better understanding of the utilization of tests appropriate to the problem at hand."

> - Greg Magarian, M.D., Director, 3rd Year Internal Medicine Clerkship, Oregon Health & Science University

"It provides an excellent practical approach to abnormal labs."

> - Northwestern University Feinberg School of Medicine Internal Medicine Clerkship website.

The Successful Match website

Our website, TheSuccessfulMatch.com, provides residency applicants with a better understanding of the residency selection process. There, you will find:

- Match statistics for every specialty
- Conversations with program directors about the selection process
- Important information about the future of each specialty, including current challenges
- Factors that led physicians to pursue different specialties
- Resources to help you succeed in clerkships

Consulting services

We also offer expert one-on-one consulting services to medical students. Whether you seek an overall strategy for match success, accurate assessment of your candidacy for a particular specialty or program, review of your curriculum vitae or personal statement, or thorough preparation for interviews, you can rest assured that we have the knowledge, expertise, and insight to help you achieve your goals.

If you are interested in our consultation services, please visit us at www.TheSuccessfulMatch.com.

MD2B Titles

The Successful Match: 200 Rules to Succeed in the Residency Match

Success on the Wards: 250 Rules for Clerkship Success

Clinician's Guide to Laboratory Medicine: Pocket

Internal Medicine Clerkship: 150 Biggest Mistakes And How To Avoid Them

Surgery Clerkship: 150 Biggest Mistakes And How To Avoid Them

Psychiatry Clerkship: 150 Biggest Mistakes And How To Avoid Them

Pediatrics Clerkship: 101 Biggest Mistakes And How To Avoid Them

Available at www.MD2B.net

Bulk Sales

MD2B is able to provide discounts on any of our titles when purchased in bulk. The discount rate depends on the quantity ordered. For more information, please contact us at info@md2b.net or (713) 927-6830.

The Successful Match: 200 Rules To Succeed in the Residency Match

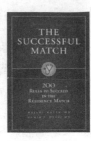

By Rajani Katta, MD and Samir P. Desai, MD

ISBN # 9780972556170

What does it take to match into the specialty and program of your choice?

The key to a successful match hinges on the development of the right strategy. This book will show you how to develop the optimal strategy for success.

Who actually choose the residents? We review the data on the decision-makers. What do these decision-makers care about? We review the data on the criteria that matter most to them. How can you convince them that you would be the right resident for their program? We provide concrete, practical recommendations based on their criteria.

At every step of the process, our recommendations are meant to maximize the impact of your application. This book is an invaluable resource to help you gain that extra edge.

"In this book, the authors do a wonderful job of addressing many myths and rumors that exist out there. They don't merely provide their opinions, but instead provide hard data — the results of surveys and studies, as well as direct quotes from important decision makers such as residency program directors."

> - A. Mallik (Amazon review)

"Drs. Rajani Katta and Samir P. Desai provide the medical student reader with detailed preparation for the matching process. The rules and accompanying tips make the book user-friendly. The format is especially appealing to those pressed for time or looking for a single key element for a particular process."

> - Review in the American Medical Student Association journal, *The New Physician*